TREATING DISORDERED SPEECH MOTOR CONTROL

KIM WILCOX

To Dr. Frederic L. Darley, the outstanding teacher and author who more than any other individual clinician has influenced approaches to evaluation and treatment of disordered speech motor control.

> Cover portrait of Frederic L. Darley by
> John Wilson of Austin, Texas.

FOR CLINICIANS BY CLINICIANS
Harris Winitz, Series Editor

This book, *Treating Disordered Speech Motor Control,* is the sixth volume in the For Clinicians by Clinicians series of texts on the diagnosis and clinical management of speech, language, and voice disorders. Each text provides a contemporary perspective on one major disorder or clinical area and is designed for use in clinical methodology courses and continuing education programs. Authors have been selected who represent a broad spectrum of clinical interests and theoretical positions and who hold the common belief that their viewpoints, experiences, and successes should be shared in order to provide a forum for clinicians by clinicians.

Volumes already published in this series are *Treating Language Disorders, Treating Articulation Disorders, Case Studies in Aphasia Rehabilitation, Treating Cerebral Palsy,* and *Alaryngeal Speech Rehabilitation.*

TREATING DISORDERED SPEECH MOTOR CONTROL

For Clinicians by Clinicians

Edited by
**Deanie Vogel and
Michael P. Cannito**

pro·ed
8700 Shoal Creek Boulevard
Austin, Texas 78758

© 1991 by PRO-ED, Inc.

All rights reserved. No part of this book may be reproduced in any form or by any means without the prior written permission of the publisher.

Printed in the United States of America

Library of Congress Cataloging-in-Publication Data

Treating disordered speech motor control / edited by Deanie Vogel and Michael P. Cannito.
    p.   cm. — (For clinicians by clinicians)
  Includes bibliographical references and index.
  ISBN 0-89079-299-2
  1. Speech disorders. 2. Motor cortex.   I. Vogel, Deanie.
II. Cannito, Michael P. III. Series.
  [DNLM: 1. Movement Disorders—physiopathology. 2. Movement Disorders—therapy. 3. Speech Disorders—physiopathology.
4. Speech Disorders—therapy.   WL 340 T7836]
RC423.T72 1990
616.85′5—dc20
DNLM/DLC   90-9167
for Library of Congress   CIP

pro·ed
8700 Shoal Creek Boulevard
Austin, Texas 78758

1 2 3 4 5 6 7 8 9 10   95 94 93 92 91

This book is dedicated to the women in my life:

> *my mother, Rose*
> *my sister, Joyce*
> *my daughter, Caitlin*

and especially my patient wife, Sherye. Without their love and support it would not have been possible.

M.P.C.

To	My parents, Meyer and Molly
To	My children, Robin, Phil, and Autumn
	And
To	Arnie

D.V.

Contents

Contributors ix

Preface xi

PART I
INTERDISCIPLINARY BACKGROUND

CHAPTER 1
Treating Disordered Speech Motor Control: An Overview 3
    Donnell F. Johns

CHAPTER 2
Comanagement of Disordered Speech Motor Control:
The Roles of the Neurologist and the Speech Pathologist 17
    Robert Lozano

CHAPTER 3
Structural and Functional Brain Imaging in Disorders
of Speech and Motor Control 43
    Delaina Walker-Batson and Phillip D. Purdy

PART II
GENERALIZED MOVEMENT DISORDERS AFFECTING SPEECH

CHAPTER 4
A Top-Down Approach to Treatment of Dysarthric Speech 87
    Deanie Vogel and Lynda Miller

CHAPTER 5
Pharmacologic Approaches to Speech Motor Disorders 111
    David B. Rosenfield

CHAPTER 6
Dysarthria: A Breakdown in Interpersonal Communication 153
    Rosemary Lubinski

PART III
PREMOTOR DISORGANIZATION OF SPEECH

CHAPTER 7
Apraxia of Speech Versus Phonemic Paraphasia:
Theoretical, Diagnostic, and Treatment Considerations 185
    Robert S. Pierce

CHAPTER 8
Acquired Neurogenic Dysfluency 217
    Jon Deal and Michael P. Cannito

CHAPTER 9
Neurogenic Disorders of Prosody 241
    Donald A. Robin, Gayle V. Klouda, and Linda N. Hug

PART IV
IDIOPATHIC SPEECH-SPECIFIC DISORDERS

CHAPTER 10
Neurobiological Interpretations of Spasmodic Dysphonia 275
    Michael P. Cannito

CHAPTER 11
Noninvasive Instrumentation in the Treatment of Stuttering ...319
    Ben C. Watson and Peter J. Alfonso

CHAPTER 12
Developmental Apraxia of Speech: Theory and Practice 341
    Thomas P. Marquardt and Harvey M. Sussman

Index 391

Contributors

Peter J. Alfonso, PhD
Haskins Laboratories
New Haven, CT 06501

Michael P. Cannito, PhD
Department of Speech
 Communication
University of Texas at Austin
Austin, TX 78712

Jon Deal, PhD
Audiology and Speech Pathology
 Service
Veterans Affairs Medical Center
Columbia, MO 65201

Linda N. Hug
Department of Speech Pathology
 and Audiology
Wendell Johnson Speech and
 Hearing Center
University of Iowa
Iowa City, IA 55242

Donnell F. Johns, PhD
Department of Surgery
University of Texas Southwestern
 Medical Center
Dallas, TX 75235

Gayle V. Klouda, PhD
2248 Danbury Street
Iowa City, IA 52240

Robert Lozano, MD, PhD
Neurological Clinic
Corpus Christi, TX 78404

Rosemary Lubinski, PhD
Department of Communicative
 Disorders and Sciences
University at Buffalo
Buffalo, NY 14260

Thomas P. Marquardt, PhD
Department of Speech
 Communication
University of Texas at Austin
Austin, TX 78712

Lynda Miller, PhD
Department of Speech
 Communication
University of Texas at Austin
Austin, TX 78712

Robert S. Pierce, PhD
School of Speech Pathology and
 Audiology
Kent State University
Kent, OH 44242

Philip D. Purdy, MD
Radiology, Neurology and
 Neurosurgery
University of Texas Southwestern
 Medical Center and Parkland
 Memorial Hospital
Dallas, TX 75235

Donald A. Robin, PhD
Laboratory of Speech and
 Language Neuroscience
Department of Speech Pathology
 and Audiology
Wendell Johnson Speech and
 Hearing Center
University of Iowa
Iowa City, IA 52242

David B. Rosenfield, MD
Stuttering Center and Speech
 Motor Control Laboratory
Department of Neurology
Baylor College of Medicine
Houston, TX 77030

Harvey M. Sussman, PhD
Department of Linguistics and
  Department of Speech
  Communication
University of Texas at Austin
Austin, TX 78712

Deanie Vogel, PhD
Audiology and Speech Pathology
  Service
Department of Veterans Affairs
  Medical Center
Reno, NV 89520
and University of Nevada School
  of Medicine
Reno, NV 89557

Delaina Walker-Batson, PhD
Department of Communication
  Science
Texas Woman's University
Denton, TX 76204
and Department of Radiology
University of Texas Southwestern
  Medical Center
Dallas, TX 75235

Ben C. Watson, PhD
Callier Center
University of Texas at Dallas
Dallas, TX 75235

Preface

This is a book about neuromotor disturbances of speech production. Its purposes are (1) to look at the phenomena in question somewhat more broadly than is typically done in books about "motor speech disorders"; (2) to address some current issues that have been neglected in the clinical literature; and (3) to integrate recent clinical information from various disciplines, most particularly speech pathology and neurology. It is not our purpose to provide a comprehensive textbook on normal and disordered speech neurophysiology. Much of the material contained herein is therefore highly technical and specialized, and is aimed primarily at a practicing professional readership. It should also be quite useful, however, to advanced graduate students in the area of neuropathologies of communication, perhaps as supplemental reading to a more basic text.

The term "speech motor control" in the title of this book refers to a process that we view quite broadly to include premovement organization (i.e., linguistic formulation), not merely motoric execution and modulation; in our view, without organization there can be no control. As a consequence of this orientation, we have included substantial content not only from the phonological domain of language, but from the affective and pragmatic arenas as well.

The book is organized into four major subdivisions. The first provides general background information including a historical retrospective (Johns), a cross-disciplinary perspective (Lozano), and a review of nervous system organization and methods for studying its structure and function (Walker-Batson and Purdy). The second section deals with assessment and management of generalized movement disorders affecting speech, that is, the dysarthrias. Included in this section are the pharmacological approach (Rosenfield), patient and family counseling (Lubinski), and a metalinguistic "knowledge-driven" orientation toward functional communication for dysarthric speakers (Vogel and Miller). Third is a section encompassing the higher-order disturbances of premotor organization of speech, their differential assessment, and their management. These disturbances include phonemic paraphasia and apraxia of speech (Pierce), right and left hemisphere dysprosody (Robin et al.), and acquired neurogenic dysfluency (Deal and Cannito). Last are the idiopathic speech-specific disorders of stuttering (Watson and Alfonso), spasmodic dysphonia (Cannito), and developmental apraxia of speech (Marquardt and Sussman). These latter speech disturbances remain enigmatic but bear many striking resemblances to the more clearly delineated neuromotor pathologies discussed in the preceding chapters.

Several relevant areas are not covered in this volume. Their omission reflects the editors' attempt to focus on contemporary issues that have not been discussed extensively elsewhere. For example, numerous studies on speech therapy for dysarthria have appeared recently and have been reviewed repeatedly in a number of excellent secondary sources (Rosenbek & LaPointe, 1985; Netsell, 1986; Yorkston, Beukelman, & Bell, 1988; Yorkston & Beukelman, 1989). Because several reviews of this area have already appeared in the For Clinicians by Clinicians series (Dworkin, 1984; McDonald, 1987), we have not included reviews on speech therapy for dysarthria.

Another area we opted to omit is that of augmentative communication. The book by McDonald (1987) published in this series presents an extensive description of augmentative communicative devices used by cerebral palsied individuals and contains excellent chapters by Musselwaite (1987) and Vanderheiden (1987). In addition, the volume by Beukelman, Yorkston, and Dowden (1985) provides an excellent resource for clinicians wishing to learn about the latest in augmentative communication equipment. Finally, we chose not to include a chapter on surgical and prosthetic management. Extensive and superior discussions of these topics are found in chapters by Rosenbek and LaPointe (1985), Rosenbek (1984), and Johns (1985), and in the recent book by Yorkston, Beukelman, and Bell (1988).

A number of content themes underlie and link the various chapters in this volume. For instance, neuroanatomy is outlined in Chapter 3 by Walker-Batson and Purdy, who focus on structural and functional brain imaging. This theme is expanded upon in Chapter 10 in Cannito's description of spasmodic dysphonia. Rosenfield's treatment of neuroanatomy and neurophysiology in Chapter 5 concentrates in part not only on underlying causes of specific disorders of speech motor control but also deals with the effects of pharmacology on speech disorders.

Another theme, assessment of certain disorders of speech motor control by means of instrumentation, is described by Watson and Alfonso in Chapter 11. Assessment procedures are also introduced in Chapter 2 by Lozano and in Chapter 7 by Pierce. Lozano is both a neurologist and a speech-language pathologist; he describes assessment of the patient with disordered speech motor control from the point of view of both professions. Pierce, from the point of view of a psycholinguist, writes of assessment procedures that can be used to differentiate apraxia of speech from phonemic paraphasias.

Therapeutics is a frequently occurring content theme in this text. In Chapters 4–9, 11, and 12, contributors offer suggestions for treatment. Vogel and Miller describe a "top-down" communication-oriented approach to the treatment of dysarthria, while Lubinski writes of the roles the dysarthric patient, the family, and the speech-language pathologist play in the therapeutic process. Pierce presents descriptions of treatment programs designed to remediate apraxia of speech or to decrease or eliminate phonemic paraphasias. Robin et al. focus on treatment of disordered prosody; Marquardt and Sussman suggest methods for treating developmental apraxia of speech. Deal and Cannito outline general schema within which to approach treatment of neurogenic dysfluency. All of these chapters are supported with extensive case study material.

Two additional content themes in this volume are neuromotor dysfunction and communication. In Chapter 5, Rosenfield discusses neuromotor disorders in general, while in Chapter 9 Cannito writes of neuromotor dysfunction in spasmodic dysphonia. Watson and Alfonso, in Chapter 11, discuss the use of instrumentation in cases in which there is neuromotor dysfunction. In Chapter 7 Deal and Cannito concentrate on neuromotor dysfunction in neurogenic dysfluency. Focusing on the communication process, in Chapter 4, Vogel and Miller offer an approach to improve the dysarthric patient's overall communicative ability, and Lubinski in Chapter 6 suggests how families can improve their communication with the dysarthria patient. In Chapter 2 Lozano presents his views on communication from a slightly different perspective: he offers suggestions for clearer communication between speech-language pathologists and physicians.

The editors of this volume wish to acknowledge the contribution of Dr. Harris Winitz, the series editor, whose concept of this series, "For Clinicians by Clinicians," has led to the publication of a rich variety of suggestions for treating disordered communication. These suggestions have proven to be of great value to clinicians who have read the books and are influenced by them.

REFERENCES

Beukelman, D. R., Yorkston, K. M., & Dowden, P. A. (1985). *Communication augmentation: A casebook of clinical management.* Austin, TX: PRO-ED.

Dworkin, J. P. (1984). Specific characteristics and treatment of the dysarthrias. In H. Winitz (Ed.), *For clinicians by clinicians: Vol. 1. Treating articulation disorders* (pp. 263–288). Austin, TX: PRO-ED.

Johns, D. F. (1985). Surgical and prosthetic management of neurogenic velopharyngeal incompetency in dysarthria. In D. F. Johns (Ed.), *Clinical management of neurogenic communicative disorders* (pp. 153–177). Austin, TX: PRO-ED.

McDonald, E. T. (1987). Speech production problems. In E. T. McDonald (Ed.), *For clinicians by clinicians: Vol. 4. Treating cerebral palsy* (pp. 171–190). Austin, TX: PRO-ED.

Musselwaite, C. R. (1987). Augmentative Communication. In E. T. McDonald (Ed.), *For clinicians by clinicians: Vol. 4. Treating cerebral palsy* (pp. 209–238). Austin, TX: PRO-ED.

Netsell, R. (1986). *A neurobiologic view of speech production and the dysarthrias.* Austin, TX: PRO-ED.

Rosenbek, J. C. (1984). Selected alternatives to articulation training for the dysarthric adult. In H. Winitz (Ed.), *For clinicians by clinicians: Vol. 1. Treating articulation disorders* (pp. 249–262). Austin, TX: PRO-ED.

Rosenbek, J. C., & LaPointe, L. (1985). The dysarthrias: Description, diagnosis, and treatment. In D. F. Johns (Ed.), *Clinical management of neurogenic communicative disorders* (pp. 97–152). Austin, TX: PRO-ED.

Vanderheiden, G. C. (1987). Advanced technology aids for communication, education and employment. In E. T. McDonald (Ed.), *For clinicians by clinicians: Vol. 4. Treating cerebral palsy* (pp. 257–273). Austin, TX: PRO-ED.

Yorkston, K. M., & Beukelman, D. R. (1989). *Recent advances in clinical dysarthria.* Austin, TX: PRO-ED.

Yorkston, K. M., Beukelman, D., & Bell, K. R. (1988). *Clinical management of dysarthric speakers.* Austin, TX: PRO-ED.

PART I
Interdisciplinary Background

CHAPTER 1

Treating Disordered Speech Motor Control: An Overview

Donnell F. Johns

In considering the subject of treating disordered speech motor control, one must recognize that the communication process and resultant human communicative behavior are both dependent upon and the product of a complex nervous system. Subsystems, traditionally labeled an "input, central, and output" sequence, have been proposed to segment the study of complex human communicative disorders. I recognize the artificiality of these categorical distinctions, since the nervous system functions in a unified and interconnective fashion, and have used this postulation for convenience. The overlapping and interlocking sequencing that is required for our most distinctive characteristic, the ability to communicate with verbal symbols, however, requires fractionation of the system to allow for systematic investigations of portions of the communication sequence. The admittedly simplistic sensory-neural-motor division offers a convenient and useful approach to study this unitary and complex process. It allows for classification of various functions and disorders and permits investigation of the parts of the totality. This classification scheme, while imperfect, is also of some value when one considers that no one discipline can assume the responsibility of explaining completely the communicative process. Interdisciplinary inquiry permits scrutiny of the parts, so that a start may be made toward the organization of the parts relative to the whole. It is recognized that normal or deviant speech behavior is inextricably linked to and cannot be separated from the functions that collectively comprise the central process of communication.

A HISTORICAL PERSPECTIVE

The subject of disordered vocal motor control—motor speech disorders associated with neurologic deficits—is generously reflected in the neurological literature of the past century, the speech and hearing literature of the past six decades, and the neurolinguistic literature in the past quarter century. A review of that combined literature clearly demonstrates that speech deficits associated with neuropathologic lesions have been a fertile area for controversy. An examination of that literature also reveals a relative paucity of systematic research designed to increase the understanding of neurogenic motor speech disorders based on empirically derived data. This paucity is largely due to the misunderstandings and confusions among past and contemporary researchers and clinicians. Such confusion has often led to mismanagement of patients resulting in frustrations for the patient, family members, significant others, and certainly the clinician.

Within the past decade, major advances in diagnostic tests have been followed by an increasing number of studies designed to reappraise existing data or to obtain new data on the clinical course of various motor speech disorders and the extent to which they are affected by therapeutic intervention. Speech-language pathologists, classically trained and oriented in the artful science of diagnosis, prognosis, and therapy, have found that every decision in diagnosis, prognosis, and therapy involves an assessment of probabilities—and thus a type of statistical exercise. We have been challenged to perform systematic and replicable investigations for individuals and groups of patients. Investigators have been asked to conduct clinical experiments that satisfy the standards of science while answering the burning questions asked in clinical practice. These scientific challenges in the performance and evaluation of diagnosis, as well as the strategy of therapy and the arrangements used to deliver remedial treatment to individual patients with increased clinical sophistication and scientific rigor, have been referred to as cause-effect or "impact" research (Feinstein, 1985). Changes that occur as outcomes during and after the intervention of the procedures or techniques under scrutiny have been the focus of single-case studies. Such studies are a crucial prelude to, and provide the empirical foundation for, follow-up replication studies that may employ larger sample sizes and the power of statistics. Dworkin, Abkarian, and Johns (1988) indicate that, "given this precursor role, case studies are bound to specify the clinical procedures that are associated with the obtained results . . . by exerting a high level of rigor in the description and evaluation of the treatment protocols employed" (p. 291).

Objective measurement of relevant behavioral changes is considered by Darley (1972) to be a fundamental consideration in studying the effectiveness of therapy. He suggested that supplementary physiological or psychophysical measurements of behavioral change should be considered whenever possible. He further admonished that "there is no use in even beginning this sort of investigation unless research can be more than an interested clinician's artistic and intuitive reporting of change observed in his patients. Reliable quantitative data must be gathered with rigorous objectivity" (p. 11). Darley also urged clinical speech pathologists to measure changed aspects of the patient's psychological status—that is, "his adaptation to his problem and his environment"—as objectively as possible. This volume accepts and meets these challenges, as will be revealed to the reader in the next 11 chapters.

We have come a long way and take pride in our sophisticated diagnostic repertoire, employing bio-electric-acoustic-kinematic-neuro invasive and noninvasive procedures. We have begun to include these procedures in our treatment armamentarium. It is often considered unscholarly to cite historical references; the preference is to reference only works that are "hot"—that is, in press or not more than two to three years old—and refereed journals are preferred. My thesis, however, is that we must acknowledge our rich and instructive history, learn from it, and build upon it, so as not to be doomed to repeat it and cyclically reinvent the wheel. With particular reference to disordered motor control, a person whom we would certainly respect as a bona fide contemporary neuroscientist—C. S. Sherrington (1906)—stated: "By combining methods of comparative psychology with the methods of experimental physiology, investigations may be expected ere long to furnish new data of importance toward the knowledge of movement as an outcome of the working brain" (p. 7).

It was Lashley in 1961 who hypothesized, "The translation from the spatial distribution of memory traces to temporal sequence seems to be a fundamental aspect of the problem of serial order" (p. 180). Along the same lines, he stated that temporal integration of motor control seems to be "the most important and also the most neglected problem of cerebral physiology" (Johns, 1975, p. 176).

An obvious disorder of speech motor control is stuttering. There is a plethora of literature to support a neurologic basis for stuttering. Stuttering is found universally among humans and has been described since the days of early recorded history. Accounts of it can be found in clay tablets of Mesopotamia that were made centuries before the birth of Christ. Van Riper (1971) relates that Aristotle described stuttering in 384 B.C., but only in the 19th century did writers begin to attribute stuttering to a malfunctioning or damaged brain. I offer this early definition for the reader's consideration: "Stuttering is a syllabic dysarthria produced by lack of coordination of voice, respiration and articulation, due to neurological deficits." That definition was made by Kussmaul in 1877 (Johns, 1975, p. 162).

Although we should not forget the early studies in the late 1920s and the 1930s by Orton, Travis, Bryngelson, West, and Van Riper, and others of that time period, Luchsinger and Arnold (1965) have summarized their shortcomings: "During the third and fourth decades of our century, psychological explanations predominated. These are not completely satisfactory however—because history has shown many drastic changes in the interpretation of disease. With the progress of medicine, many 'functional' ailments have proved to be caused by organic changes within various anatomic, neurological, or via chemical alterations" (p. 109).

In 1970, Masland presented a well-written and scholarly report on brain mechanisms underlying language function and concluded that "the work which Dr. Orton did so many years ago was well recognized at that time . . . recent experiments serve even more to accentuate how far ahead of his time he was and how perceptive were his comments regarding cerebral dominance" (p. 109).

A CROSS-DISCIPLINARY PERSPECTIVE

The efficacy of speech therapy regimens designed to treat patients with disordered speech motor control secondary to neurologic impairment has been questioned by many, as pointed out by Lozano in Chapter 2 of this work, despite recent reports to the contrary (Wertz, LaPointe, & Rosenbek, 1984; Dworkin et al., 1988). When presented with evidence that specifically devised management strategies have been demonstrated to be effective in treating such individuals, there are those who reserve or maintain their "lofty" opinions, such as that held by an observer who upon first watching Watts' steam engine in operation said, "Yes, it works in practice, but will it work in theory?" (DiSimoni, 1989, p. 2).

While increasingly sophisticated physiologic-anatomic descriptions of neuromotor speech disorders provide a strong basis for assessment techniques and hold promise for more specific and sophisticated focus for treatment, the controversy over preferred treatment approaches continues. This situation exists in large part because anecdotal clinical reports form the base of support for the treatment effect and only very recently have methods of treatment been subjected to formal experimental evaluation. In short, the vast majority of treatment methods in current use have not been subjected to formalized, systematic research investigations, although such inquiry could provide critical information that would be of substantial value in treating disordered speech motor control. Lozano, in this volume, points out the great need for the development and experimental documentation of new treatment techniques including the effectiveness of these methods compared to no treatment or to one or more of the more traditional behavioral methods that have been described. A speech-language pathologist and neurologist, Lozano stresses interdisciplinary cooperation between neurology and speech-language pathology for improved patient management. He discusses patient management sequences from the point of view of each discipline and presents assessment outlines and treatment procedures conducted by practitioners from both professional areas.

REVIEW OF NERVOUS SYSTEM ORGANIZATION; STUDY OF STRUCTURE AND FUNCTION

Basic knowledge of anatomic and neurophysiologic aspects of speech and language processing both in the normal state and in the state of neurological dysfunction is critical to the clinician in formulating a rationale for treatment of patients who present with disordered speech motor control. The various imaging techniques that enhance this knowledge are presented in Chapter 3 by Walker-Batson and Purdy, who demonstrate in their overview the use of current brain-imaging technologies in normal subjects and patients with neurogenic communicative disorders. Concrete evidence is beginning to emerge describing neurological dysfunction not previously documented, and the use of the information provided by various neuroimaging techniques appears to be on the threshold of clinical utility. Walker-Batson and Purdy present a cogent overview of six current brain-imaging technologies; they describe both their clinical and research use. This information is enhanced by case presentations utilizing these technologies that provide new insight regarding the nature of neurological disorders affecting speech motor control. X-ray computed tomography (CT) and magnetic resonance imaging (MRI) describe the cerebral structure in living individuals. Functional assessment of brain activity includes magnetic resonance spectroscopy (MRS), single-photon emission tomography (SPECT), positron emission tomography (PET), and topographic mapping of brain electrical activity that provides information regarding neurophysiological and neurochemical aspects of speech-language processing. Presently the primary application of neuroimaging technologies is in their clinical utility in terms of medical management; nonetheless, the use of this information in formulating treatment programs gained from brain-imaging technologies is indeed exciting. Recently Zhang, Wilson, Levesque, Harper, and Engel (1989) presented a multimodal stereotactic imaging system for mapping brain functional imaging to anatomic structure that allows for simultaneous displays from PET, MRI, CT, and digital subtraction angiography (DSA) that has been applied to localizing tissue functions.

These rapidly evolving technologies are providing new insights into the organization, function, and dynamics of speech processes and are exciting for both basic scientists and clinical researchers. Such revelations also hold promise for hands-on professionals by providing new information which may permit the formulation of novel and increasingly sophisticated clinical interventions.

GENERALIZED MOVEMENT DISORDERS AFFECTING SPEECH

Two of the more perplexing disorders of speech motor control are stuttering and spasmodic dysphonia. In Chapter 5 of this work, Rosenfield presents an in-depth discussion of pharmacologic approaches to speech motor disorders, comparing the various medications that are helpful in treating these disturbances as well as the side effects of these drugs. The fundamental concepts pertinent to an understanding of pharmacology including principles of therapeutics, sources of drug information, and neurotransmitters are presented with a focus on patients with movement disorders—the largest impaired population—for whom pharmacologic therapy might be of interest.

Regarding stuttering in the framework of neurogenic motor speech disorders, in 1975 I stated: "It is known, for example, that there are subclasses of stuttering which are indisputably related to neuropathology. At this point in time, however, the etiology or etiologies that are causal or maintain stuttering in the vast number of stuttering persons are not known. If there is a neurologic basis of stuttering, significant new management strategies and approaches and preventive programs could be designed. Moreover, if a neurological cause for stuttering is found, other methods of controlling this movement disorder, perhaps through chemical therapy, could be approached with new vigor, analogous to controlling epilepsies through drug therapy" (p. 177).

Rosenfield points out, however, that it can be misleading to discuss pharmacologic therapies for motor speech disorders because of the questionable assumptions that these therapies exist and that therefore cures are available; he emphatically states that none of these assumptions are true. However, he goes on to state that understanding the effects of such medications should enhance the interaction between speech-language pathologists and neurologists in treating patients with speech motor control disorders. The fact of the matter is that currently many patients with movement disorders affecting speech routinely are being treated with pharmacologic agents. In this regard, Rosenfield presents information about the efficacy of pharmacologic treatment for a broad range of patients presenting with disordered speech motor control: he includes not only stuttering and spasmodic dysphonia but a wide variety of movement disorders associated with extrapyramidal diseases that result in involuntary movements whether they be patterned or nonpatterned, predictable or unpredictable, or repetitive or nonrepetitive as exemplified by patients with hypo- and hyperkinetic dysarthrias. However, he also focuses on the treatment of patients who stutter or present with spasmodic dysphonia. Regarding the latter, Rosenfield not only presents pharmacotherapeutic treatments but additionally describes related surgical interventions such as intralaryngeal muscle botulinum toxin injection, blocking out recurrent laryngeal nerves with local anesthetics, and unilateral surgical sectioning of the recurrent laryngeal nerve for symptom amelioration. He points out that while medical or surgical treatments may decrease the symptoms considerably, patients with these treatments have some residual voice compromises. Moreover, he categorically states that no patient has been totally cured by either of the medical or surgical regimens.

In contrast to Rosenfield's pharmacologic approach, Vogel and Miller in Chapter 4 describe a top-down approach to management that involves the study of the relationships between language and the context in which language is used to resolve communication breakdowns between dysarthric speakers and their listeners. This process is contrasted with a symptomatology approach, or as they indicate, a bottom-up process in which the organization of language is largely ignored. The latter orientation focuses on the physiologic system underlying motor speech production—such as respiration, phonation, resonance, articulation, or prosody—in which a symptom is treated and the resultant effect is noted (e.g., velopharyngeal incompetency/palatal lift prosthesis-reduction in hypernasality). Vogel and Miller indicate that bottom-up processing can be thought of as analogous to inductive thinking in that this process utilizes available information to collect a group of details before constructing a general pattern. Bottom-up processing is contrasted with a top-down approach, which addresses the cognitive processes and utilizes cognitive information to construct a gestalt or whole—that is, the top-down process is analogous to deductive thinking in which a general hypothesis is formulated that infers specific outcomes on the basis of the general pattern or principle. The authors point out that clinicians treating patients with dysarthria may find it beneficial to discover the patients' level of knowledge regarding language and communication and then determine whether treatment should be focused on the top-down process, which provides the cognitive scaffolding for effective communication by making dysarthric patients aware of how language is communicated, or the bottom-up symptomological approach. Vogel and Miller do not discount the importance of regimens that employ instrumental procedures, physical interventions such as palatal lift prostheses, bite-block techniques, or other behavioral therapies; they recognize that many of these remedial approaches are basic to the treatment of dysarthric patients. The authors also acknowledge that improved results utilizing the top-down approach have not been substantiated by systematic investigations, but based on their observations they indicate that this approach can be used effectively with patients who demonstrate an understanding of the characteristics of how language is communicated.

While there is a modicum of existing literature addressing the psychosocial consequences associated with long-term disabilities, chronic illness, and specific disorders such as aphasia, there is no information substantiated by research regarding the breakdown in the patient's social system as a result of impaired interpersonal communication due to dysarthria. In Chapter 6, Lubinski examines the role of the speech-language pathologist in identifying and remediating psychosocial problems of dysarthric adults. This chapter is divided into four main sections, the first of which focuses on the individual with dysarthria and the resultant psychosocial impact on interpersonal functioning and communication. The second part explores how this disorder may affect the individual in a family context. The third section describes the impact and effects of institutionalization of dysarthric patients. Part 4 discusses the stress that the speech-language pathologist may incur in working with dysarthric individuals, particularly those with progressive degenerative disorders. This last section provides an insightful assessment of the personal and professional consequences that a speech pathologist might experience as a result of working with severely dysarthric adults over a long period of time: emotional exhaustion, depersonalization, and feelings of reduced personal accomplishment or burnout. The effects of burnout are numerous and Lubinski describes a number of positive actions that can be taken to prevent or ameliorate stress and burnout among those of us who practice in the helping professions.

DISTURBANCES OF PREMOTOR DISORGANIZATION OF SPEECH

In Chapter 7 Pierce presents theoretical, diagnostic, and treatment considerations for patients with apraxia of speech and those patients with phonemic paraphasias. The specific speech and language impairments in adults are reviewed with special emphasis on differentiating apraxia of speech from phonemic paraphasia. Patient behaviors that differentiate between the two are described, and treatment considerations for each disorder are presented; the treatment approaches for these disorders are different. Available therapies are reviewed and their techniques are contrasted, which again highlights the dramatic difference between therapeutic regimens used in the treatment of apraxia of speech and those used to treat paraphasic errors. Pierce rightly points out that many of the behaviors displayed by apraxic and paraphasic speakers are similar, but the approach to treatment is distinctly different for the two disorders.

I have already indicated in this chapter that there is a plethora of literature to support a neurologic basis for stuttering. In 1975 I stated: "It would appear unscientific to dismiss a hypothesis of a neurogenic basis for stuttering, or conversely to accept such a hypothesis uncritically. I believe that there are compelling reasons to systematically study the disorder of stuttering within a neurologic framework in an attempt to add to the knowledge regarding the nature of this particular disorder which has eluded our understanding since the beginning of recorded history" (p. 173). In Chapter 8, Deal and Cannito present, in my view, a masterful exposition that defines the characteristics of neurogenic dysfluency. They deftly differentiate neurogenic dysfluency from other types of dysfluency. The authors identify etiologies and delineate different forms of neurogenic dysfluency, which logically leads into suggested treatment strategies. They note that they use *neurogenic dysfluency* in lieu of *neurogenic stuttering* because they question the appropriateness of the term *stuttering* in a neurogenic context.

Deal and Cannito present evidence that neurogenic dysfluency can occur in association with a variety of neuropathologic disease processes as well as with stroke, head trauma, space-occupying neoplasms, and other conditions. While they indicate that neurogenic dysfluency is unlikely to be a unitary disorder, they refer to a number of descriptive reports and discussions in the literature to make the case that neurogenic dysfluency occurs as an isolated disorder, without concomitant aphasia, apraxia, or dysarthria. They also do a masterful job of bringing order out of the chaos of the bewildering, confusing, and inconsistent terminology that has been used to describe the disorder.

Deal and Cannito review the major neurogenic speech and language disorders in which a form of neurogenic dysfluency might be (and is often) found, such as in aphasia. To this disorder they apply the term "nonfluency," implying a linguistic deficit. They then review dysfluency as a component of motor speech disorders and indicate that dysfluency "implies a nonlinguistic motor control problem." In this regard they concisely review disorders such as apraxia of speech, dysarthria, and palilalia.

A description of profiles that differentiate types of acquired neurogenic dysfluency from developmental stuttering and psychogenic dysfluency is presented as a guideline for clinicians. The description can be especially helpful to clinicians attempting to determine whether a dysfluency is of neurogenic or psychogenic origin. Deal and Cannito present descriptive literature reports of neurogenic dysfluency being associated with single left hemisphere vascular episodes, bilateral or multiple vascular episodes, nonvascular etiologies, and progressive disorders such as Parkinson's and Alzheimer's diseases. They also present case reports of neurogenic dysfluency associated with various brain tumors, polysystemic central nervous system degeneration, and drug usage.

Treatment approaches are grouped under two broad headings: managing the underlying pathology and direct symptom modification. In the section on managing the underlying pathology, Deal and Cannito refer to the 1976 case report by Donnan as the only one reporting that surgical intervention for acquired neurogenic dysfluency was the management procedure of choice. In fact, left carotid endarterectomy was performed to ameliorate carotid artery stenosis, and while it resolved the patient's stuttering the surgery was undoubtedly designed to restore cerebral blood flow. I would like to add two fascinating reports by R. K. Jones, published in 1966 and 1967. In 1967 Jones published an article entitled "Dyspraxic Ambiphasia—A Neurophysiologic Theory of Stammering," which was prompted by a clinical report (1966) in which he described four patients who had stuttered severely since childhood and who had presented to him having recently developed brain pathology. Jones reported that after surgery on the damaged hemispheres he observed complete remission of stuttering in all of his patients. He had performed the Wada sodium amytal technique prior to and following surgery and found that "the results of stammering of a one-sided operation for unrelated lesions in these four patients was quite startling and can only be explained by the view that stammering is associated with an interference by one hemisphere with the speech performance of the other" (1966). He found no recurrence of stuttering after periods ranging from 15 months to 3 years.

Deal and Cannito describe prosthetic or assistive devices that have proved useful in the management of some forms of neurogenic dysfluency. They describe direct modifications of dysfluent symptoms and divide these "stuttering therapies" into two general classes, fluency-shaping therapy and stuttering modification therapy. They counsel that an eclectic approach toward treating acquired neurogenic dysfluency would seem to be advisable and indicate that the available literature "provides a fertile basis for clinical experimentation with a variety of potential combinations and permutations." The authors conclude with a classification scheme of approaches that have been employed in treating acquired neurogenic dysfluency patients. Their purpose is to bring order to the diverse array of treatment approaches, and I feel that they succeed admirably. Ending on an encouraging note, they indicate that controlled clinical experimentation that will expand our knowledge of acquired dysfluency is beginning to emerge. They further note that there is no shortage of field-tested approaches for remediation of acquired neurogenic dysfluency, and that "all of them have contributed successfully to the management of selected cases."

Robin, Klouda, and Hug discuss disorders of prosody in patients with focal cerebral lesions in Chapter 9. After presenting a review of the relevant literature, the authors discuss the steps involved in the diagnosis of prosodic disturbances. Their discussion focuses on the importance of acoustic measures to complement perceptual judgments, and the need to examine both the production and comprehension of prosody by patients. A description of various treatment approaches for disorders of prosodic comprehension and prosodic production deficits is presented with detailed profiles of cases possessing different prosodic profiles.

IDIOPATHIC SPEECH-SPECIFIC DISORDERS

One of the most variable disturbances of motor control is spasmodic (spastic) dysphonia (SD). The dinosaur was common but is now extinct;

in contrast, spasmodic dysphonia is an uncommon but real and current disorder that clinically presents as a disturbance of phonation. While the precise incidence and prevalence of SD remains unknown, both "its apparent focality and function specificity make it one of the most puzzling and controversial disorders of human communication." In Chapter 10, Cannito provides a coherent basis for interpretation: a neurogenic model involving the pyramidal-extrapyramidal voluntary motor system. This model implicates the supranuclear (upper motor neuron) system, and the author presents evidence that infranuclear explanations involving lower motor neurons or peripheral nerves are inadequate to account for vocal and other symptoms exhibited in this enigmatic disorder. The implications of this model for clinical management are discussed in a case study. Management of spasmodic dysphonia is considered within a motor speech disorder framework that emphasizes enhancement of the physiologic substrate; the focus is on compensated intelligibility rather than traditional voice therapy techniques. Cannito brings into bold relief the value of intelligibility testing in both assessment and ongoing management of this disorder.

Monitoring Physiologic Events

The use of noninvasive instrumentation for monitoring physiologic events during speech production has been confined primarily to laboratory settings involved in research of normal subjects and in populations who demonstrate dysfunctions of speech motor control. In Chapter 11 Watson and Alfonso present a rationale for incorporating noninvasive instrumentation into the clinical environment to identify and treat movement abnormalities associated with disorders of speech motor control, especially stuttering. They present illustrative examples that demonstrate the potential value of kinematic monitoring devices in identifying physiologic abnormality and in facilitating training of therapeutic targets. A description of clinical and laboratory evidence indicating that abnormalities in control of the respiratory and laryngeal systems may be associated with stuttering is offered. The development of Watson and Alfonso's rationale has emerged from research findings and clinical observations of stuttering individuals. This chapter demonstrates that noninvasive instrumentation is appropriate for treatment of deficits in a variety of clinical populations. It further illustrates that application of noninvasive instrumentation as a shared technology between clinic and laboratory can facilitate the transfer of laboratory findings and can be successfully applied in the clinical treatment of patients. This interface not only provides a more meaningful interaction between clinic and laboratory, but ultimately benefits persons with disordered speech motor control associated with stuttering, spasmodic dysphonia, and head trauma.

Developmental Apraxia of Speech

In the concluding chapter, Marquardt and Sussman offer a neuromorphology theory to account for developmental apraxia of speech. Their chapter provides an attempt to explain some of the disparate characteristics that have been proposed. The authors note that treatment for the disorder is based on approaches for children with articulation disorders, but emphasize that differential diagnosis of the disorder often proves difficult due to overlapping characteristics shared with phonological disorders and childhood aphasia. Although the disorder has been defined in similar terms for more than 30 years, a neurological construct to account for this disorder had not been suggested heretofore. Marquardt and Sussman propose a neurologically based model that accounts for important observed behavior characteristics of the disorder and also provide a framework for appraisal and differential diagnosis. They review and evaluate the relative merits of a variety of treatment regimens, finding a lack of evidence to support the effectiveness of these treatment approaches. A case study is presented that exemplifies the diversity of therapy approaches for children with developmental apraxia of speech and provides direction for therapeutic intervention through a series of highly individualized treatment approaches that address various aspects of the disorder. A review of techniques for functional articulation disorders that are adaptable to treating developmental apraxia of speech is presented, as well as several organized systems of therapy evolved from other disorders that appear to have value for working with these children.

SUMMARY

Desired outcomes have resulted from employing clinical management interventions consisting of appropriate and specific remedial procedures that have emerged from empirical studies. Reports of such studies provide valuable insights leading to a comprehensive understanding of the nature of disordered vocal motor control and enhance mutual scientific communication regarding human communicative ability, the product of the human nervous system that underlies the overt expression of verbal communication with which we are familiar.

This text, *Treating Disordered Speech Motor Control,* provides the reader a clear understanding of the structure and function of the peripheral and central nervous system of humans. It reaffirms that functional human communication has a physical reality in the human brain by presenting convincing evidence supported by electrophysiological, psychophysical, and neuroimaging findings. The relative merits of specific treatment programs are examined by presenting detailed clinical analyses and psychosocial outcomes. A wealth of empirical data are generated as the basis for proposing clinical strategies designed for the establishment of treatment programs and implementation of specific therapeutic techniques in a systematic and rational manner.

REFERENCES

Darley, F. L. (1972). The efficacy of language rehabilitation in aphasia. *Journal of Speech and Hearing Disorders, 37*, 1.
DiSimoni, F. G. (1989). *Apraxia of speech: Theoretical and practical considerations.* Dalton, PA: Praxis House.
Dworkin, J. P., Abkarian, G. G., & Johns, D. F. (1988). Apraxia of speech: The effectiveness of a treatment regimen. *Journal of Speech and Hearing Disorders, 53*, 280–294.
Feinstein, A. R. (1985). *Clinical epidemiology: The architecture of clinical research.* Philadelphia: W. B. Saunders.
Johns, D. F. (1975). *Speaking out on neurogenic and "neurogenic" disorders of output processing.* In M. D. Sullivan & M. S. Kommers (Eds.), *Central auditory processing disorders* (pp. 148–182). Omaha: University of Nebraska Medical Center Press.
Jones, R. K. (1966). Observations on stammering after localized cerebral injury. *Journal of Neurology, Neurosurgery, and Psychiatry, 29*, 192.
Jones, R. K. (1967). Dyspraxia ambiphasia—A neurophysiologic theory of stammering. *Transactions of the American Neurological Association*, p. 197.
Lashley, K. S. (1961). The problem of serial order and behavior. In S. Saporta (Ed.), *Psycholinguistics: A book of readings* (pp. 180–198). New York: Holt, Rinehart and Winston.
Luchsinger, R., & Arnold, G. E. (1965). *Voice-speech-language.* Belmont, CA: Wadsworth.
Masland, R. L. (1970). Brain mechanisms underlying the language function. In *Human communication and its disorders—An overview* (NINDS Monograph), pp. 85–109.
Sherrington, C. S. (1906). *The integrative action of the nervous system.* New Haven, CT: Yale University Press.
Van Riper, C. (1971). *The nature of stuttering.* Englewood Cliffs, NJ: Prentice-Hall.
Wertz, R. T., LaPointe, L. L., & Rosenbek, J. C. (1984). *Apraxia of speech in adults.* New York: Grune and Stratton.
Zhang, J. X., Wilson, C., Levesque, M., Harper, R. M., and Engel, J. (1989). Multimodal stereotactic imaging for mapping brain functional imaging to anatomic structure. *Society for Neuroscience Abstracts, 15*, 1239.

CHAPTER 2

Comanagement of Disordered Speech Motor Control: The Roles of the Neurologist and the Speech Pathologist

Robert Lozano

> *Lozano is a speech-language pathologist and a neurologist. He discusses patient management from the point of view of each discipline, and outlines assessment and treatment procedures conducted by the professionals from both areas. Finally, he underscores the need for cooperation between professionals from each discipline in order to provide the best care available for the communicatively impaired patient.*

1. What is the most important part of the neurologic examination?
2. How does the speech pathologist's approach differ from the neurologist's approach to patient management?
3. Which skills did Lozano find easy to transfer from speech pathology to medical practice?

As I rounded the corner to enter the hospital room I could hear my next patient before I could see him. He was complaining to his roommate that he wished that he had never mentioned "it" because now more doctors would be coming to see him and probably they would "do more tests." "It" was a momentary visual blurring that occurred as he was walking and turning round, and "it" was the reason I was consulted. I had not seen the patient yet, but already I knew from hearing him speak that his neurologic examination would be abnormal. His speech was marked by prominent ataxic dysarthria with monopitch, an occasional pitch break, and an explosive quality. I could hear the dysmetria in his articulation. I had learned to recognize it when I was a speech pathologist.

It was extremely flattering to be asked to write a chapter for this book. "We want you to contribute because of your unique perspective," I was told. I suppose the foundation of my "uniqueness" was laid when I completed my master's degree in speech pathology, entered the doctoral program at Wayne State University, and was awarded a traineeship in speech pathology at the Allen Park, Michigan, Veterans Hospital. There I developed an interest in the acquired speech and language disorders of neurologically impaired adults. Later I received my Certificate of Clinical Competence in Speech Pathology from the American Speech-Language-Hearing Association (ASHA).

Still later, I completed my Ph.D. degree in speech pathology and became the director of speech and language pathology at the Rehabilitation Institute in Detroit, Michigan. For a while, things were going pretty well. Then for various reasons I left the Institute and went to medical school. I received my M.D. degree from Michigan State University and completed a year of internal medicine residency. Then I finished a 3-year residency in neurology at the University of Texas Health Science Center in San Antonio and started private practice in Texas.

If I am unique, I suppose it is because of my experience on both sides of the street. I was a clinical speech-language pathologist working with neurologically impaired adults, and now I am a physician diagnosing and treating neurologic illness of which aphasia or dysarthria may be a symptom or a sign.

When I made the transition from speech pathology to medicine, one speech pathologist friend of mine dubbed me a defector. What gave that endearing nickname meaning was the sense of rivalry and competition that may exist between speech pathology and neurology. I had gone over to the other side. But rather than experiencing defection, I feel more like a person who has undergone a personal evolution, one that began in speech pathology and continued to grow in neurology. For me the two professions represent different parts of the same continuum. Caring for the patient is the desire of both professions. Of course there are differences as well as similarities in the two professions, and I will discuss a number of them in this chapter.

PREPARATION

Academic Preparation

The academic preparation for speech pathology is slightly different from the academic background needed for medicine. In speech pathology there is an undergraduate core curriculum designed to prepare the student for the graduate courses necessary to obtain the master's degree and certification by ASHA. Academic courses are required in areas such as anatomy of the speech and hearing mechanism, neuroanatomy, speech physiology, acoustics, phonetics, linguistics, psychology, and psycholinguistics. The doctorate in speech pathology basically is a science degree. At this time there is no clinical doctorate. To pursue the doctorate is a personal decision; the doctoral degree is not a requirement for certification or state licensure.

The traditional undergraduate preparation for medicine includes courses in biology, general chemistry, organic chemistry, physics, physiology and biochemistry. In part, some medical schools want a measure of how well an individual was able to handle several science classes simultaneously. Medical schools accept students with a variety of undergraduate majors so long as the student has completed the prerequisite science classes satisfactorily and so long as the school feels that the candidate will make a valuable contribution as part of that particular medical school's class. It seems, however, that students with a major in science are preferred by committees selecting candidates for medical school.

Clinical Preparation

Clinical training in speech pathology usually begins at the undergraduate level and continues as part of the graduate curriculum. Supervised clinical practica in a range of speech and language disorders are required. In most medical schools, the medical student enters the clinical practicum years after spending two years studying basic science (microbiology, pharmacology, pathology, physiology, etc.). During the third and fourth years of medical school, the student enrolls in courses in internal medicine, pediatrics, psychiatry, obstetrics-gynecology, and surgery. Here the abstract of classroom science merges with the reality of the sickness, disease, and pestilence found in the clinic-hospital setting.

In almost every state in the United States, at least one year of postgraduate training is required before a physician can be licensed. The trend in American medicine has been for the recent medical graduate to select a multiyear training program in a specific area of medicine, for example, in internal medicine, obstetrics-gynecology, family medicine, or pediatrics. At least a year of internal medicine or its equivalent must be completed prior to entering a 3-year neurology residency. Postgraduate medical training is vigorous and includes long periods of being on call during which the resident may have a continuous work period of 30 hours or more.

In speech pathology, after completing a graduate program, the student must undergo a supervised work experience during the clinical fellowship year (CFY). The specialization that occurs in speech pathology depends not only on the student's academic training program but also heavily on the type of work place the student selects to complete the CFY. School-based speech pathologists develop more experience and expertise in articulation disorders and language delay, while hospital-based speech pathologists learn more about neurogenic communication disorders such as aphasia and dysarthria. Speech pathology specialization is driven by the experiences of the individual clinician.

I think speech-language pathologists know more about what neurologists do than vice versa. Usually the speech pathologist must educate the physician regarding the benefits of speech and language therapy for the patient with communication disorders. This is necessary so that physicians will make the appropriate patient referrals. Speech pathologists should know that physicians also must educate. For example, a physician arriving at a hospital for the first time must make the existing medical staff aware of what the physician can do for the patients at that facility. Speech pathologists should remember that they offer important and beneficial services to patients and that they need to communicate this fact to physicians.

I believe my experience in speech-language pathology has been extremely valuable to me as a physician. There are several skills which I learned as a speech pathologist that I continue to use as a neurologist. The interviewing skills I used as a speech pathologist transferred easily to my medical practice. And listening skills are crucial in both speech pathology and medicine. Listening to the patient and caring about those things that are important to the patient are the most valuable skills the health-care provider can possess. The ability to observe patient behavior critically is a skill learned by speech pathologists and used extensively by neurologists. I learned to appreciate how illness or disability impacts on the patient as a person and on the patient's position in the family and in society during the years I was a speech pathologist. From the perspective of seeing patients as people, compassion for others may grow. I learned to set aside the goals of a treatment session to comfort a distraught patient when I was a speech pathologist.

THE NEUROLOGIST'S APPROACH TO PATIENT MANAGEMENT

For the neurologist, the knowledge of the anatomy, physiology, and pathophysiology of the nervous system provide the conceptual framework for problem solving. Each patient presents a unique set of circumstances and complaints which are dissected out by careful history taking. The neurologist's goals are to provide answers to the questions "Where is the lesion?" and "What is the nature of the lesion?" After the diagnosis is made, appropriate treatment can begin or appropriate referral can be made.

The History

The history is the most important part of the neurologic evaluation. While the history is taken, the neurologist forms a set of hypothetical diagnoses, and with selected follow-up questions each hypothetical diagnosis is tested and ranked according to the likelihood of its occurrence. This has been referred to as "hypothesis driven" history taking. Information is gathered on essential basic factors including the age and sex of the patient, onset of the problem, progression of symptoms, duration and course of the problem, and predisposing conditions. This information is used by the neurologist to decide the level of the nervous system at which the lesion is located and the disease process most likely involved.

Neurologic Examination

The neurologic examination provides a detailed evaluation of the integrity of the nervous sytem. Generally, the complete neurologic examination consists of an evaluation of the patient's mental status, cranial nerves, motor system, sensory system, and gait. The mental status examination tests alertness, orientation, attention, memory, and speech and language functions. This examination may include determining if the patient is aware of the time, date, and place of the examination and asking the patient to do mathematical calculations, to interpret proverbs, and to solve hypothetical problems such as "What would you do if you smelled smoke in a crowded theater?" The cranial nerve examination involves evaluation of the function of nerves with nuclei located above the spinal cord. Cranial nerves important to speech motor control, their functions, and methods for testing them are listed in Table 2.1.

An evaluation of the motor system includes noting appearance of the muscles and an examination of muscle tone and strength. Some neurologists include coordination and deep tendon reflex testing in their evaluation of the motor system. Passive movements are evaluated while

TABLE 2.1
Cranial Nerves Involved in Speech Motor Control, Their Functions, and Methods of Evaluation

Cranial Nerve	Function	Method of Evaluation
V Trigeminal	Sensation from masseters, palate, and pharynx	With a pin, examiner pricks patient's face first on one side, then on the other, and asks patient to identify location of pinprick.
	Motor to mandibular muscles	Patient is asked to simulate a bite while examiner attempts to pry patient's jaws apart. Examiner checks for weakness of jaw.
		Patient relaxes and opens jaw slightly. Examiner taps on jaw to test for jaw jerk.
VII Facial	Sensation from anterior tongue; motor to face	Examiner observes for facial movement, tics, and tremors, and asks patient to look upward while wrinkling forehead.
		Patient blows out cheeks; examiner squeezes cheeks in to force expulsion of air.
IX Glosso-pharyngeal	Sensation from posterior tongue, soft palate, and pharynx; motor to pharynx	Elevation of palate and contraction of pharyngeal wall are observed during phonation.
X Vagus	Motor to larynx, pharynx, and soft palate	As in IX, also assess phonatory capabilities.
XII Hypoglossal	Motor to tongue	Patient presses tongue to inside of right, then left, cheek while examiner palpates from outside.
		Patient flexes tongue in and out of mouth rapidly while examiner checks alternate motion rate.

moving the patient's limb as the patient maintains the limb in a state of relaxation. Active movements are evaluated as the patient carries out movements described by the examiner.

Sensory testing involves assessing temperature, pain, light touch, vibration, and proprioception throughout the body. The examiner may pinch the patient's muscles or press on structures that are sensitive to pressure, for example, the larynx. Or the examiner may test the ability to identify light touch as the patient's skin is stroked or touched with a light pinprick. Gait and station are also tested as the patient performs a number of standing and walking exercises.

There are several branching steps that can be included in the neurological examination. These steps are used to evaluate a possible abnormality further or to better define the level in the nervous system at which a dysfunction may be present. Specific maneuvers are used to elicit pathologic signs, many of which have been named for dead neurologists. For example, when stroking the lateral aspect of the sole of the patient's foot, the examining neurologist is attempting to observe whether the patient's big toe moves up or down. An upward moving toe (dorsoflexion) is a pathologic sign of an upper motor neuron lesion affecting that extremity and is referred to as the Babinski reflex.

A further description of the clinical neurological examination seems to be beyond the scope of the information appropriate to present here. The interested reader is encouraged to consult Brookshire (1986) or Rodnitzky (1988) for more information on this topic.

As a speech pathologist, I was never favorably impressed with the speech and language evaluations conducted by a neurologist. I found these evaluations to be too brief and lacking in depth and detail. Please spare me "Say Methodist-Episcopal"! As a neurologist, I find myself thinking how long, detailed, and burdensome are the evaluations conducted by the speech-language pathologist. Please spare me "Say /pa/ta/ka/"! The point here is that the speech evaluation serves a different function for each discipline. The neurologist is conducting a screening of speech functions, looking for errors that will confirm the suspicion of a lesion. Speech and language is just a portion of a complete neurologic examination. The speech pathologist's evaluation, on the other hand, involves taking an inventory of communication skills, analyzing errors, and forming a basis for diagnosing and treating the patient's communication disorder.

In general, there should be no real surprises during the neurologic exam. Examination results should confirm the verbal hypotheses formed during the history taking. If the examination results do not fit the hypotheses formed from the existing history, further information must be obtained.

Neurologic Diagnosis

The neurologist who conceptually applies the neuroanatomical grid to the results of the patient's history and neurological examination is attempting to answer the question "What is the lesion?" To answer the question "Where is the lesion?" the neurologist references the probable location of the lesion against those neuropathologic processes which can occur at that site. The possible etiologies arising from this cross-referencing are the differential diagnoses of the patient's problem.

Neurologists relish differential diagnoses. A "differential" is a list of the possible diagnoses that may account for the patient's neurologic condition. The spectrum of etiologies of a particular condition are held up for scrutiny. For example, the neurologist considers the question "Is the patient's neurologic deficit compatible with dysfunction caused by tumor, ischemia, degenerative processes, infection, or metabolic dysfunction?" In a sense, the neurologist approaches the patient's problem as a marvelous intellectual puzzle that can be solved with information from the history; knowledge of neuroanatomy, neurophysiology, and neuropathology; logic; and confirmation from the results of the neurologic examination. Typically the level of the lesion is determined first and then the neurologist speculates about which disease processes are present at that location. In neurology circles, great accolades are given to those neurologists who can produce a range of possible diagnoses. Although the list should be complete and include uncommon diseases, emphasis should be placed on typical presentations of common diseases. There is a saying among neurologists in South Texas that goes, "When you're out on the ranch and you hear hoofbeats, the first thing you think of should *not* be zebras."

Diagnoses that may be considered in conditions producing disordered speech motor control are listed in Table 2.2.

Laboratory Tests

Once the differential diagnoses have been determined, additional laboratory tests may be ordered. Needed information may come from blood analysis, examination of the cerebrospinal fluid, neurologic electrophysiology evaluations, and special imaging procedures (see Walker-Batson and Purdy, this volume). The added information is obtained in order to exclude some diagnoses and to support the most likely diagnosis. The choice of laboratory tests selected is based on information regarding the suspected disease and the pathologic findings. Table 2.3 contains a list of some laboratory tests used to diagnose conditions for which disordered speech motor control is a symptom.

Many tests are performed so frequently that they are considered routine; the complete blood count (CBC) is an example. The CBC provides

TABLE 2.2
Neurologic Causes of Disorders of Motor Control of Speech

Myasthenia gravis
Eaton-Lambert syndrome
Parkinson's disease
Alzheimer's disease
Multiple sclerosis
Encephalopathies—toxic/metabolic, progressive multifocal
   leukoencephalopathy
Cerebellar degeneration—idiopathic, toxic
Olivopontocerebellar degeneration
Amyotrophic lateral sclerosis
Wilson's disease
Huntington's disease
Thryoid disease
Parathyroid disease
Ischemia
Stroke
Encephalitis
Meningitis
Lues
Jakob-Creutzfeldt disease
Trauma, closed head injury
Toxins—alcohol, lead, mercury, drugs
Cerebral palsy
Tumors—carcinoma: primary, metastatic; benign
Metabolic derangements—hyponatremia, hypokalemia, hypoglycemia,
   vitamin deficiencies

the physician with a quantitative and qualitative analysis of the patient's blood. The number of leukocytes, or white blood cells (WBCs), will increase with infection and stress. The differentiation of WBCs into types also is helpful in diagnosis. The number of red blood cells (RBCs) provides a measure of the body's ability to produce blood cells and also is used to identify the presence of anemia. Further hematologic measures can provide information regarding the amount of hemoglobin (the oxygen-carrying component in the RBCs) and the hematocrit (the percentage of RBC mass compared to the blood volume). The average size of the RBCs is referred to as the mean corpuscular volume (MCV). Increased MCVs are detected in certain disease states.

The CBC can yield important information. For example, a man who had undergone stomach surgery several years previously developed symptoms of difficulty walking and dysarthric speech. A CBC revealed a normal WBC and decreased numbers of RBCs with decreased hemoglobin and hematocrit. MCV was enlarged. Based on the results of the CBC together with the history of stomach surgery, the physician checked

TABLE 2.3
Laboratory Tests Used in Diagnosis of Patients with Disorders of Motor Control of Speech

Complete Blood Count (CBC)
  White Blood Cells (WBC), Red Blood Cells (RBC), Hemoglobin, Hematrocrit, indices including Mean Corpuscular Hemoglobin (MCH) and Mean Corpuscular Volume (MCV)

Serum Metabolic Tests
  Sodium
  Potassium
  Chloride
  Bicarbonate
  Glucose
  Blood Urea Nitrogen (BUN)
  Creatinine
  Magnesium
  Calcium
  Uric acid
  Cholesterol
  Triglycerides
  Total bilirubin
  Serum glutamic-pyruvic transaminase (SGPT)
  Serum glutamic-oxaloacetic transaminase (SGOT)
  Gamma-glutamyl transpeptidase (GGTP)
  Lactic dehydrogenase (LDH)
  Alkaline phosphatase
  Creatine phosphokinase (CPK)

Special Serum Tests
  Gamma immunoglobin (IgG)
  Serum protein electrophoresis
  Ceruloplasmin
  Copper
  Vitamin B_{12}
  Thyroid functions
  Ammonia
  Acetylcholine receptor antibody
  Rapid plasma reagin (RPR)

Cerebrospinal Fluid (CSF) Studies
  Cell count and differential—WBC, RBC
  Glucose
  Protein

Special CSF Tests
  IgG
  Oligoclonal bands—electrophoresis
  Fungal, bacterial, viral studies
  Veneral Disease Research Laboratories (VDRL)

---

the patient's vitamin B_{12} level and reviewed the patient's history of alcohol intake. The physician reasoned that results of the previous surgery had resulted in impaired vitamin B_{12} absorption and that the patient was suffering neuronal damage secondary to vitamin B_{12} deficiency. That was a possible cause of the patient's walking and speech difficulties.

Metabolic screening is another laboratory test used frequently. This procedure varies from community to community and is based on the capability of the laboratory equipment available in a particular locale. The following example illustrates how the metabolic screen was helpful in treating an elderly person who was taking oral hypoglycemic medication for diabetes. The patient was brought into the emergency room of a local hospital after developing slurred speech and confusion. As part of a metabolic screen, the patient's serum glucose was checked and was found to be abnormally low. After adjustment of the glucose level, the patient's speech and mental functioning returned to normal.

There are patients for whom special blood studies may be indicated. For example, serum ceruloplasmin (a transport protein for copper) and serum copper levels should be checked in the patient for whom Wilson's disease is suspected.

Examination of the cerebrospinal fluid (CSF) may be necessary in some cases. Essential examination of CSF must include cell count and differential glucose and protein. The cells are identified and quantified. The specific findings in the CSF may be very important for the confirmation of the proposed diagnosis. Increased WBCs in the CSF may mean infection. An excessive number of RBCs in the CSF may indicate the presence of a subarachnoid hemorrhage. Glucose is actively transported in the CSF. An abnormally low CSF glucose level often is indicative of inflamed meninges. In classic tuberculosis meningitis, the CSF glucose also is extremely low. Central nervous system syphilis often is revealed by hundreds of WBCs in the CSF with a predominance of lymphocytes. So it becomes obvious that the specific findings in the CSF may be very important for the confirmation of the proposed diagnosis.

Depending on the anticipated diagnosis, additional special tests on the CSF may be needed. For example, in suspected multiple sclerosis, most neurologists would request the determination of gamma immunoglobins (IgG) for evidence of increased levels. In such patients, examination of the CSF with electrophoresis may reveal the presence of oligoclonal bands which tend to support the diagnosis of multiple sclerosis.

Special imaging techniques are very useful for diagnosis. In multiple sclerosis, magnetic resonance imaging (MRI) has been extremely useful in detecting white matter plaques. MRI also has been helpful in demonstrating the presence of occult tumors. Computerized tomography (CT) is another imaging technique that contributes to the confirmation of the diagnosis of stroke, hemorrhage, and tumor. For an extensive discussion of brain imaging techniques, see Walker-Batson and Purdy, Chapter 3 of this volume. Examples of MRI and CT scans of patients who exhibited disordered speech motor control are shown in Figures 2.1 and 2.2.

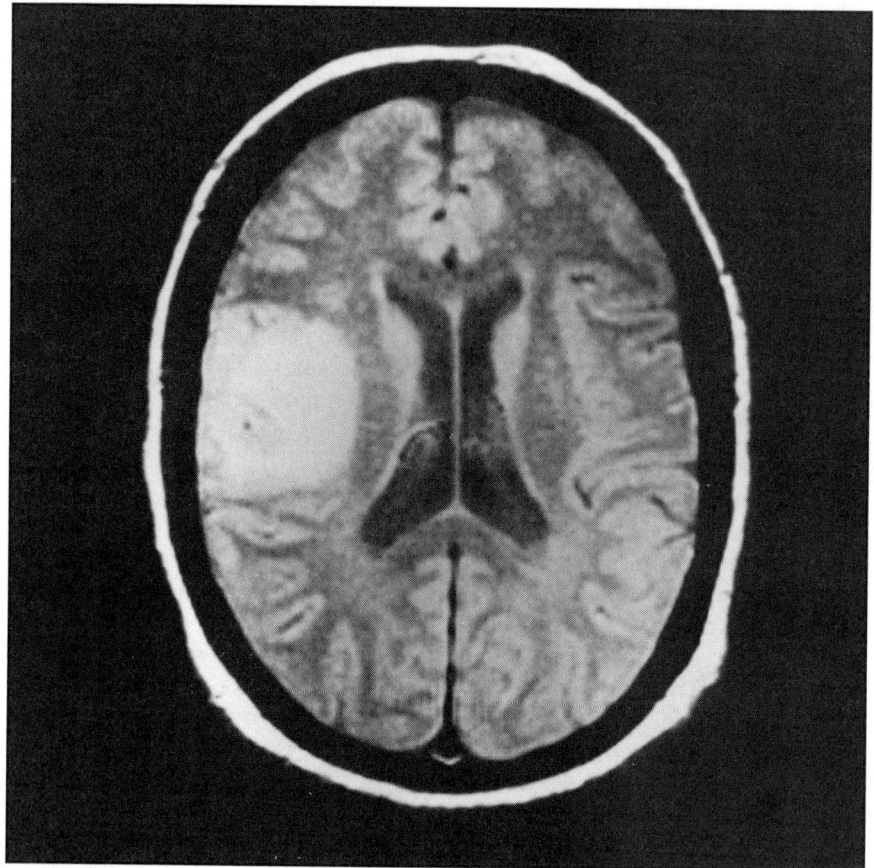

Figure 2.1 Head MRI, T1 image. A 53-year-old female with history of breast cancer presented with seizure, mild left facial palsy and mild dysarthria. Diagnosis: Single metastatic tumor in right hemisphere.

In patients with neuromuscular disorders, specific electrophysiologic studies may be required. Nerve conduction velocities (NCV) and electromyography (EMG) may be used in diagnosis. The recording of muscle fasciculations and denervation potentials may substantiate denervation changes found in amyotrophic lateral sclerosis (ALS). A biopsy of muscles may be needed to determine correct neuromuscular diagnosis.

Treatment

For the neurologist, arriving at a diagnosis may be easier than selecting the most effective treatment. There can be a wide range of acceptable

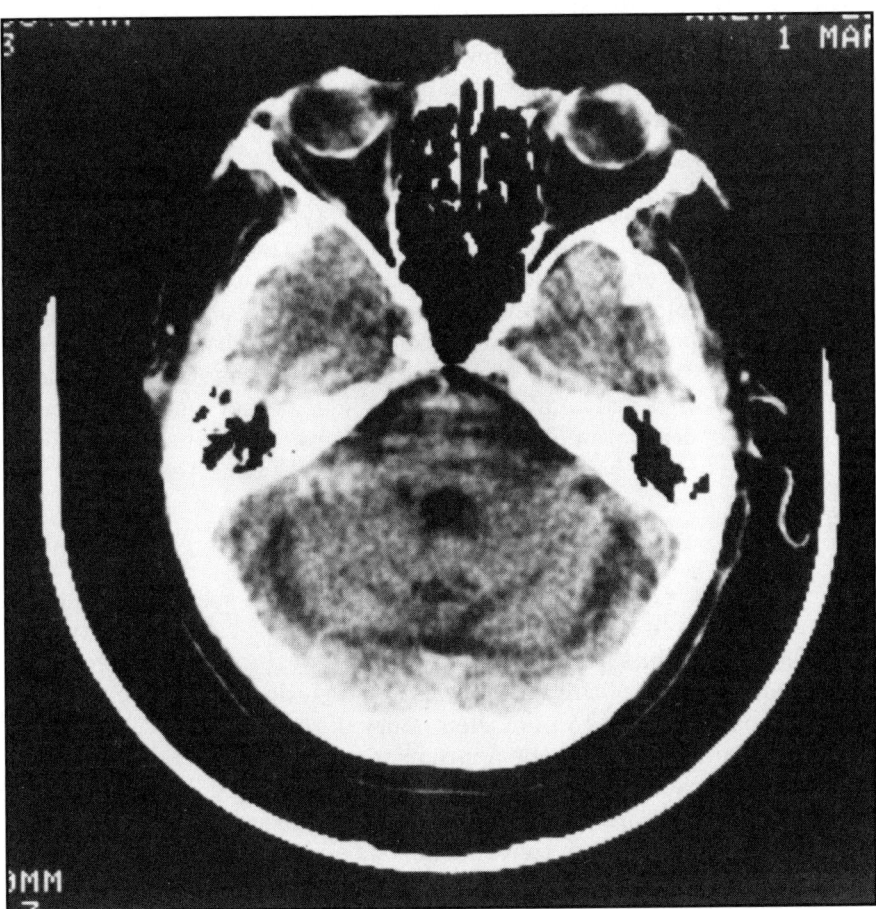

Figure 2.2 CT-scan image. A 65-year-old male with long-standing gait ataxia, extremity dysmetria, and ataxic dysarthria. Diagnosis: Marked cerebellar atrophy, possible cerebellar stroke.

medical therapies for some disorders, due in part to the seemingly continuous introduction of new therapeutics. This is highly praised by some as medical progress. Sometimes when a new medication or surgery is found to be efficacious for treating a certain disease, the news appears in the lay press and public interest is aroused. If the new cure is not available in the United States due to restrictions set by the Food and Drug Administration, for example, some patients will travel to countries outside the United States where they can obtain the cure. In reality, these new cures may not be any more effective than the existing "tried and true" therapies which, because of their easy availability, also may be less expensive. As a rule, the experimental trials comparing one therapy with another lag long behind the excitement generated by the lay press. To be sure, new instrumentation and treatment programs become available in speech pathology that improve the quality of a patient's life. In medicine, new treatment programs, if effective, can extend that life.

Typically the physician begins the patient on a therapeutic trial of medication or refers the patient for another type of therapy or for surgery. The neurologist makes adjustments to the treatment regime pragmatically, based on the success or failure of the current treatment. Usually a neurologist who refers a patient to a speech pathologist has identified the patient's neurologic problem and the referral is part of an overall treatment plan. Most neurologists categorize the speech pathologist as an allied health professional just as they would categorize the physical or occupational therapist. These professionals are considered by the physician to be members of the rehabilitation team.

Referral to a Speech Pathologist

A consultation request from the neurologist to the speech pathologist may read: "Patient had stroke, has slurred speech; evaluate and treat." Now the patient has been placed in the care of the speech pathologist for the remediation of the communication disorder. The speech pathologist has been trained to take the history of the patient's communication impairment, to select the appropriate diagnostic measures, and to design and carry out the plan for the treatment of the disorder. I have found that many neurologists have no idea that speech pathologists have a master's level education, that there exists a national organization with criteria for certification of speech pathologists, and that in many states speech pathologists must be licensed to practice. When a neurologist has a patient with a speech disorder for which there is no effective medical therapy, however, there exists the hope that the speech pathologist can improve the patient's ability to communicate and therefore improve the quality of the patient's life.

The efficacy of speech-language therapy has been questioned by some physicians. As a speech pathologist, at times I felt there were hordes of demonic physicians roaming the countryside chanting, "Why bother with therapy? It doesn't work!" Despite evidence that speech therapy for disordered speech-motor control *does* work (Wertz, LaPointe, & Rosenbek, 1984; Dworkin, Abkarian, & Johns, 1988), many neurologists continue to question its efficacy. There is doubt, also concerning the value of language therapy for facilitating recovery from aphasia even though there is evidence that language therapy is efficacious (Sparks, Helm, & Albert, 1974; Kushner & Winitz, 1977; Wertz et al., 1981; Wertz et al., 1986; Marshall, 1986; Albert & Helm-Estabrooks, 1988; Marshall et al., 1989). I think this "no benefit" attitude also has been dispelled by the fact that third-party payers have recognized the benefit of speech-language therapy and have offered reimbursement for the services of a speech-language pathologist.

It is my hunch that the assumption that language therapy doesn't work is based in part on the speech and language examination conducted by the neurologist. The typical neurologist—that is, one who does not have a special interest in higher cortical functioning in general or in speech and language in particular—evaluates the patient only for the purpose of determining the presence of aphasia versus dementia or confused mental state. The neurologist usually makes a modest effort to classify the type of aphasia for anatomic correlation, then refers the patient to a speech pathologist for a thorough evaluation and subsequent treatment for the communication disorder. Eventually the patient returns to the neurologist, who reevaluates the communication disorder and determines whether residual speech or language impairment is present. Usually it is. Although the patient's speech intelligibility and language skills may have improved with therapy, residual speech or language impairment may persist. The presence of this residual deficit may account for the skepticism.

I believe that almost all patients who have a speech or language problem secondary to neurologic impairment should be evaluated by a speech pathologist. I also believe that a competent speech pathologist can decide who may and who may not benefit from a trial of treatment. Furthermore, it is my belief that not all patients need speech therapy. There are some who will achieve good recovery without intervention and there are some who will never be capable of effective communication. It is also important to recognize that not all patients want speech therapy. Time is spent most effectively with patients who are motivated. Rather than treatment, a reevaluation at a later time is appropriate for some patients. Just as physicians are skeptical of referring patients to surgeons who always recommend a specific operation, they tend to be somewhat wary of referring a patient to a speech pathologist who recommends therapy for all patients regardless of how dismal the prospects for a successful outcome may be.

THE SPEECH PATHOLOGIST'S APPROACH TO PATIENT MANAGEMENT

Diagnosis and Treatment

Although I believe this is happening less frequently now than it has in the past, there are some patients who arrive for a speech evaluation who don't know just why they are there. Often a patient will express great relief upon meeting a professional whose purpose is to focus on remediation of the communication disorder. During the initial interview when obtaining information about the patient's background, the speech pathologist also gathers a spontaneous speech and language sample and estimates the patient's mental status and ability to comprehend. The speech pathologist is concerned with answers to the questions "Does the patient have a speech and/or language disorder?" "What are the patient's residual capabilities?" and "How can I facilitate the improvement of the patient's communication skills?" To answer these questions, diagnostic assessment is completed.

The speech pathologist selects diagnostic instruments to establish and record the patient's communicative abilities. In the formal evaluation, standardized procedures are employed for obtaining samples of the patient's speech and for scoring those samples. The formal speech and language evaluation administered by the speech pathologist is much more detailed and quantifiable than the screening administered by the neurologist. A partial list of tests and instruments that may be used by speech-language pathologists to identify and assess various speech and language disorders is provided in Table 2.4.

After the speech and language is assessed, often the disorder is classified. It is interesting that there appear to be lumpers and splitters among both neurologists and speech-language pathologists. Many neurologists tend to split language disorders—that is, aphasia—into groups by type while lumping speech disorders—that is, dysarthria—together. Many speech-language pathologists, on the other hand, tend to lump aphasia while splitting dysarthria into groups by patterns of characteristics. Tables 2.5 and 2.6 list types of dysarthria and aphasic syndromes.

Once the level of residual function has been determined, the speech pathologist can design a treatment program. Most therapy for neurologically based speech disorders involves providing stimulation and teaching compensatory strategies. The patient's residual communicative strengths can be used to improve impaired communication skills. The structuring of individualized treatment is not a trivial task. The best speech clinicians are those who are resourceful and imaginative in designing treatment programs.

In summary, neurologists have a "disease-state" orientation to patient management. They obtain a history and conduct an examination to discover features of dysfunction as evidence of lesions in the patient's nervous system. Then they attempt to localize and determine the etiology of the lesion; and this information aids them in making decisions regarding the treatment to follow.

The speech pathologists' approach to management of the patient with disordered speech motor control is a functional one. They must deter-

TABLE 2.4
Methods for Evaluating Adult Neurogenic Communication Disorders

Motor-Speech Disorders

  Auditory Perceptual Methods
    Assessment of the Intelligibility of Dysarthric Speech (AIDS)
    Computerized Assessment of the Intelligibility of Dysarthric Speech
    Mayo Clinic Motor Speech Evaluation
    Frenchay Dysarthria Test
    Dabul Apraxia Battery
    Informal tests of nonspeech behaviors, e.g., vowel prolongation, alternate motion rate

  Acoustic Methods
    Instrumentation, e.g., oscilloscope, spectrograph, Visi-Pitch, PM Pitch Analyzer

  Imaging Methods
    Stroboscopy
    Endoscopy
    Videofluoroscopy

  Aerodynamic Methods
    Oral-Nasal Airflow Measures

Language Disorders
  Porch Index of Communicative Abilities
  Minnesota Test for the Differential Diagnosis of Aphasia
  Boston Diagnostic Aphasia Examination/Boston Naming Test
  Western Aphasia Battery
  Communicative Abilities in Daily Living
  Token Test
  Auditory Comprehension Test for Sentences
  Arizona Battery of Communication

mine not only what the patient cannot do but also what the patient can do. After determining a patient's communicative strengths and weaknesses, speech pathologists design speech therapy utilizing the strengths to improve the weaknesses. Their goal is to restore speech intelligibility to a level as near to premorbid ability as is possible, and, if effective verbal communication cannot be restored, the patient must be taught alternate methods of communication.

CASE STUDIES

In this section, I will describe three patients with neurologically based speech disorders. In the first case the speech pathologist was an integral part of the patient's management plan.

TABLE 2.5
Dysarthria Types and Their Highest Ranked Symptoms

Dysarthria Type	Highest Ranked Symptoms
Flaccid	Hypernasality Imprecise consonants Breathiness
Spastic	Imprecise consonants Monopitch Reduced stress
Ataxic	Imprecise consonants Excess and equal stress Irregular articulatory breakdown
Hypokinetic	Monopitch Reduced stress Monoloudness
Hyperkinetic (Chorea)	Imprecise consonants Prolonged intervals Variable rate
Hyperkinetic (Dystonia)	Imprecise consonants Distorted vowels Harsh voice quality
Mixed (ALS)	Imprecise consonants Hypernasality Harsh voice quality
Mixed (MS)	Impaired loudness control Harsh voice quality Defective articulation
Mixed (Wilson's disease)	Monopitch Monoloudness Reduced stress

Note. Adapted from *Motor-Speech Disorders* by F. L. Darley, A. E. Aronson, and J. R. Brown, 1975, Philadelphia: W. B. Saunders Company. Copyright 1975 by W. B. Saunders Company. Adapted by permission.

Case 1

One night while at a party, I was approached by the wife of an attorney who knew I was both a physician and a speech pathologist. She wanted me to meet her husband, a 28-year-old man who had no significant past medical history but who recently had been experiencing some speech difficulties. When I met him I noted that his speech was slow and labored. He said that people were beginning to notice that he "sounded

TABLE 2.6
Contemporary Classifications of Aphasic Syndromes

Type	Task	Symptom
Broca's	Spoken discourse	Nonfluent
	Auditory language comprehension	Relatively normal
	Sentence repetition	Abnormal
Global	Spoken discourse	Nonfluent
	Auditory language comprehension	Poor
	Sentence repetition	Poor
Transcortical Motor	Spoken discourse	Nonfluent
	Auditory language comprehension	Relatively normal
	Sentence repetition	Relatively normal
Mixed Transcortical	Spoken discourse	Nonfluent
	Auditory language comprehension	Abnormal
	Sentence repetition	Relatively normal
Wernicke's	Spoken discourse	Fluent[a]
	Auditory language comprehension	Poor
	Sentence repetition	Poor
Conduction	Spoken discourse	Fluent[a]
	Auditory language comprehension	Relatively normal
	Sentence repetition	Poor
Transcortical Sensory	Spoken discourse	Fluent[a]
	Auditory language comprehension	Poor
	Sentence repetition	Relatively normal
Anomic	Spoken discourse	Fluent
	Auditory language comprehension	Relatively normal
	Sentence repetition	Relatively normal

[a]Although output is fluent, it is paraphasic and may convey low information content.

different" and that often he was asked if he had a cold. He was concerned especially because his profession demanded good communication skills.

The attorney told me that in general he had been feeling weak and that his hands had become clumsy. In addition, he reported that occasionally he felt as if fluid were beginning to regurgitate through his nose. As I listened to him, I noted that his speech was slow and deliberate with a suggestion of mild hypernasality and mild imprecise articulation. I recommended that he consult a neurologist and a speech pathologist for evaluation.

Results of the neurological evaluation revealed weakness and fasciculations in his extremities and that mild spasticity and hyperreflexia (exaggeration of the deep tendon reflexes) were present. Sensation was intact.

The patient had no higher cortical dysfunction, but he did have inadequate velopharyngeal closure and slowed tongue movements, which are evidence of cranial nerve motor impairments. His mild spasticity and increased deep tendon reflexes were signs of upper motor neuron dysfunction, while the fasciculations that were evident were indicative of lower motor neuron disease. There were signs of mixed upper and lower motor neuron lesions at the level of and below the medulla.

When a neurologist is confronted with this constellation of symptoms and signs, he must include motor neuron disease in the differential diagnosis. Treatable causes of motor system dysfunction such as thyroid disease and heavy metal poisoning must be considered and ruled out. Other possible causes of similar dysfunction include bulbar-cervical spinal cord diseases such as bulbomyelia. Tumor and multiple sclerosis must be considerations also.

Laboratory and imaging techniques were ordered. Electromyography supported the clinical suspicion of denervation changes. Blood chemistry and special tests were not diagnostic. Imaging did not reveal a tumor or changes consistent with structural pathology. A presumptive diagnosis of amyotrophic lateral sclerosis (ALS) was made. This motor neuron disease is progressive and devastating and, to date, incurable.

Results of the patient's speech evaluation revealed a severe dysarthria. Initially treatment for the speech impairment focused on tongue-strengthening exercises, but as the patient's condition gradually worsened the focus of therapy was changed to speech rate control. Eventually, despite the patient's efforts to talk, he could no longer use verbal communication effectively and a letter and word board and an electric printer were introduced. Unfortunately these augmentative communicative devices were not totally successful, and his communication remained severely impaired.

The patient experienced progressive deterioration of strength throughout his body. He lost his job. He became wheelchair bound. Swallowing became increasingly difficult for him. After several years of debilitation and emotional distress, the patient died.

The neurologist's role in the management of this patient was to establish the correct diagnosis with special emphasis on ruling out treatable causes of denervation and motor dysfunction. The speech pathologist's role was to diagnose the speech problem, attempt to preserve communication, introduce compensatory techniques, and ultimately facilitate the use of methods of communication that were alternatives to speech. In other words, the speech pathologist's responsibility was to help the patient achieve optimum communication despite the debilitating neurologic condition.

When faced with a patient with an incurable disease, the physician may feel powerless to help the patient and so may resort to therapies that have questionable effectiveness or that have been reported successful by anecdote rather than by results of controlled treatment studies. The physician may think, "What harm can it do?" and encourage the patient to try an unproven therapy. Unfortunately, the patient's hopes of being cured are raised, then crushed, with each unsuccessful therapeutic trial. It is my opinion that honest communication between the patient and physician should guide the therapeutics. Supportive care is essential. The plight of patients with ALS is this: their bodies are wasted; they have no strength to perform basic self-care; it is likely that they are unable to speak so that they can be understood; and they may have significant swallowing and feeding difficulties. At the same time, they have retained sensation so that they may have physical pain, yet are unable to move; and they have retained their mental functions so that they are aware of what is happening to them.

In this case, the speech pathologist's task was a formidable one. The goals of speech therapy had to be altered as the patient deteriorated, until ultimately the patient was forced to abandon verbal communication. Alternate methods of communication were attempted and the method was selected that was the most effective for allowing the patient to express his needs. How can anyone overestimate the value of being introduced to a communication system that is the debilitated, dependent patient's only way to express himself, to communicate with others? I believe that all such patients should be referred to a speech pathologist.

Case 2

In this case study, I did not refer the patient to a speech pathologist. He was a 67-year-old right-handed man who had been admitted to the hospital for futher evaluation of a pleural effusion and possible open lung biopsy. About 12 years previously he had developed a sudden unsteadiness and weakness in his left leg. This eventually improved; over the years, however, his ability to walk in a steady manner had gradually declined, and when I first saw him he was using a walker for assistance. His speech was affected; I recognized the characteristics of ataxic dysarthria. His handwriting had deteriorated, and he had difficulty coordinating his hands and fingers to do fine work. As he spoke, I noticed that his grammar and syntax were appropriate and that he had no word retrieval difficulties. He denied memory loss. He had experienced an episode of blurred vision while using his walker when he had attempted to turn around; this episode had lasted approximately one or two seconds. He denied tinnitus, vertigo, diplopia (double vision) or amaurosis fugax (transient monocular blindness), weakness, or sensory loss.

At this point my hypothesis was a lesion in the cerebellum and I asked some follow-up questions to probe for a possible etiology. Although he was a smoker, he had no history of cancer, but he did have a pleural effusion from undiagnosed disease. He had used alcohol excessively 12 years before, at the time when he had noticed his first symptoms, but he had quit drinking and had abstained for several years. There was no family history of neurological disturbances similar to those he reported, nor of metabolic disease.

The pertinent findings of his neurologic examination were the following: nystagmus on lateral gaze and preserved strength throughout. Appendicular dysmetria (inability to gauge the distance, speed, and power of a movement) and dysdiadochokinesis (inability to perform and sustain rapid alternating movements) were present bilaterally. He could not stand with his feet together and his gait was wide-based. He had difficulty when he attempted to turn, and he nearly fell each time he tried to do so.

Laboratory examination revealed normal metabolic parameters including thyroid functions. CT scan of the head showed marked diffuse cerebellar atrophy. No tumor or infarction was seen.

The most likely diagnosis was a form of idiopathic or nonfamilial cerebellar degeneration. Alcoholic cerebellar disease and a form of cerebellar paraneoplastic syndrome (tumor) were possibilities also. As I considered referring him to a speech pathologist, I asked him how he felt about his speech. Although he recognized his speech was "not like it used to be," he said he was not especially disturbed by it and felt that by speaking slowly he could be understood by others. However, he was very stressed by his decreased ability to walk. I referred the patient to a physical therapist but did not refer him to a speech pathologist. At that point, I wondered if the defector was also a traitor.

Later this patient underwent open lung biopsy, which diagnosed carcinoma. At that time, further staging procedures were to be considered.

Case 3

Sometimes it is difficult to know whether to refer a patient to a speech pathologist—or indeed just what to do. The final case study illustrates this dilemma.

Once I received a telephone call from a friend who said that he had tried several ways to solve his speech problem. He was a 45-year-old right-handed man with a history of hypertension and headaches. His speech problem had begun about 5 years before his phone call to me. At that time he had developed a persistent cough and a tickling sensation in his throat. After two months he discovered that a steroid inhaler and oral medication provided some relief from his cough; however, his voice did not return to normal and continued to sound slightly strained. During the next few years, the strained sound continued. At the patient's insistence, his internist referred him to an ear-nose-throat (ENT) specialist; results of the ENT examination revealed no laryngeal pathology. Eventually he was examined by a second ENT physician who performed a direct laryngoscopy, but again no laryngeal pathology was found. The second ENT physician referred him to a speech pathologist who recommended voice therapy.

Treatment for the voice disorder did not produce significant change. My friend then went to a second speech pathologist, who referred him back to the internal medicine specialist for suspected allergies. The internist detected serologic evidence of an active allergic response and referred my friend to an allergy specialist. The allergist identified several environmental allergies and began a series of allergy shots. Subsequently, my friend's voice began to sound even more strained than before the allergy shots were administered.

My hapless friend reported that for about two years, which was three years after his problems started, he experienced pitch breaks and voice squeals. Indeed, to me the overall quality of his voice seemed strained and strangled. He had sought the opinion of a third ENT physician who had referred him to a fourth ENT specialist. The fourth doctor diagnosed my friend's problem as spastic dysphonia and referred him to a neurologist who agreed with the diagnosis. The neurologist found that, aside from the dysphonia, my friend's neurologic examination was normal. Subsequent to the neurological evaluation, the fourth ENT physician offered him the options of laryngeal nerve resection or botulinum toxin nerve blockade. (See Chapter 10, this volume, for a discussion of these procedures.)

My friend was contacting me to ask for my opinion. He wanted to know what to do next. I was certain that his voice problem was not psychiatric in origin, although it should not be surprising to find that a person who has been evaluated for the same problem by multiple physicians and speech pathologists for many years with no resolution to his misery is exhausted emotionally. It takes a great deal of personal courage, not to mention a great deal of money, to live a life with a strained, strangled-sounding voice and to continue to seek help for years. Unfortunately this course of multiple referrals is typical for patients with spastic dysphonia. There is ongoing research attempting to provide information regarding treatment for spastic dysphonia (see Chapter 10, this volume). Neither physicians nor speech pathologists have a simple solution at this time. In the meantime, my friend and others like him sit and wait.

SOME CONCLUDING REMARKS

In summary, the best care for the patient with a communication disorder is achieved when the neurologist and the speech pathologist realize that each offers different yet competent services that benefit the patient and agree to cooperate in patient management. Successful comanagement of the patient is accomplished more efficiently when the speech pathologist and the neurologist realize that there are strengths and shortcomings in both professions.

The speech and language disorders of neurologically impaired adults sparked my interest in medicine and neurology. I have cared for patients both as a speech pathologist and as a neurologist, and as a member of both professions I have learned this: Listen to your patients, attend to their concerns, maintain open communication with them, give them your best and most honest effort, and you will help them.

REFERENCES

Albert, M. L., & Helm-Estabrooks, N. (1988). Aphasia therapy works [Letter to the editor]. *Archives of Neurology, 45*, 372–373.

Brookshire, R. H. (1986). *An introduction to aphasia.* Minneapolis, MN: BRK Publishers.

Dworkin, J. P., Abkarian, G. G., & Johns, D. F. (1988). Apraxia of speech: The effectiveness of a treatment regimen. *Journal of Speech and Hearing Disorders, 53*(3), 280–293.

Kushner, D., & Winitz, H. (1977). Extended comprehension practice applied to an aphasic patient. *Journal of Speech and Hearing Disorders, 42*(2), 296–305.

Marshall, R. C. (1986). *For clinicians by clinicians: Vol. 3. Case studies in aphasia rehabiliation.* Austin, TX: PRO-ED.

Marshall, R. C., Wertz, R. T., Weiss, D., Aten, J., Brookshire, R. H., Garcia-Bunuel, L., Holland, A., Kurtzke, J., LaPointe, L. L., Millianti, F. J., Brannegan, R., Greenbaum, H., Vogel, D., Carter, J. E., Barnes, N. S., & Goodman, R. (1989). Home therapy for aphasic patients by trained and non-professionals. *Journal of Speech and Hearing Disorders, 54*(3), 262–270.

Rodnitzky, R. L. (1988). *Van Allen's pictorial manual of neurologic tests* (3rd ed.). Chicago: Year Book Medical Publishers.

Shewan, C. M., & Kertez, A. (1984). Effects of speech and language treatment on recovery from aphasia. *Brain and Language, 23*, 272–299.

Simmons, N. (1978). Finger counting as an intersystemic reorganizer in apraxia of speech. In R. H. Brookshire (Ed.), *Clinical aphasiology: Conference proceedings* (pp. 174–179). Minneapolis, MN: BRK Publishers.

Sparks, R., Helm, N., & Albert, N. (1974). Aphasia rehabilitation resulting from melodic intonation therapy. *Cortex, 10*, 303–313.

Wertz, R. T., Collins, M. J., Weiss, D., Kurtzke, J. F., Friden, T., Brookshire, R. H., Pierce, J., Holzapple, P., Hubbard, D. J., Porch, B. E., West, J. A., Davis, L., Matovich, V., Morely, G. K., & Resurreccion, E. (1981). Veterans Administration cooperative study on aphasia: A comparison of individual and group treatment. *Journal of Speech and Hearing Research, 24*, 580–594.

Wertz, R. T., LaPointe, L. L., & Rosenbek, J. C. (1984). *Apraxia of speech in adults: The disorder and its management.* New York: Grune & Stratton.

Wertz, R. T., Weiss, D., Aten, J. L., Brookshire, R. H., Garcia-Bunuel, L., Holland, A. L. Kurtzke, J. F., LaPointe, L. L., Milianti, F. J., Brannegan, R., Greenbaum, H., Marshall, R. C., Vogel, D., Carter, J. E., Barnes, N. S., & Goodman, R. (1986). Comparison of clinic, home, and deferred language treatment for aphasia: A Veterans Administration cooperative study. *Archives of Neurology, 43*, 653–658.

CHAPTER 3

Structural and Functional Brain Imaging in Disorders of Speech and Motor Control

Delaina Walker-Batson and Phillip D. Purdy

> Walker-Batson and Purdy provide a comprehensive discussion of the imaging technologies used to identify and confirm pathologies that underlie speech and language disorders. They discuss the limitations of these imaging tools in assessment.
>
> 1. What are the differences between functional and structural brain-imaging technologies?
> 2. According to Walker-Batson and Purdy, which imaging technologies are the backbone of medical management in neurological disorders?
> 3. What are some of the limits of the use of these imaging tools in assessing brain-speech mechanisms?

Brain imaging is increasingly being applied in disease states that affect both speech motor control and language. The rapidly evolving technologies of these new imaging techniques challenge the clinician to keep abreast not only of the nomenclature but of the clinical and research applications of these tools. This chapter provides an overview of six current brain-imaging technologies, their clinical and research use, and case presentations demonstrating these technologies in neurological disorders affecting speech motor control.

Over the past 30 years techniques have evolved for evaluating various aspects of cerebral structure and function in living individuals. Structural assessments include X-ray computed tomography (CT) and magnetic resonance imaging (MRI). Functional assessments include magnetic resonance spectroscopy (MRS), single-photon emission tomography (SPECT), positron emission tomography (PET), and topographic brain electrical activity mapping (BEAM).

Whereas the earliest understanding of cortical function related to speech and language was based on postmortem examination of lesions, recently the structural approach to lesion location has been enhanced by computerized tomography; biological or functional imaging technologies are providing information on neurophysiological and neurochemical aspects of speech and language processing. These tools are also providing beginning data bases regarding regional cerebral blood flow (rCBF), oxygen, glucose and phosphate metabolism, neurotransmitter function, and cortical electrical activity imaging in normal and neurologically impaired subjects. These tests can be applied not only at rest but during a variety of linguistic activation conditions as well.

In acquired language disorders, functional brain-imaging technologies have demonstrated areas of cortical dysfunction as determined by glucose metabolism (Metter, Hanson, Kempler, Squire, Wasterlain, & Benson, 1983), rCBF (Walker-Batson, Devous, Bonte, & Oelschlaeger, 1987; Tikofsky et al., 1985), and corticoelectrical activity (Nagata, Tagawa, Shishido, & Uemura, 1986) in areas remote from the primary lesion site as depicted on CT. In a variety of neurologic disorders affecting speech motor control, physiological brain-imaging tools have demonstrated central nervous system dysfunction not evident with anatomic-structural techniques (Bromfield, Ludlow, Bassich, & Theodore, 1988; Calne et al., 1985; Cannito, Pool, Freeman, & Finitzo, 1985; Devous et al., 1990; Kushner, Reivich, Alavi, Greenberg, Stern, & Dann, 1987). Collectively these studies suggest that brain speech-language theory based on structural damage alone needs to be enlarged to account for neurophysiologic and neurochemical changes observed after brain damage or in disease states. Recent papers suggesting neurobiologic models of speech motor control (Kent, 1984) reflect physiologically based approaches.

Current models of neural coding for all information processing, including speech and language, posit complex dynamic interactions of neuronal network ensembles dedicated to specific functions located throughout the brain. Theoretical models of information processing for machine representation in artificial intelligence (Shaw, Silverman, & Pearson, 1985; Grossberg, 1987) have been developed stemming from work over the past 20 years from basic neuroscience and supported by recent human brain-imaging studies (Posner, Petersen, Fox, & Raichle, 1988; Petersen, Fox, Posner, & Raichle, 1988). Using a subtraction technique with a PET scanner during various language-processing tasks in normal subjects, neuroscientists at Washington University, Saint Louis, have postulated that elementary operations of human information processing are strictly localized; however, numerous brain areas interact even during very simple tasks (Posner et al., 1988).

Postulated models of speech and language processing emphasizing integration of cortical and subcortical systems (Brown, 1980; Crosson, Novack, & Trenerry, 1988; Gordon, 1985; Kornhuber, 1977) extend classical cortical connectionist theory and suggest inclusion of neurotransmitter pathways. These models will, no doubt, undergo numerous revisions as more data are acquired regarding neurophysiologic and neurochemical coding for language and all information processing from brain imaging of animals and humans and basic neuroscience.

While the information gained from brain imaging for validating neural models of information processing is exciting, it should be remembered that the primary application of the neuroimaging technologies is clinical utility in terms of medical management. The physician orders an imaging assessment to aid in determining a medical diagnosis. Because the nervous system involves integration of information from many systems simultaneously, a brief review of functional neuroanatomy and neurochemistry will orient the reader to some clinical principles.

FUNCTIONAL NEUROANATOMY AND NEUROCHEMISTRY

Functional Neuroanatomy

Functionally, the brain can be divided into five major subgroups: brain stem, cerebellum, diencephalon, basal ganglia, and the lobes of the telencephalon. These groups will be discussed separately, though necessarily superficially. The reader is referred to textbooks of neuroanatomy and neurophysiology for more detailed discussion (Carpenter, 1985; Gilman & Newman, 1987).

Brain stem. The brain stem is comprised of three structures, extending inferiorly to superiorly: the medulla, the pons, and the midbrain (see

Figures 3.1–3.2). The brain stem generally serves three major functions. First, it is the part of the brain that is necessary for maintenance of basic life functions. Among these are respiration and the maintenance of consciousness. Lesions in different parts of the brain stem will result in different respiratory patterns. However, a large lesion in the lower medulla may result in respiratory arrest. This is incompatible with life without mechanical support. Animal studies indicate that a lesion in the central upper pons or lower midbrain results in a permanently comatose state. This is verified in human experience (Plum & Posner, 1980). Additionally, some control over cardiac function resides in the medulla.

The brain stem secondly serves as the output station for cranial nerves. These include the 3rd to 12th nerves, excluding only the optic nerve and olfactory nerve, controlling vision and smell. Other special sensory nerves controlling balance and hearing (the 8th cranial nerve) and taste (the 9th and 12th cranial nerves) pass through the brain stem on their way to sensory areas of the cerebral cortex responsible for their perception. Cranial nerves responsible for control over eye movements (the 3rd, 4th, and 6th nerves) arise from the midbrain and upper pons. Those responsible for control over facial movements and for perception of sensation from the face (the 5th and 7th nerves) arise from the pons.

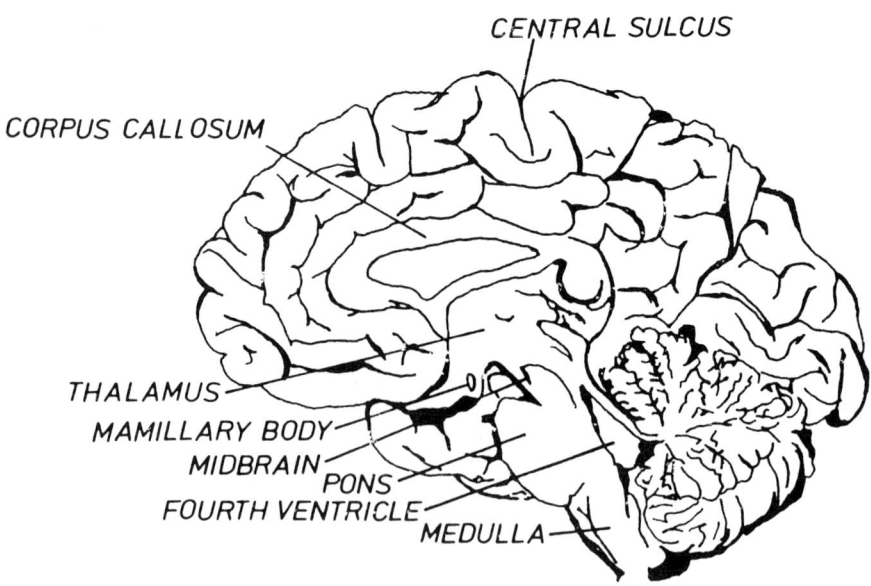

Figure 3.1 Midsagittal section of brain stem, cerebellum, and cerebrum. Redrawn from *Neurosciences for Allied Health Therapies* (p. 15) by D. R. Brown, 1980, Saint Louis: C. V. Mosby. Copyright 1980 by C. V. Mosby. Adapted by permission.

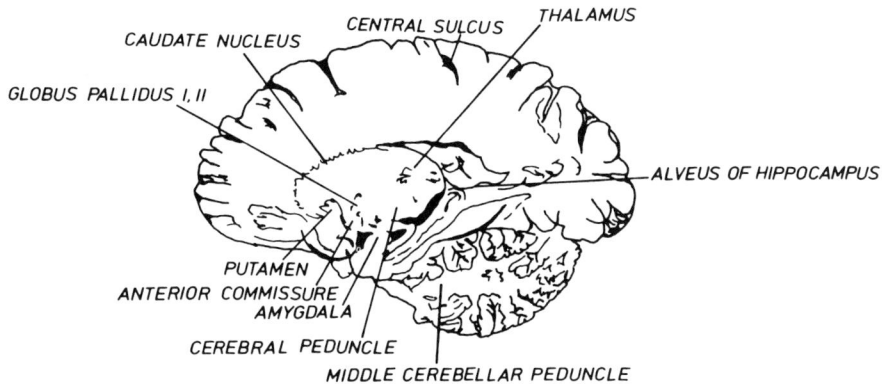

Figure 3.2 Saggital section through thalamus showing middle cerebellar peduncle of cerebellum.

The brain stem anatomy of the 5th nerve is complex and beyond the discussion here. The cranial nerves in the medulla, including the 9th through 12th nerves, function in motor control over the tongue and pharynx. The vagus nerve (10th cranial nerve) also functions in control over heart rate and rhythm.

The third major function of the brain stem is as a relay station between the cerebral cortex, basal ganglia, diencephalon, cerebellum, and spinal cord. As such, it constitutes the way that the rest of the body communicates with the cerebral hemispheres. There are many pathways within the brain stem that serve different sensory and motor functions. In humans, an example of the importance of these pathways is demonstrated in the "locked-in" syndrome. Patients with lesions in the base of the pons (basis pontis), which transmits motor signals from the brain to the spinal cord, can have complete paralysis from the neck down, along with inability to move facial muscles. Sensation can be preserved, resulting in a patient who can feel but cannot talk or move. Communication with these patients is possible only because their eye movements are preserved. They have no impairment of consciousness or thinking.

The function of the brain stem in communication with the cerebellum cannot be overstated. The three major tracts (the superior, middle, and inferior cerebellar peduncles) through which the cerebellar outflow occurs pass through the midbrain, pons, and medulla, respectively (see Figures 3.1–3.3).

Cerebellum. The cerebellum functions in the motor system to modify outputs originated elsewhere and coordinate muscle groups so that movements wind up having smooth, purposeful character. It receives input

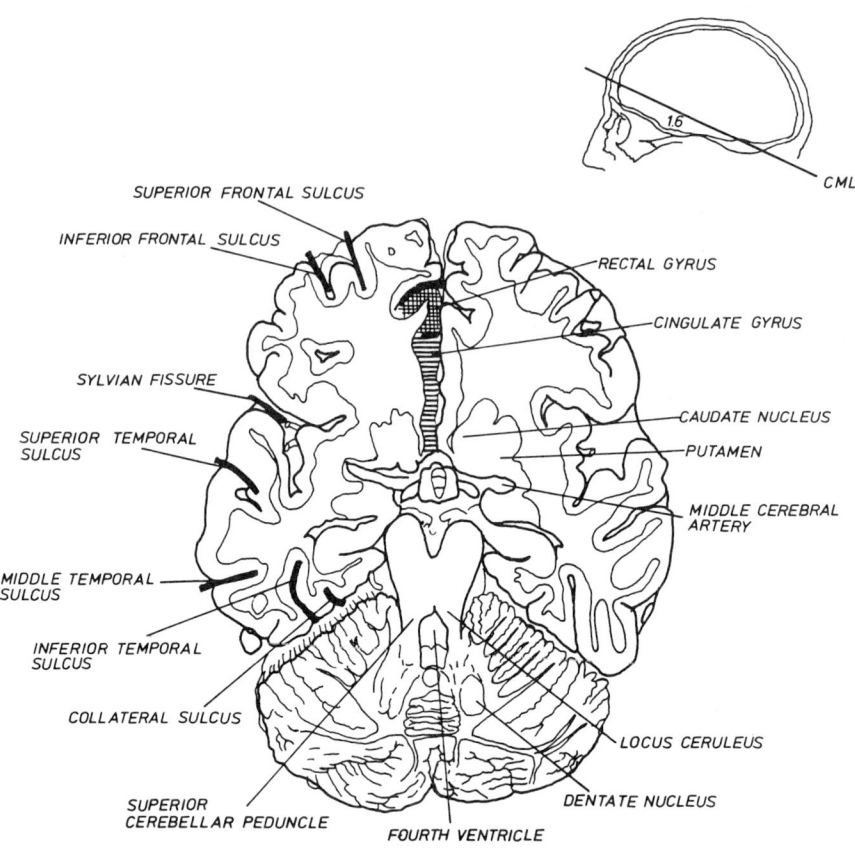

Figure 3.3 Axial section showing brain level and prominent structures 15° parallel to the canthomeatal line (CML), 13th section from the vertex, upper surface. Redrawn from *An Atlas of the Human Brain for Computerized Tomography* (p. 63) by T. Matsui and A. Hirano, 1978, Tokyo: Igaku-Shoin. Copyright 1978 by Igaku-Shoin. Adapted by permission.

mainly from sensory fibers concerned with proprioception (position sense) in tendons and joints and from vestibular inputs concerned with the position of the head. Using these inputs as to the positioning of the body in space, the cerebellum generates outputs to the motor system which pass to the midbrain (red nucleus). From there, they decussate to pass to the thalamus on the other side of the brain. From the thalamus, they are projected to the motor cortex to modify the outputs from the motor cortex to the spinal cord. Thus information as to where joints and tendons are in space is modified on an ongoing basis to create smooth and coordinated motor actions. The importance of the cerebellum is seen in the various ataxic syndromes that result from lesions in it and in the actions of individuals intoxicated by the cerebellar toxin ethanol.

The diencephalon. The diencephalon is comprised of four major parts: the epithalamus, the thalamus, the hypothalamus, and the subthalamus. Generally these are nuclear structures that are extremely complex in their organization and serve as modifiers in both motor and sensory functions. The hypothalamus is critical in endocrine function and secretes numerous hormones that regulate basic body metabolism. Other biological drives, such as hunger and thirst, also originate there. Of particular interest to the speech-language clinician is the presence in the thalamus of the major relay stations for both hearing and vision between the sensory organs (the cochlear and optic nerves from the ears and eyes) and the cortex where they are perceived (see Figures 3.4–3.5). For hearing this takes place in the medial geniculate body in the thalamus. For vision it takes place in the lateral geniculate body. From there impulses are projected to the superior temporal lobes for hearing and to the occipital lobes for vision.

The basal ganglia. The basal ganglia are comprised of the caudate nucleus, the putamen, the globus pallidus, and the amygdala. These are all large nuclei that are closely related structurally to the cerebral cortex (see Figures 3.2–3.5). Generally the caudate, putamen, and globus pallidus function to modify motor outputs. They are part of the extrapyramidal system. Lesions in them result in varying degrees of movement dysfunction. Their importance to the motor system is reflected in such diseases as Parkinson's disease and Huntington's chorea, both of which are primarily movement disorders.

Though the amygdala (see Figure 3.2) is considered to be one of the basal ganglia by some neuroanatomists, its function is somewhat separate. Its inputs are primarily olfactory, and its outputs project to the hypothalamus to function in endocrine control and to modify behavioral responses in such basic emotions as fear and rage. The amygdala has other functions relating to emotional and hormonal responses, some of which vary from species to species and are not fully understood in humans. The amygdala is integrally related to the limbic lobe to form part of the limbic system, which functions extensively in regulation of emotional and hormonal reactions.

The cerebral lobes. There are four major lobes comprising the cerebral cortex: the frontal, the parietal, the occipital, and the temporal (see Figure 3.6). In the depth of the sylvian fissure, lateral to the basal gan-

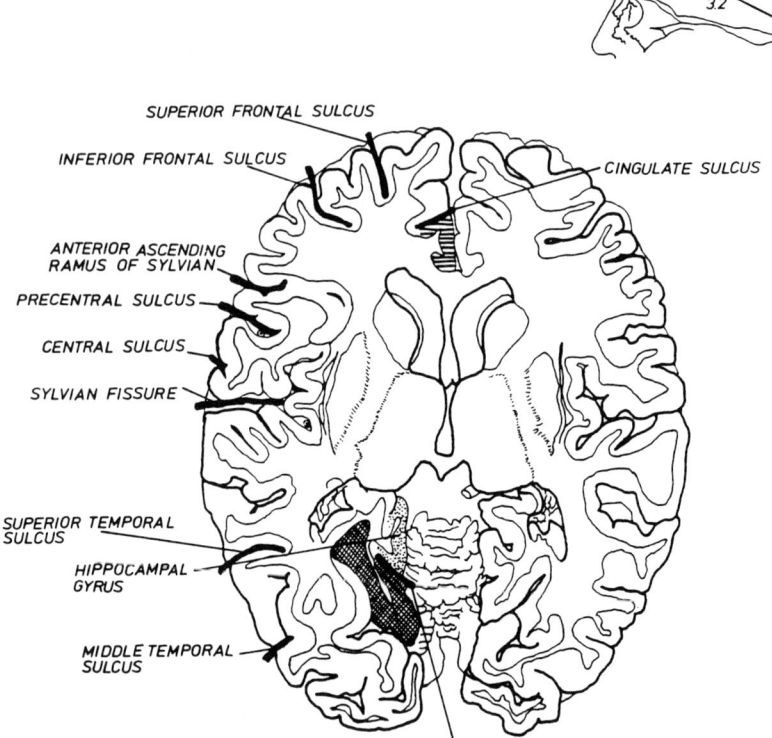

Figure 3.4 Axial section showing brain level and prominent structures 15° parallel to the canthomeatal line (CML), 10th section from the vertex, upper surface. Redrawn from *An Atlas of the Human Brain for Computerized Tomography* (p. 53) by T. Matsui and A. Hirano, 1978, Tokyo: Igaku-Shoin. Copyright 1978 by Igaku-Shoin. Adapted by permission.

glia, lies the insula. Another so-called lobe, the limbic lobe, lies on the medial surface of the brain and consists primarily of the cingulate gyrus and the parahippocampal gyrus. The limbic lobe functions in emotional regulation and in regulation of many body or visceral functions. It is not a true lobe because it is made up of parts of the temporal, parietal, and frontal lobes, but forms a conceptual lobe in the sense that the complex of brain that it encompasses acts together in the performance of its role.

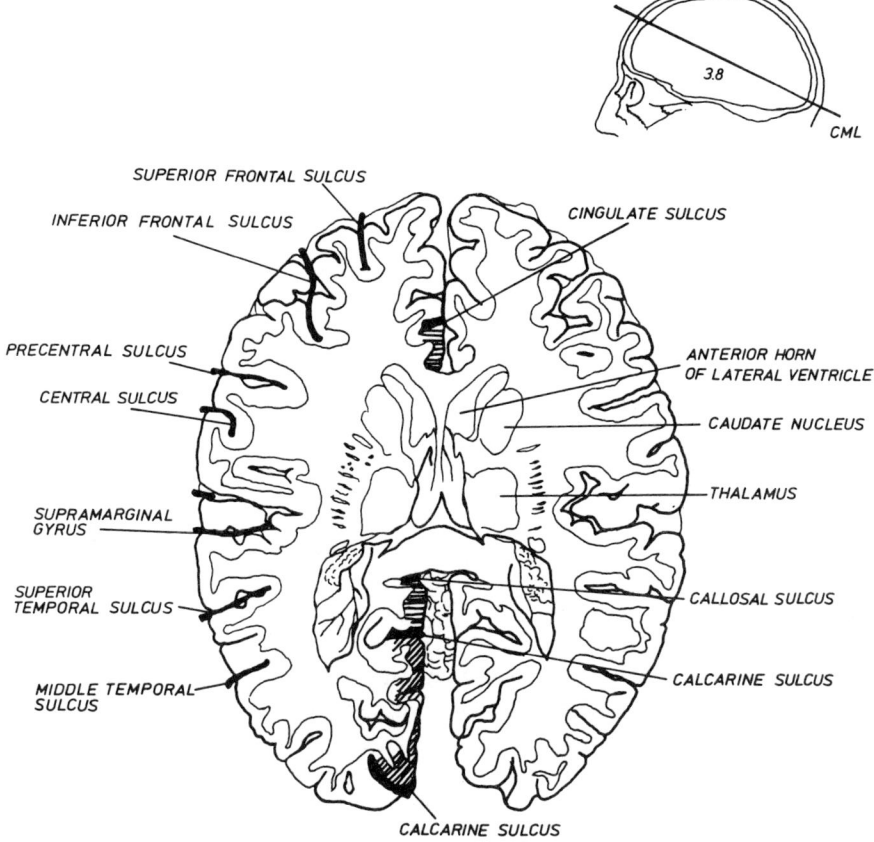

Figure 3.5 Axial section showing brain level and prominent structures 15° parallel to the canthomeatal line (CML), 9th section from the vertex, upper surface. Redrawn from *An Atlas of the Human Brain for Computerized Tomography* (p. 49) by T. Matsui and A. Hirano, 1978, Tokyo: Igaku-Shoin. Copyright 1978 by Igaku-Shoin. Adapted by permission.

All of the major lobes contain association areas that integrate sensations and responses and provide the substrate for thought. There is a high degree of redundancy in association areas, so that it is often possible to have significant lesions in these regions unilaterally without significant clinical deficit. As the largest lobe of the brain, the frontal lobe contains large association areas anteriorly. Posteriorly, the frontal lobe is separated from the parietal lobe by the central sulcus. Along the anterior margin of the central sulcus is the precentral gyrus. This strip of

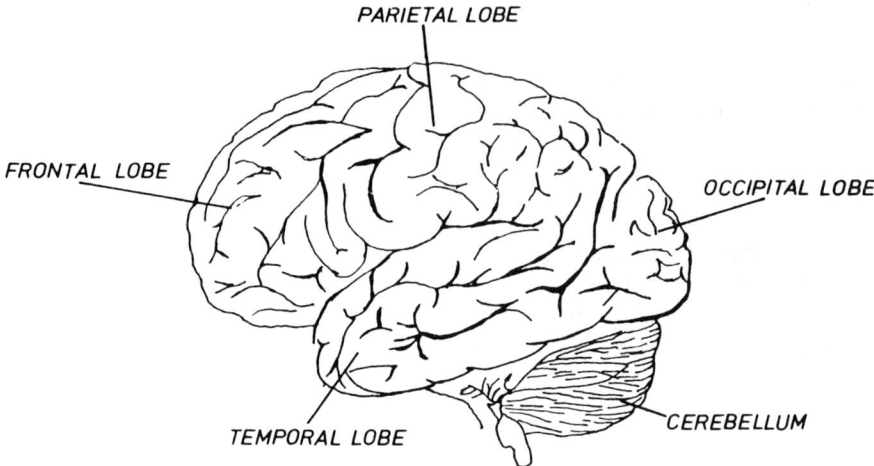

Figure 3.6 Lateral view of cerebral cortex showing four major lobes and cerebellum.

gray matter contains the primary motor cortex. It is organized in accordance with an inverted homunculus, or little man. This results in control of facial and head muscles taking place adjacent to the sylvian fissure. Control over the hand and arm lies immediately above the control over the face. The trunk follows next, near the vertex in the precentral gyrus. Control over the hip and leg is at the vertex and along the medial surface of that gyrus. The motor strip gives rise to fibers that descend in the posterior limb of the internal capsule to the cerebral peduncle in the midbrain. From there the motor fibers descend in the pons (in the basis pontis) to the medulla, where they form a bundle of fibers referred to as the medullary pyramids. This gives rise to the term *pyramidal tracts* to refer to the bundles of motor fibers which then, at the junction of the medulla and the cervical spine, cross from left to right or right to left to descend in the opposite side of the spinal cord. Adjacent to the motor strip are supplementary motor areas. Anterior to these, on the lateral surface of the brain, is an area that functions to control eye movements. Additional association areas control vocalization and speech output in the dominant hemisphere. Emotive aspects (prosody) of speech output arise, to some extent, from the nondominant hemisphere. The anatomy of language function is complex and is known now to include not only the cortex but the thalamus and basal ganglia as well.

On the medial surfaces of the frontal lobes are areas that control sphincter tone in the bowel and bladder. It is involvement of these areas bilaterally that results in incontinence as a late symptom of dementia.

Patients with midline tumors (megingioma of the falx, for example) will also present with leg weakness (involvement of the medial motor strip) and incontinence, and can clinically mimic spinal cord lesions.

The parietal lobe begins at the central sulcus and extends posteriorly to a poorly defined margin on the lateral surface and to the parieto-occipital sulcus on the medial surface of the brain. Inferiorly, it is demarcated from the temporal lobe by the sylvian fissure anteriorly and by a more poorly defined margin posteriorly. The parietal lobe contains the primary sensory cortex responsible for perception of such sensations as touch, pain, and temperature. The primary sensory cortex is adjacent to the central sulcus and is again organized according to an inverted homunculus. Supplementary sensory cortex is adjacent to the primary sensory cortex. More posteriorly there are association areas and areas that are responsible for recognition of body parts. Patients with right parietal lesions will frequently not recognize the left side of their body. When shown their left hand, they may recognize it as a hand but deny that it is theirs. They may also ignore not only their own left side but all events occurring to the left of the midline. In general, organization in space seems to be largely represented in the parietal lobe. Additionally, calculation and the naming of objects are functions which are parietal, usually in the dominant hemisphere. Posteriorly, the parietal lobe blends into the occipital lobe and there is an area that functions in control of slow, pursuit eye movements.

The occipital lobes are responsible for vision and integration of visual inputs for visual pattern recognition. As such, there are primary visual areas and visual association areas. Generally the central or "macular" vision is perceived in the tips of the occipital lobe and the more peripheral visual areas are represented more anteriorly.

The temporal lobes are another highly redundant area of the brain. They function in memory and audition, with the primary auditory sensory areas lying in the superior temporal lobes. Audition is represented bilaterally from each ear, though it is more strongly represented in the contralateral temporal lobe. Also, in the dominant hemisphere, the primary receptive areas for language function resides in the posterior superior temporal lobe.

In addition to the major lobar organization, there are extensive interconnections between lobes and between hemispheres. The interconnections take place via axons projecting extensively throughout the "white matter" in the brain. The major communication between left and right hemisphere takes place via the corpus callosum. This large bundle of white matter crosses the midline at the level of the lateral ventricles and is easily visualized on MRI.

Chemical Neuroanatomy

Many disorders of speech motor control co-occur, with basal ganglia disease resulting from various neurochemical abnormalities. Synaptic transmission occurs by means of chemicals called neurotransmitters. Neuromodulators can alter signal transmission without doing it through the synaptic mechanism. To function effectively as a neurotransmitter, certain chemical actions must occur. A compound must be synthesized in the presynaptic neuron, released from the presynaptic neuron, be bound to a receptor on the postsynaptic element where the membrane potential is altered, and finally be removed from the synaptic site or destroyed biochemically (Gilman & Newman, 1987, p. 222). Communication between neurons is highly complex and not fully understood, as demonstrated by the role of peptides. Peptides can serve as chemical messengers like neurotransmitters or as neuromodulators and can be released at locations other than the synapse.

Chemicals that have been tentatively or definitely identified as neurotransmitters include several different classes of molecules and over 20 different substances (Gilman & Newman, 1987). Two that have been studied extensively are acetylcholine and the monoamines such as dopamine, norepinephrine, and the indolamine serotonin. Because these two classes of neurotransmitters are important in motor control, their systems will be briefly overviewed.

Acetylcholine neurons in the CNS have been found to function in motor control through the cholinergic interneurons of the striatum (see Figure 3.7). Recent studies have suggested a role of acetylcholine terminals in the CNS as a factor in spasmodic dysphonia (Miller, Woodson, & Jankovic, 1987) and stuttering (Rastatter & Harr, 1988). This system has also been found to have a role in the dementia of Alzheimer's disease. Acetylcholine is the primary neurotransmitter of the peripheral nervous system and is released at the neuromuscular junction by all alpha, beta, and gamma motor neurons of the brain stem and spinal cord (Gilman & Newman, 1987). Acetylcholine neurons within the central nervous system are found in nuclear groups in the ventral forebrain, the temporal lobe, the brain stem, and the interneurons of the striatum.

Monoamines that have been identified as neurotransmitters in the CNS include the catecholamines dopamine, norepinephrine and epinephrine, and the indolamine serotonin. The location of monoamine-containing neurons in the brain has been the subject of much study over the past 20 years. It is known that these neurons are unevenly distributed throughout the brain (Versteeg, Van der Gugten, DeJong, & Palkovts, 1976). Two primary dopaminergic systems are shown in Figure 3.8. These are the nigrostriatal dopamine system important in motor control and the mesolimbic and mesocortical systems that have been

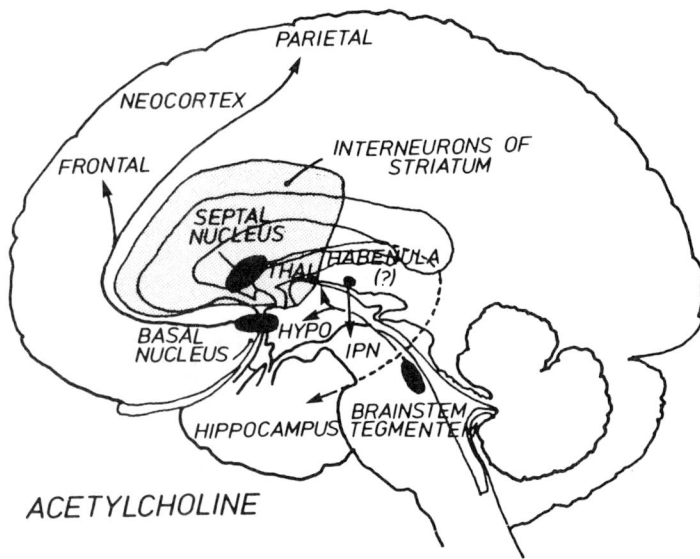

Figure 3.7 Location of acetylcholine neurons in the CNS and their projections. Areas containing cell bodies are striated gray. Projection pathways indicated with solid and broken black lines with arrows. *HYPO*, hypothalamus; *IPN*, interpeduccular nucleus; *THAL*, thalamus. Redrawn from *Manter and Gatz's Essentials of Clinical Neuroanatomy and Neurophysiology* (p. 223) by S. Gilman and S. W. Newman, 1987, Philadelphia: F. A. Davis Company. Copyright 1987 by F. A. Davis Company. Adapted by permission.

linked to the schizophrenias. Parkinson's disease is the result of damage to the nigrostriatal system due to the loss of the inhibitory input to caudate and putamen neurons. The mesolimbic and mesocortical dopamine system is thought to selectively inhibit transmission of sensory information, therefore enhancing the signal-to-noise ratio. This process is known as lateral inhibition and is important in information processing of all sensory systems (Gilman & Newman, 1987).

Norepinephrine in the CNS is thought to be functionally related to inhibition of spontaneous activity. That is, like dopamine, norepinephrine may enhance the signal-to-noise ratio in its terminal field. Norepinephrine cell bodies are confined to the brain stem, but their axons extend to all parts of the CNS (see Figure 3.9). A strongly lateralized distribution of norepinephrine in the human thalamus has been reported in the left pulvinar (Oke, Keller, Mefford, & Adams, 1978).

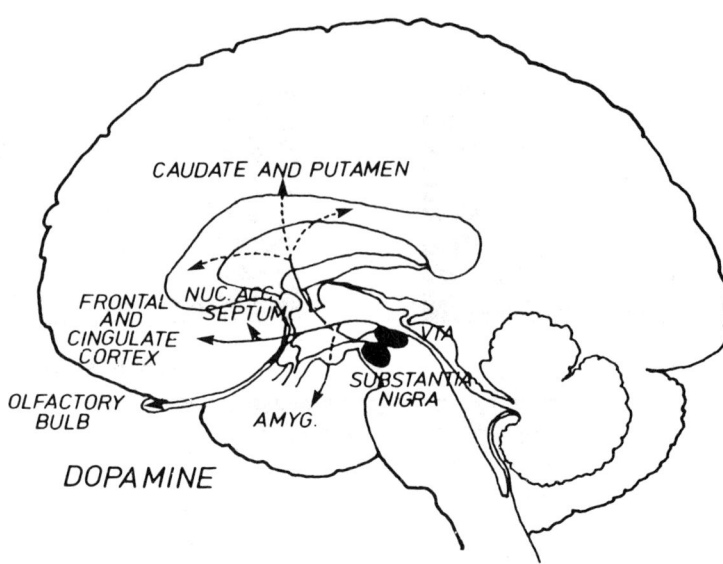

Figure 3.8 Locations and projections of two of the major dopaminergic systems in the brain are shown with solid and broken black lines with arrows. *AMYG*, amygdala; *NUC ACC*, nucleus accumlens; *VTA*, ventral tegmental area. Redrawn from *Manter and Gatz's Essentials of Clinical Neuroanatomy and Neurophysiology* (p. 225) by S. Gilman and S. W. Newman, 1987, Philadelphia: F. A. Davis Company. Copyright 1987 by F. A. Davis Company. Adapted by permission.

DESCRIPTION OF NEUROIMAGING TECHNOLOGIES

Imaging technologies to be reviewed in this section include X-ray computed tomography, magnetic resonance imaging, magnetic resonance spectroscopy, single-photon emission tomography, positron emission tomography, and brain mapping of cortical electrical activity. These techniques are grouped into two primary categories: anatomic or structural and physiologic or functional.

Structural Assessments

X-ray computed tomography (CT). Over the past 15 years, CT scanning has dramatically changed the diagnosis and treatment of neurological disorders. It is often the first test ordered by the physician because it is widely available and noninvasive. CT provides useful information in the study of brain structure, anatomy, and pathology. Many pathological conditions that at one time had to be determined by neurological and behavioral clinical assessments can now be objectively defined with CT. Because disorders of speech motor control and language often result

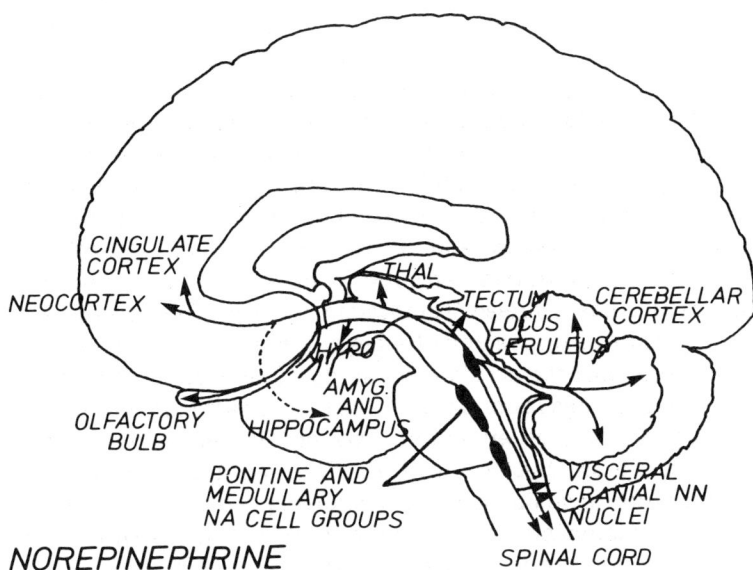

Figure 3.9 Norepinephrine (noradrenaline) neurons in the brain stem and their projections are indicated with solid and broken black lines with arrows. *AMYG*, amygdala; *HYPO*, hypothalamus; *NA*, norepinephrine; *THAL*, thalamus. Redrawn from *Manter and Gatz's Essentials of Clinical Neuroanatomy and Neurophysiology* (p. 226) by S. Gilman and S. W. Newman, 1987, Philadelphia: F. A. Davis Company. Copyright 1987 by F. A. Davis Company. Adapted by permission.

from brain lesions of various etiologies (vascular diseases, trauma, tumors), CT scanning has provided a large body of literature correlating cerebral lesions with various clinical profiles of speech and language disorders. The technology of X-ray CT employs transmission tomography combining the techniques of standard radiography and computerized tomography to produce a cross-sectional image of the subject. Transmission tomography derives information from the distribution of tissue density or attenuation coefficients (Brownell, Budinger, Lauterbur, & McGeer, 1982). Contrast between structures offered by CT is dependent on the X-ray absorbed and on the thickness, density, and atomic number of the structures imaged (Metter & Hanson, 1985). That is, tissue that has high absorption, such as bone with its high level of calcium, is more clearly defined than other tissues. Because electron density differences between adjacent structures are small, distinctions between various structures within the brain are more difficult to image.

CT images represent a display on a monitor screen of an X, Y coordinate system contained within the computer with values assigned in accordance with the calculated tissue densities in the plane of the scanned tissue. In current scanners, that coordinate system typically is a grid 512 squares wide and 512 squares high. Each square is referred to as a pixel. Each pixel within the computer is assigned a value based on a standard reference point selected by the manufacturer. In most cases, water is assigned a value of zero. Other standard values may vary somewhat. However, in most current CT scanners, the density of brain ranges between 40 and 60. The attenuational coefficient that is assigned to a pixel is determined by a number of properties, including not only tissue density but the energy of the X-ray beam as well. The size of each pixel is determined by the size of the field examined. A pixel will be smaller, for instance, if the field of view is 20 cm wide rather than 40 cm wide. This field size is set by the operator at the time the scan is obtained.

The CT image is an axial slice that is usually around 10 mm in thickness; thus the term *computerized axial tomography* or *CAT scan* is often used instead of *CT scan*. These axial images vary from 5° to 20° above and parallel to the canthomeatal line. Brain images can be seen from the perspective that the viewer is above and looking down or below and looking up depending on the scanner, but usually the patient's left is on the viewer's right in most modern scanners. Figure 3.10 is a CT axial section without intravenous contrast of an infarction in Broca's area in a patient with nonfluent aphasia.

Magnetic resonance imaging (MRI). This structural imaging technology is complementing or replacing CT scanning in many settings because of its excellent sensitivity and ability to display lesions in multiple planes (see Figure 3.11). Compared to CT, MRI provides better contrasts between gray and white matter and greatly improved ability to examine the posterior fossa. Additionally, the ability in higher magnetic field strengths to examine iron concentrations in the brain enables some biochemical imaging with proton MRI. The clinical utility of this technology is evolving.

MRI uses analysis of the behavior of atomic nuclei with odd numbers of protons in magnetic fields. It utilizes radiofrequency signals to determine the energy released as nuclei alternate in strong and varying magnetic fields. The orientation of these fields and the signed frequencies created in them localize energy sources that are then analyzed by a computer and constructed into multiple planar images that can then be stacked to achieve three-dimensional representations.

The sequences of the radiofrequency signal are set by the operator and can be varied to look at different properties of the tissue. Specifically, two "relaxation times" labeled T1 and T2 as well as "spin density" information can be examined. Therefore, in contrast to CT, MRI can examine multiple tissue characteristics.

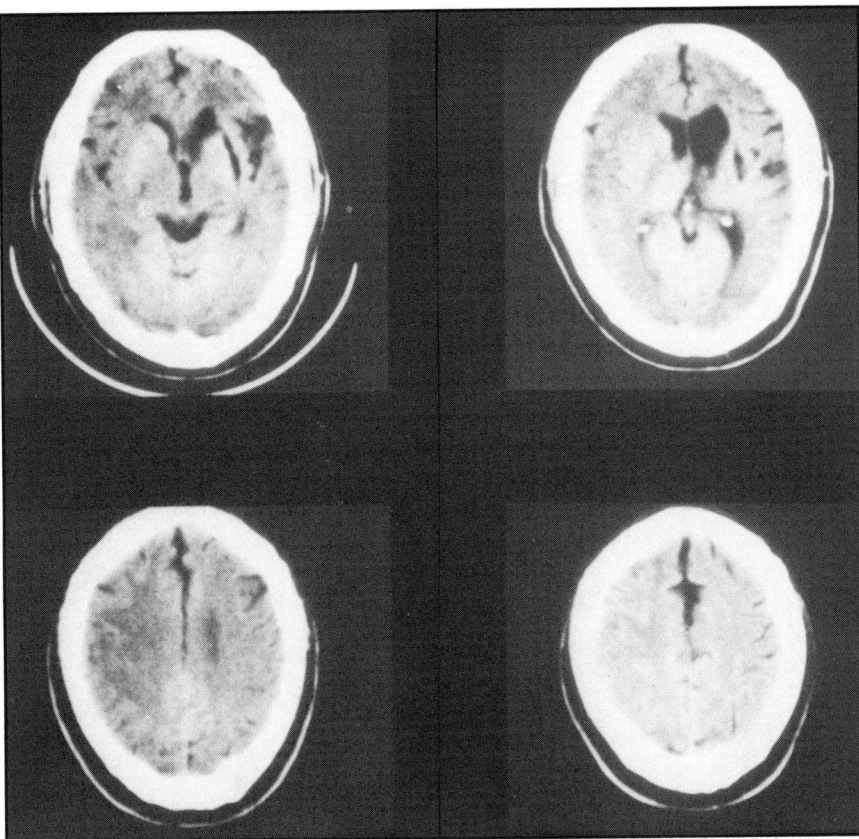

Figure 3.10 CT axial section without contrast agent of an infarction in the left anterior motor speech area in a patient with nonfluent aphasia. The patient's left side is on the viewer's right in this image.

Functional Brain-imaging Assessment

While CT and MRI have greatly enhanced our understanding of structural anatomy in pathologic states, physiological brain-imaging technologies have been developed that can give quantitative information about brain blood flow and blood volume, glucose metabolism, oxygen uptake, cortical electrical activity, and the concentration of neurotransmitter receptors (Gilman & Newman, 1987). Almost 10 years ago David Caplan asked: "Do language systems depend on some neurotransmitters and not others?" (1980, p. 237). Future functional brain-imaging technologies may help provide answers to such complex questions regarding biochemical and physiological coding for speech motor control and language.

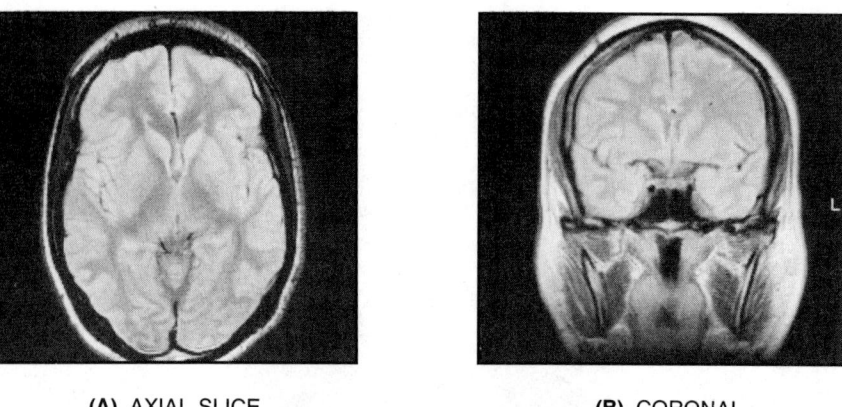

(A) AXIAL SLICE   (B) CORONAL

(C) SAGGITAL

Figure 3.11 MRI T2-weighted images demonstrating multiple planes: (A) axial, (B) coronal, and (C) saggital. MRI scanner operating at 0.35 tesla.

Magnetic resonance spectroscopy (MRS). MRS represents one of the most recent developments in cerebral metabolic research and extends the MRI technology to include analysis of such characteristics as phosphate metabolism and pH of tissues in various pathologic states. This technique, like MRI, employs a large magnetic field. Since true "images" are not currently acquired and since chemical processes are being examined, it represents a combined approach of structural and functional brain assessments. Studies with MRS in humans are just beginning (Radda, 1986; James et al., 1987), but initial efforts indicate that important biochemical processes can be monitored in vivo at the molecular level with deviations detected in various pathological states (Bottomley, Drayer, & Smith, 1986; Walker-Batson, Bonte, Devous, Ajamani, Nunnally, & Babcock, 1987; Welch et al., 1987). Thus far this technique has been used to study the phosphorus (31-P) signal, primarily because it is present in sufficiently high concentrations to be detectable by MRS.

The MRS technology uses a surface coil with a spectrometer interfaced to a very strong magnet. Although MRS is not yet available for clinical use, it has the potential to provide information about biochemical aspects of recovery from various disorders of speech motor control and language due to infarction and trauma.

Positron emission tomography (PET). PET utilizes emission tomography with radionuclides and has evolved from technology recognized 35 years ago (Brownell et al., 1982). Positron isotopes give off positively charged electrons. On annihilation with a negative electron, two photons that travel in exactly opposite directions are produced. Two detectors in coincidence positioned around a patient's head can then detect both photons. Positron-emitting compounds must be produced in a cyclotron. Carbon, nitrogen, oxygen, and fluorine can be developed as positron emitters. When synthesized into compounds such as glucose and injected intravenously, the radioactive material is taken up by brain tissue. This results in the emission of gamma rays which can be detected with photomultiplier tubes (Gilman & Newman, 1987). Computer processing then constructs an image of the concentration (uptake) of the injected element. To the extent that the uptake reflects metabolism, PET images constitute images of metabolic processes.

PET imaging of dopamine receptors in normal subjects has been reported (Wagner et al., 1983) as well as imaging of damaged striatal dopaminergic terminals in induced parkinsonism (Calne et al., 1985; Chiueh et al., 1987). PET scanning has also indicated ictus location in seizure disorders (Bromfield et al., 1988) and metabolic depression in acquired speech disorders not shown on CT (Kushner et al., 1987).

One of the primary disadvantages of PET scanning is the expense. For most institutions the cost to set up a PET scanner is prohibitive because of the need for a cyclotron and the expensive scanner cost. Thus this tool is found primarily in research environments.

Single-photon emission computed tomography (SPECT). Differences between SPECT and PET are based on the technology and the emitters employed. Whereas PET uses radioisotopes that decay by the emission of positrons, SPECT uses single-photon radionuclides. The isotopes employed with SPECT are more readily available than those employed with PET. Their half-lives are longer than those of the positron emitters, and therefore even cyclotron-produced compounds can be manufactured elsewhere. Thus an on-site cyclotron is not necessary. Although the isotopes used with first-generation SPECT machines lacked the resolution and specificity of PET radioisotopes, second-generation SPECT machines have much-improved resolution capabilities and studies can be performed at a small fraction of the cost of PET scans. Single-photon techniques have been used to study brain blood flow primarily because of its autoregulatory link to brain metabolism (Devous, Stokely, & Bonte, 1985). The early SPECT machines used both rotating (Stokely, Sveinsdotir, Lassen, & Rommer, 1980) and stationary (Kanno & Lassen, 1979) detector techniques with xenon-133, Tc-99, or N-isopropyl-p (IMP-123)-iodoamphetamine and I-123-trimethyl-propanediamine as tracers.

Images from a prototype rotating machine (Medimatic 64, Copenhagen) employing xenon-133 as the tracer (Bonte & Stokely, 1981) are shown in Figures 3.12–3.13. This particular technique uses four banks of sodium iodide detectors arranged in a hollow configuration that rotates around the patient's head. Xenon is administered in air-oxygen mixture by inhalation during the first minute of the 4-minute procedure. Three tomographic sections are generated at 2, 6, and 10 cm above and parallel to the canthomeatal line. Regional cerebral blood flow (rCBF) is measured in milliliters per minute per 100 g of tissue and is displayed quantitatively in a 16-shade black-and-white or color scale.

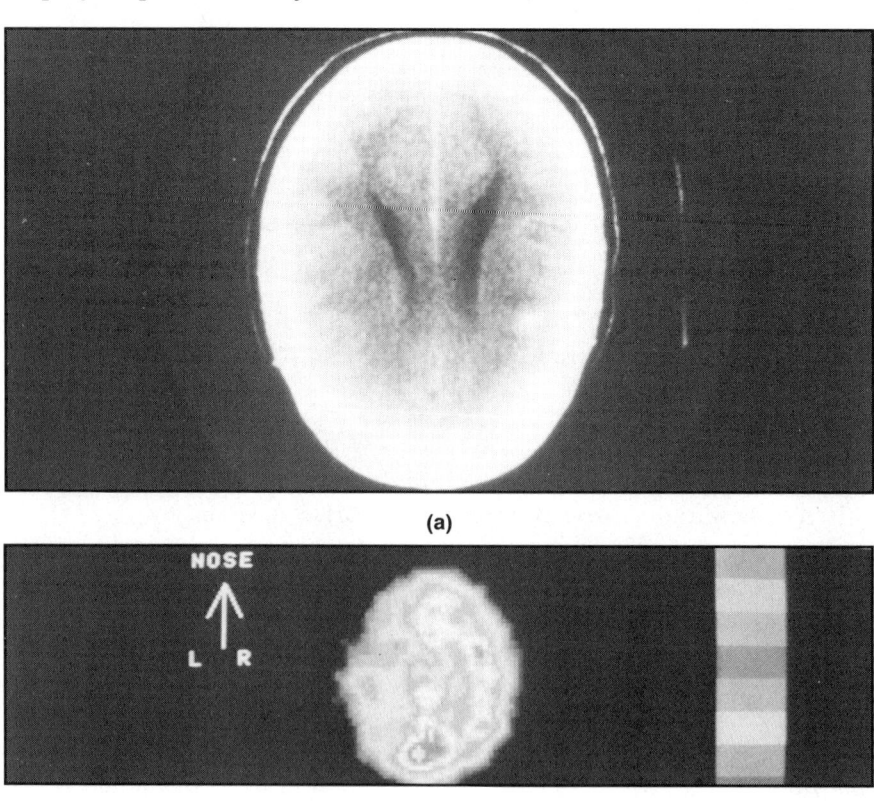

Figure 3.12 CT and xenon-133 SPECT regional cerebral blood flow images of Case 1. (*a*) CT scan shows a very small left frontal lesion; (*b*) SPECT shows reduced blood flow in most of the left hemisphere.

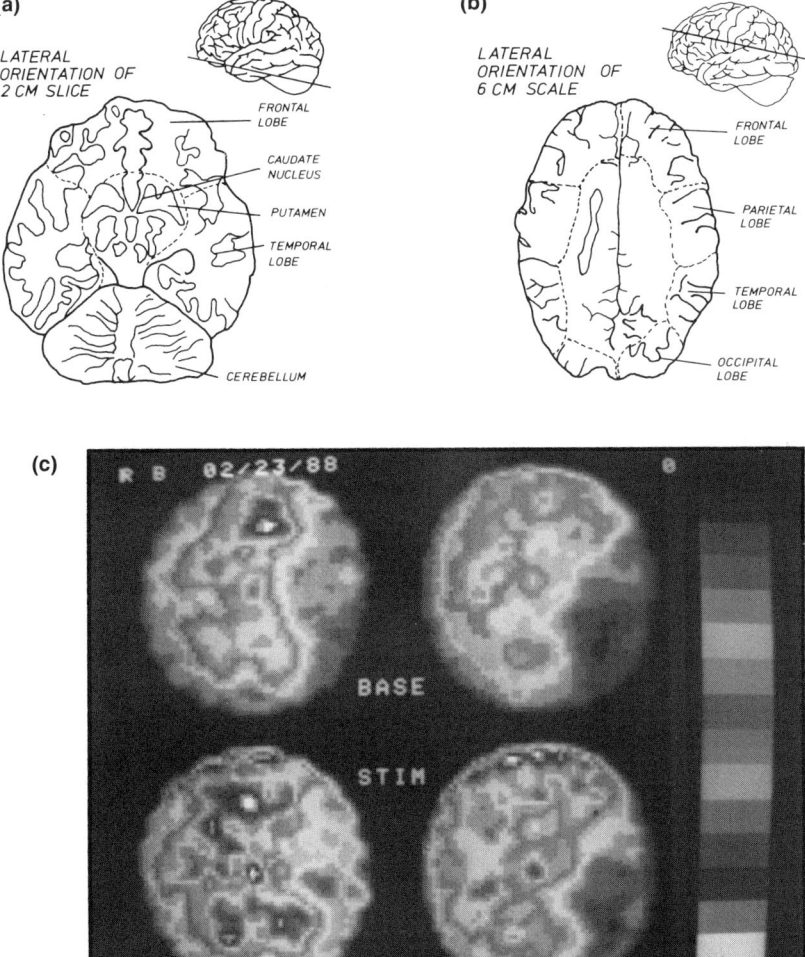

Figure 3.13 Cerebellar (slice 1) and cortical (slice 2) xenon-SPECT images at rest and during linguistic activation of Case 2. Templates showing tomographic sections at (a) 2 cm (slice 1) and (b) 6 cm (slice 2) above and parallel to the canthomeatal line. (c) Xenon-SPECT images at rest (left) and during linguistic activation (right). There is little change in cortical flow during the linguistic activation but marked increases in cerebellar regions, particularly on the right.

Second-generation SPECT machines, which are just emerging, can provide whole brain images at multiple angles much like MRI and have greatly improved resolution capabilities over the first-generation machines. The most recent SPECT machines provide sequential dynamic imaging of rCBF and are currently employing technetium-99 and I-123 iodoamphetamine as the tracers. With further development of appropriate radiopharmaceuticals, it is anticipated that receptor function will be possible with some SPECT systems.

One second-generation SPECT system (PRISM, Ohio Imaging, 1988) in research use at the University of Texas Southwestern Medical Center consists of three detectors equipped with a fan beam collimator that matches the detector size to the head. Three rectangular scintillation cameras are arranged at 120° increments to form a triangle around the head. Photons are collected over 360° which permits high sensitivity. This system has been used thus far to study stroke and epilepsy (see Figure 3.14).

Topographic mapping of brain electrical activity. This technology is an outgrowth of standard electroencephalography (EEG) and, like the other brain-imaging technologies, its development has been made possible by computer technological advances. This technique is referred to by various commercial names (BEAM [brain electrical activity mapping], Nicolet; BRAINMAP, Cadwell). While still in the initial stages, this technology shows promise for distilling and displaying electrophysiological data from the brain with more sophistication and accessibility than standard EEG recordings, and is becoming an established tool in the diagnosis and treatment of various neurological and cognitive disorders (see Figure 3.15). Neurometric analysis allows collection and quantification of EEG data for comparison to normative data bases. Mapping of cortical electrical activity includes somatosensory, visual, and auditory stimulation and is sometimes referred to as brain wave cartography.

The preliminary work in speech and language disorders with this technology was done by Frank Duffy and his associates at Boston Children's Hospital (1979, 1980, 1985, 1986). Numerous laboratories, however, are now using this technology for both research and clinical application (Pool & Finitzo, 1987; Finitzo et al., 1987). Brain mapping can complement standard EEG, long-latency cortical-evoked potentials, CT, MRI, PET, and SPECT to aid in identifying cognitive and organic neurological abnormalities. Studies that have compared brain blood flow and oxygen metabolism to electrical cortical activity have found differences in the cortical electrical activity not seen on the tomographic vascular and metabolic measures (Nagata et al., 1986). It has been suggested that this may reflect deafferentation in sites remote from the primary lesion.

CLINICAL USE OF NEURODIAGNOSTIC TECHNIQUES

Much of the growth in the clinical neurosciences over the last 15 years can be related to the development of new imaging tools with which to

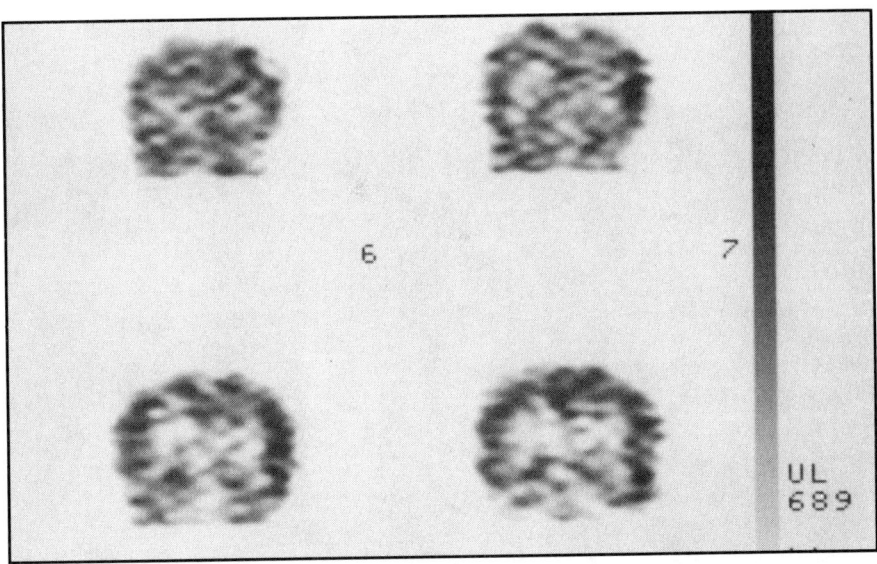

Figure 3.14 Image from second generation IMP-SPECT machine demonstrates an area of high regional cerebral blood flow during ictal SPECT study of Case 3. There are increases on three coronal sections in right parietal cortex extending into right temporal regions.

examine patients. One need only realize that CT, MRI, SPECT, PET, clinical MR spectroscopy, and BEAM were all nonexistent until the early 1970s to recognize the challenge facing the clinician who wants to remain abreast of this field. Common to these modalities and the progress in their development is the explosive evolution of computer technologies which enable the rapid data processing that is central to image reconstruction. Prior to 1970, structural brain assessment was made by evaluation of the ventricles (pneumoencephalography) via instillation of air in the subarachnoid space and examination with plain X-rays. Also, structural assessment was made by examination of the cerebral blood vessels (angiography) via injection of contrast in the arteries and the use of plain X-rays to photograph the passage of contrast through the arterial system and into the venous system. Though many inferential data could be obtained, it was not until the development of these newer modalities that direct imaging of the brain became possible. From a clinical perspective, the progress of the last 15 years in neuroimaging has largely been in the area of structural assessment. However, as functional assessments evolve to provide better resolution and broader informational possibilities, they also are beginning to occupy a role in clinical patient care.

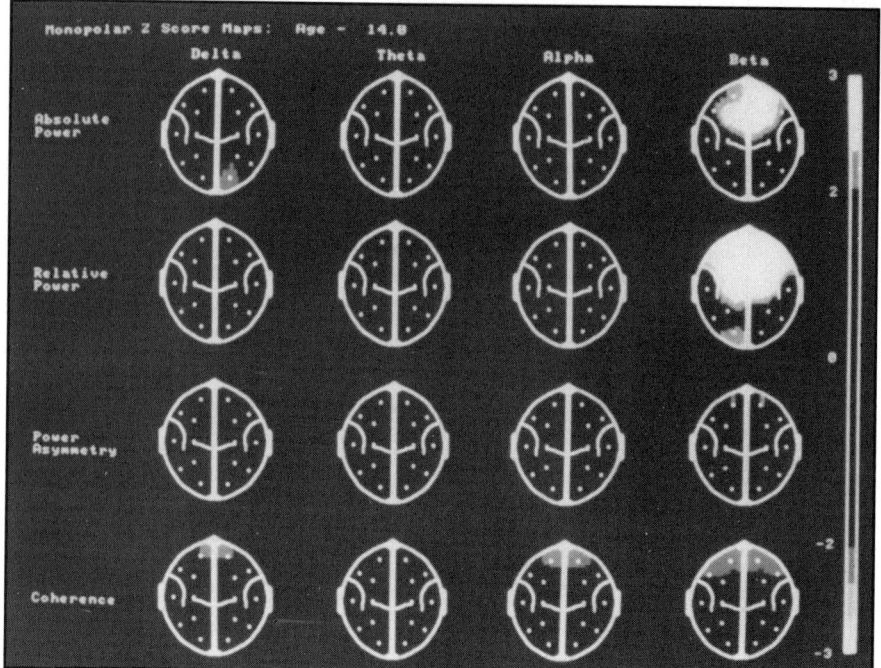

Figure 3.15 Brainmap of 14-year-old male diagnosed as having language and learning disorder. Z-score map demonstrates how patient deviates from normal.

Structural Assessments

No diagnostic modality since the introduction of the use of X-rays has had as much impact on the practice of neurology or neurosurgery as CT scanning. CT still forms one cornerstone of clinical neurologic practice. However, the introduction of MRI in the early 1980s substantially modified the way CT is used in ordinary practice.

Because CT and MRI examine different physical properties, there is some difference in the types of information that can be derived from CT and MR images. In addition, coronal and sagittal acquisitions are possible with MRI, which gives greater flexibility in anatomic examination. As the technologies have advanced, the cost of a CT scanner has been substantially reduced. Generally speaking, a CT scanner now is approximately half as expensive as an MR scanner.

Because it examines density to radiation transmission, CT remains the diagnostic procedure of choice for examination of bony abnormalities, calcifications, or the presence of blood (subarachnoid hemorrhage, subdural hematoma, or parenchymal hematoma). Since it is best for visualizing fractures and hemorrhages, this means CT remains the better modality in a setting of trauma. It is also the best in the postoperative setting, where one is often looking for hemorrhages. This is especially true when metallic objects, such as aneurysm clips, have been placed intracranially and may be subject to the creation of artifacts in the magnetic fields used for MRI. For examination of the ventricular system in hydrocephalus, either CT or MRI is adequate.

Diseased white matter emits a signal that is different from that of healthy white matter; thus MRI is the technology of choice for examination in various white matter diseases, the most well-known of which is multiple sclerosis. Since there are frequent artifacts in the posterior fossa (brain stem or cerebellum) on CT examination, MRI is the procedure of choice when pathology in that location is suspected.

For examination in strokes, CT or MRI is adequate. MRI may be more sensitive, although this view is controversial. In brain tumors, either CT or MRI is adequate. MRI has the advantage of coronal and sagittal displays but the disadvantage of difficulty distinguishing tumor from surrounding edema. With the development of contrast agents for MRI such as gadolinium, this disadvantage is disappearing.

Functional Assessments

As SPECT and PET technologies evolve, radionuclide chemistry for examination of cerebral blood flow and glucose metabolism has become available. Cerebral blood flow imaging has been used for evaluation of language function and in the study of visual processing, since this method shows change when the eyes are closed and when they are open. Additionally, emotional disturbances such as schizophrenia and dementing diseases such as Alzheimer's disease show changes that may be characteristic on cerebral blood flow examination. In arteriovenous malformations, stealing of blood supply from the surrounding brain has been shown. Blood flow imaging may also provide the earliest means to image strokes. If so, it may be increasingly prominent as new therapies become available for early intervention. At present, however, this is still speculative. In epilepsy, changes in blood flow have been shown to help localize seizure foci. Likewise, with PET, areas of increased metabolism have been shown in seizing foci.

As metabolic imaging with PET or MRS becomes more readily available, new applications will undoubtedly be discovered. The ability of MR spectroscopy to image phosphate metabolism, lactate concentrations, acid concentrations, and possibly other chemical processes is intriguing and as yet unexplored.

The use of standard electroencephalography remains a mainstay in neurologic evaluation. With the advent of brain-mapping technologies, image processing has been applied to EEG data. The availability of images has enabled anesthesiologists to more closely monitor brain waves during surgery. Additionally, the use of images rather than paper tracings may ease the interpretation of frequency data that are collected in EEGs. However, this technique is not yet in widespread clinical use.

Although the field of neuroimaging in some aspects seems revolutionary in terms of studying speech-language mechanisms, as with any rapidly developing technology much of the research is preliminary. Van Lackner (1985) cites several limitations to the use of the new imaging technologies in neurolinguistic research. These include (1) difficulty in acquiring normative data bases due to the individual variability in linguistic processing; (2) the global nature of most of the techniques, making quantification difficult; (3) the time required for analysis if more detailed quantification is applied; (4) the resolution limits of most of the first-generation imaging tools, which make correlations with speech and language processing tentative at best; (5) rapid technological advances that can make studies obsolete before they are completed; (6) significant cost; and (7) time course constraints. With these limits recognized, in the next section we will review research studies related to speech motor control conducted with these technologies.

RESEARCH FINDINGS WITH IMAGING TECHNOLOGIES

By far the largest body of literature related to speech and language function utilizing brain-imaging technologies has been in the area of acquired lesions and aphasia or aphasia-apraxia of speech (Alexander & Schmitt, 1980; Benson, 1984; Brunner, Kornhuber, Seemuller, Suger, & Wallesch, 1982; Kertesz, Harlock, & Coates, 1979; Metter, Wasterlain, Kuhl, Hanson, & Phelps, 1984; Metter & Hanson, 1985; Metter, Hanson, Kempler, Jackson, Mazziotta, & Phelps, 1987; Naeser et al., 1981; Naeser et al., 1982; Nagata et al., 1986; Walker-Batson, Devous, Bonte, & Oelschlaeger, 1987; Walker-Batson, Devous, Millay, Reynolds, Ajamani, Grant, & Bonte, 1988; Poeck, de Bleser, & von Keyserlingk, 1984; Tikofsky et al., 1985). Far fewer brain-imaging studies have been carried out in disorders of speech motor control specifically (Cannito et al., 1985; Finitzo et al., 1987; Groswasser, Korn, Groswasser-Reider, & Solvi, 1988; Horner & Massey, 1983; Kushner et al., 1987; Ozaki, Baba, Narita, Matsunaga, & Takebe, 1986; Ruff & Arbit, 1981; Schiff, Alexander, Naeser, & Galaburda, 1983; Square, Darley, & Sommers, 1982). This is due, no doubt, to the rarity of some disorders of speech motor control, such as apraxia of speech and spasmodic dysphonia, and to the fact that focal lesions present experiments that are more amenable for research than progressive neurological disorders with co-occuring dysarthrias or speech-specific disorders without definitive etiology. This section will review studies of (1) general neurological disorders affecting motor speech systems; (2) disordered premotor organization for speech; and (3) speech-specific disorders such as stuttering and spasmodic dysphonia. Research studies reviewed from the above categories will contrast types of neuroimaging technologies employed rather than being exhaustive literature reviews due to space limitations.

Neurological Disorders Affecting Motor Speech Systems

Neurological disorders such as Parkinson's disease, Huntington's disease, Wilson's disease, multiple sclerosis, amyotrophic lateral sclerosis, cerebellar ataxia, and focal epilepsy with co-occuring speech disorders have been studied with CT scanning (Adam, Fabre, Guel, Bessoles, Roulleau, & Bes, 1983; Fisher, 1984; Hirose, Kiritani, & Sawashima, 1980; Lechtenberg & Gilman, 1978; Ozaki et al., 1986) and more recently with MRI (Starosta-Rubinstein et al., 1987) to determine clinico-anatomical correlations. Studies employing physiological brain-imaging tools, including PET (Calne et al., 1985; Chiueh et al., 1987; Metter, Hanson, Phelps, Squire, Wasterlain, & Benson, 1983) and SPECT (Homan, Devous, Stokely, & Bonte, 1987), are providing information regarding metabolic-neurotransmitter-blood flow aspects of dysfunction in various neurological diseases with co-occuring speech disorders. It has been suggested that in neurologic speech disorders the degree of the speech defect is commensurate with the severity of the physical disability (Abbs, 1981). The correlation of lesion and degree of speech impairment, however, is less clear (Flowers, 1978). Neurologic disorders of both the central and peripheral nervous systems historically have been difficult to manage, treat, and understand (Darby, 1985). Brain-imaging technologies coupled with improved techniques of molecular biology and genetics have begun to provide information with clinical applications on the neural mechanisms of these disorders.

In many progressive neurological diseases, dysarthria is often the most common (Starosta-Rubenstein et al., 1987) or first presenting symptom (Herderschee, Stam, & Derex, 1987). Both structural and functional imaging studies have pointed to subcortical pathology, particularly basal ganglia pathology. In acquired basal ganglia pathology, lesion location on CT has been reported to correlate with speech symptoms (Brunner et al., 1982; Damasio, Damasio, Rizzo, Varney, & Gersch, 1982; Naeser et al., 1982). However, in progressive neurological diseases, brain-behavioral correlations with CT scanning have been less clearly related. The improved resolution of MRI provides clearer images for clinico-anatomic comparisons. In an MRI study of 41 patients with Wilson's disease, Starosta-Rubenstein et al. (1987) found 22 of the patients had dysarthria that was correlated with lesions of both the putamen and caudate. PET studies of patients with Parkinson's disease and Huntington's disease (Kuhl, Metter, Riege, & Markham, 1984; Metter, Riege, Hanson, Kuhl, & Phelps, 1983; Metter & Kempler, 1986) have reported decreases in glucose utilization in the caudate and putamen. This local hypometabolism was found to appear early before bulk tissue loss. Using an intercorrelation method, Metter, Hanson, Phelps, Squire, Wasterlain, and Benson (1983) found a decrease in cortico-cortical metabolic correlations and suggested that part of the function of the basal ganglia may be to help the cortex communicate between regions to accomplish planned or sequenced responses. Metter and Kempler (1986) emphasize the need for linguistic activation studies with PET to elaborate this mechanism. Other PET studies have identified neurotransmitter hypofunction before the appearance of clinical signs of Parkinson's disease and have monitored the effects of pharmacologic therapy (Calne et al., 1985; Chiueh et al., 1987).

Transient speech arrest and aphemia have been reported as symptoms of epileptic seizures (Peled, Harnes, Borovich, & Sharf, 1984; Rasmussen, 1974; Williamson, Spencer, Spencer, Novelly, & Mattson, 1985). The speech arrests have been reported to be caused by focal seizures of the motor cortex of either hemisphere (Caplan & Zervas, 1978) and usually do not occur in isolation but also include epileptic motor activity. SPECT imaging with a first-generation scanner in patients with partial seizures (Homan et al., 1987) found reduced blood flow in the contralateral cerebellum related to decreased blood flow in anterior temporal areas. There are few published reports of physiologic imaging during the ictal phase of seizure activity. A recent study by Bromfield et al. (1988) employed a speech perception activation task during a PET study of temporal lobe epilepsy to aid in localizing the specific area of ictus. This report suggests that linguistic activation may help in determining the area of ictus. Preliminary work with a second-generation SPECT scanner (PRISM, Ohio Imaging, 1988) using IMP as the tracer indicates that this technique may also have potential for ictus localization (see Case 3 in this chapter).

Disordered Premotor Organization for Speech

Various types of disordered premotor organization for speech have been studied with both structural and functional imaging technologies (Basso, Luzzatti, & Spinnler, 1980; Damasio & Van Hoesen, 1980; Freedman, Alexander, & Naeser, 1984; Rubens, 1975; Rubens, 1976; Schiff et al., 1983; Kushner et al., 1987; Sugishita et al., 1987). Imaging studies reviewed here are taken from a small number of descriptive studies of apraxia of speech only; no studies are reviewed that include motor initiation problems from supplementary motor area lesions or transcortical motor aphasias.

Studies of apraxia of speech without co-occuring aphasia that include imaging data are rare (Kushner et al., 1987; Schiff et al., 1983; Square et al., 1982; Sugishita et al., 1987). Many of the problems of clinico-anatomic correlation in pure apraxia of speech can be traced to problems of definition of the disorder itself (see Chapter 7) and to inadequate behavioral or imaging analysis or both. In a careful review of the literature, Schiff et al. (1983) found only 13 patients in the neurological literature could be defined as having pure aphemia or apraxia of speech. In a CT analysis of four patients, Schiff et al. (1983) found the lesion sites included the inferior primary motor cortex, the posterior portion of the pars opercularis of the inferior frontal gyrus, and the superficial deep frontal white matter. The authors concluded that the functional impairment underlying these varying locations is related to a disturbance of the organization for the motor aspects of speech.

Kushner et al. (1987) indicate the variability of anatomical and physiological imaging by comparing CT and PET scans in a patient with apraxia of speech. The CT scan showed no abnormalities in the left hemisphere, but PET revealed an area of hypometabolism in the inferior precentral gyrus and the adjacent subcortical space. Sugishita et al. (1987) describe two cases of pure "apraxia of speech," one in a left-handed patient with a subcortical hemorrhage and the other a right-handed patient suffering from a cerebral infarct. Comparison of MRI and CT showed that the left-handed patient had a lesion mainly involving the right precentral gyrus and its deep white matter. The right-handed patient has a lesion mainly affecting the lower parts of the left precentral and postcentral gyri and their deep white matter. These authors conclude that a corticosubcortical lesion of the lower part of the left precentral gyrus in most right-handers and the homologous region of the right hemisphere in some left-handers is involved in apraxia of speech.

Groswasser et al. (1988) describe a left-handed patient with apraxia of speech from right hemisphere involvement due to trauma. Lesion location on CT showed right frontoparietal pathology. The patient had buccofacial apraxia on command but not in spontaneous productions. A follow-up study 10 years after the original insult revealed no improvement in the apraxia of speech. A single case study of aphasia with co-occuring apraxia of speech in a left-handed patient with right-hemisphere pathology is described in Case 2 of this chapter. This patient was followed 8 years after a posterior right hemisphere aneurysm. Differences between resting state and a linguistic activation during SPECT rCBF are demonstrated.

Speech-Specific Disorders

Most of the published reports of brain imaging in spasmodic dysphonia and stuttering have been either single case studies or studies of patients with acquired disorders following known etiologies such as head trauma (Finitzo et al., 1987; Ludlow, Rosenberg, Salazar, Grafman, & Smutok, 1987) or cerebrovascular disease (Helm, Butler, & Benson, 1978; Nowack & Stone, 1987; Rosenbek, Messert, Collins, & Wertz, 1978; Rosenfield, 1972).

With increasing evidence of CNS involvement (Ludlow & Connor, 1987; Cannito et al., 1985) and the mixed treatment results of recurrent laryngeal nerve resection (Dedo, 1983; Aronson & DeSanto, 1983), efforts to determine focal CNS pathology with imaging technologies in spasmodic dysphonia represented a logical progression. The studies published to date demonstrate the current developmental limits of these tools.

An interdisciplinary team from the University of Texas at Dallas and the University of Texas Southwestern Medical Center have reported the most diverse imaging protocol in spasmodic dysphonia. In a series of papers (Finitzo et al., 1987; Finitzo & Freeman, 1989; Schaefer et al., 1985; Pool, Freeman, & Finitzo, 1987; Cannito et al., 1985), this group has reported on the use of MRI, SPECT, and BEAM in selected patients from a larger spasmodic dysphonia study. In an MRI study of 19 patients, Schaefer et al. (1985) reported no significant correlations between MRI and other predictors of brain stem and midbrain disease. However, small scattered supratentorial lesions were the most frequent MRI findings that emerged. The authors conclude: "The lack of a significant correlation between the MRI findings and other predictors of brainstem and midbrain disease and the current spatial resolution limitation of MRI suggest that we are visualizing the associated lesions rather than the actual foci of SD. The range of MRI findings is consistent with the concept that SD is a voice disorder in a heterogeneous patient population" (p. 595). The reader is referred to Chapter 10 by Cannito in this volume for a detailed discussion of this study. In a subsequent study of spasmodic dysphonia subsequent to head injury, this same group compared CT, MRI, ABR, BEAM, and SPECT in three patients and reported no consistent patterns among the technologies. Structural assessments of CT and MRI were normal in all three patients with the exception of one abnormal MRI. Functional assessment of ABR, SPECT, and BEAM were all abnormal in the Case 1 patient (who also had a language disorder), but only BEAM showed functional abnormalities in all three patients. BEAM visual evoked potentials demonstrated left temporal abnormalities that exceeded 5 standard deviations. Smaller differences were also found in right frontal areas with BEAM. The authors stress that no single technology can pinpoint CNS dysfunction, and that the absence of neuropathology on a single measure of CNS function should not be considered conclusive evidence that no neurologic lesions exist.

While these data do point to CNS abnormalities in some types of spasmodic dysphonia, the brain-imaging information cannot yet relate vocal pathology to a specific lesion or metabolic disturbance. Because of the nonspecific nature of the imaging technologies, it cannot be determined if these are co-occuring or causal phenomena. One contribution to our understanding of the neurophysiology of spasmodic dysphonia with imaging technologies may come from monitoring the effects of pharmocologic intervention (Miller et al., 1987).

Stuttering secondary to cerebral lesions has been described by several researchers who report structural brain-imaging data (Horner & Massey, 1983; Helm et al., 1978; Rosenbek, Messert, Collins, & Wertz, 1978). However, the question of whether acquired stuttering can be attributed to a specific lesion is debatable (Rosenbek et al., 1978; Nowack & Stone, 1987). It has been suggested that acquired stuttering is the result of numerous cerebral ischemic effects rather than one lesion site. While numerous reports reveal that an individual can develop stuttering with disease in either of the two hemispheres (see Chapter 8, this volume), Horner and Massey (1983) suggest that the disorder is more permanent with bilateral pathology. To date, no brain-imaging studies have been done on stutterers without known pathology to determine neurotransmitter abnormalities. This would appear to be indicated in view of recent findings implicating the acetylcholine system in a study of five stutterers (Rastatter & Harr, 1988).

CASE DESCRIPTIONS

The following section presents case reports illustrating use of various neuroimaging technologies in four patients with communication disorders. Differences between information obtained from structural and functional imaging techniques are contrasted.

Case 1. Nonfluent Aphasia Studied with CT and Xenon-133 SPECT

A 20-year-old right-handed woman with history of hypertension and migraine had sudden onset of mild hemiparesis and nonfluent aphasia as determined by the *Boston Diagnostic Aphasia Examination* (Goodglass & Kaplan, 1983). CT scan showed a very small frontal cortical lesion. At a follow-up examination 2 years later, the patient continued to have a moderately severe nonfluent aphasia and motor deficits. CT scan remained unchanged, yet xenon-133 SPECT rCBF demonstrated reduced blood flow in most of the left hemisphere, including Wernicke's area and the parietotemporal junction (see Figure 3.12).

Comments. This case demonstrates cortical dysfunction as determined by rCBF in areas remote from the primary lesion as imaged on CT scan.

Similar contrasts between physiologic and anatomic imaging techniques have been reported by other investigators using metabolic and electrophysiological techniques (Metter et al., 1984; Nagata et al., 1986). Studies of patients of this type challenge traditional brain language theory based on structural damage only and suggest that theoretical models of brain language processing need to be enlarged to account for physiologic aspects of brain function.

Case 2. Apraxia of Speech/Aphasia Studied with Xenon-133 SPECT

A 45-year-old strongly left-handed (Oldfield, 1971) male had suffered a right carotid artery aneurysm at the junction of the right posterior communicating artery with a subsequent subarachnoid hemorrhage 8 years previously. Speech and language evaluation 3 months post insult revealed moderate to severe apraxia of speech, mild comprehension and reading difficulties, and inability to write. Detailed follow-up speech and language evaluation 8 years later found the patient to have fluent spontaneous speech with only occasional literal paraphasias or sound repetitions. The patient conversed in complete, grammatically correct sentences. On the *Boston Diagnostic Aphasia Examination* (Goodglass & Kaplan, 1983) repetition, nonverbal agility, and verbal agility were normal. There was slight impairment in reading. Spelling to dictation and written confrontation-naming had changed little from 8 years previously with continued omission of vowels and phonemes. Drawings on command (*Mental Status Examination in Neurology,* Strub & Black, 1977) were rated from good to excellent and were not typical of right-hemisphere-lesioned subjects who are right-handed. CT scan showed areas of damage throughout the right hemisphere with no abnormalities in the left hemisphere. Xenon-133 SPECT rCBF during the resting condition correlated with the CT scan and showed reduced blood flow in much of the right hemisphere including areas homologous to Wernicke's area, extending anteriorly to include pre-Rolandic areas (see Figure 3.13). SPECT rCBF during a linguistic probe condition (Walker-Batson, Wendt, Barton, Devous, & Bonte, 1988) showed no changes in cortical blood flow; however, there were rCBF increases in both cerebellar hemispheres with the greatest increases in the right cerebellum (see Figure 3.13).

Comments. This follow-up case study demonstrates the use of a linguistic activation task during the rCBF xenon-SPECT procedure. Differences between resting state and cognitive probe conditions shown on slice 1 of the SPECT study suggest that recovery studies of speech and language function with various physiologic imaging tools should include language activation probes. It is not known whether our patient's rCBF increases in the cerebellum relate to his improved speech function. Other laboratories studying pharmocologic intervention in recovery of motor function after stroke have recently suggested that cerebellar metabolic increases (on PET scans) may involve the norepinephrine system in stroke recovery (M. Boyeson, personal communication, 1988). Our laboratory has previously observed a pattern of rCBF increases in the cerebellum ipsilateral to the infarct in a small series of chronic aphasic subjects (Walker-Batson, Devous, Millay, Reynolds, Ajamani, Grant, & Bonte, 1988).

Case 3. Seizures with Speech Arrest Studied with IMP SPECT

A 13-year-old right-handed male had normal birth history and developmental milestones until age 10 when he began to experience seizures. The seizures were stereotyped; they consisted of an abrupt right-face numbness around the corner of the mouth followed by opening of the mouth and right-arm extension. Consciousness was retained but there was speech arrest during the seizure. The patient could follow brief verbal commands during the seizure and postictally remember nonsense phrases delivered to him. Seizure duration was 30 seconds and the patient was normal immediately afterward. MRI scan and interictal EEG revealed no abnormalities; however, ictal EEG demonstrated bilateral seizure activity. Ictal SPECT rCBF using 1-123 iodoamphetamine (IMP) as the tracer demonstrated an area of high regional cerebral blood flow in the left parietal region surrounded by an area of relatively low perfusion (see Figure 3.14). Increased anticonvulsant medication dosage controlled the seizures.

Comments. This case demonstrates the use of a second-generation SPECT scanner (Ohio Imaging, 1988) to determine the area of ictus in seizure disorders. Studies of this type are only beginning. In this case the patient had speech arrest during the seizure without language comprehension deficits following seizure activity. IMP-SPECT rCBF study during the ictal phase localized abnormal blood flow areas in the left parietal lobe.

Case 4. Dysarthria Studied with MRI

A 62-year-old right-handed black female with a history of adult-onset diabetes and hypertension presented with an acute onset of an "ataxic-spastic" type of dysarthria. The patient was known to be status post multiple lacunar cerebrovascular accidents. On admission the patient also had left facial droop, left hemiparesis, and decreased sensation on the left side of her face. Neurological examination showed the reflexes to be hyperactive diffusely and there were bilateral postive Babinski signs. MRI showed an area of high signal intensity in the right pons extending into the basis pointis and the right middle cerebellar peduncle (see Figure 3.16). The MRI scan at other levels showed areas of high signal intensity scattered throughout the white matter. These abnormalities were not evident on the CT scan.

Comments. This case demonstrates the sensitivity of MRI when compared to CT scanning to show contrasts between gray and white matter. CT scan failed to show areas of abnormalities scattered throughout the white matter that were visualized on MRI. The speech pattern of this patient did not clearly fit into a characteristic subtype. The most marked finding on MRI in this case was in the brain stem and cerebellar regions.

CONCLUSION

In this chapter we have overviewed six current brain-imaging technologies, described their clinical and research use, and presented case studies demonstrating the use of these tools in neurological disorders affecting communication. To orient the clinician, a brief review of functional neuroanatomy and neurochemistry was provided. While basic

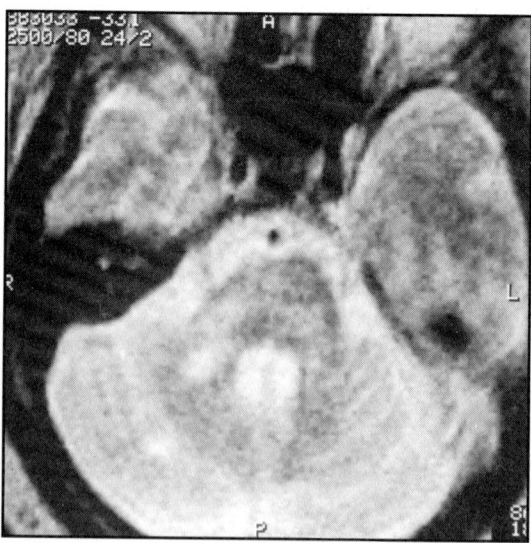

Figure 3.16 MRI axial view T2-weighted image of Case 4 showing increased signal in pons crossing midline and in the right cerebellar peduncle. These abnormalities were not evident on the CT scan.

knowledge about neuroanatomic and neurophysiologic aspects of speech and language processing in both normal and disease states is gradually being acquired with these new brain-imaging tools, their primary application is clinical utility in terms of medical management. For speech-language clinicians, an awareness of the differences in the various imaging techniques will enhance their understanding of the patient's total medical status and enable them to more effectively participate in team treatment approaches. Beginning research data from numerous imaging technologies are providing concrete evidence of neurological dysfunction in certain speech disorders not previously documented (Devous et al., 1990). The use of these advanced technologies to help in determining and monitoring appropriate medical treatments (i.e., drugs) in disorders of speech motor control is on the threshold of clinical utility.

REFERENCES

Abbs, J. H. (1981). Neuromotor mechanisms of speech production. In J. K. Darby, Jr. (Ed.), *Speech evaluation in medicine* (pp. 180–198). New York: Grune and Stratton.

Adam, P., Fabre, N., Guel, A., Bessoles, G., Roulleau, J., & Bes, A. (1983). Cortical atrophy in Parkinson disease: Correlation between clinical and CT findings with special emphasis on prefrontal atrophy. *AJNR, 4,* 442–445.

Alexander, M. P., & Schmitt, M. A. (1980). The aphasia syndrome of stroke in the left anterior cerebral artery territory. *Archives of Neurology, 37,* 97–100.

Aronson, A. E., & DeSanto, L. S. (1983). Adduction spastic dysphonia: Three years after recurrent laryngeal nerve resection. *Laryngoscope, 93,* 1–8.

Basso, A., Luzzatti, C., & Spinnler, H. (1980). Is ideomotor apraxia the outcome of damage to well-defined regions of the left hemisphere? *Journal of Neurology, Neurosurgery and Psychiatry, 43,* 118–126.

Benson, D. F. (1984). Positron emission tomography in aphasia. *Seminars in Neurology, 4,* 169–173.

Bonte, F. J., & Stokely, E. M. (1981). Single-photon emission computed tomography of regional cerebral blood flow in cerebral vascular disease and stroke: Concise communication. *Journal of Nuclear Medicine, 22,* 1049–1053.

Bottomley, P. A., Drayer, B. P., & Smith, L. S. (1986). Chronic adult cerebral infarction studied by phosphorus NMR spectroscopy. *Radiology, 160,* 763–766.

Bromfield, E. B., Ludlow, C. L., Bassich, C. J., & Theodore, W. H. (1988). Cerebral activation during speech perception in temporal lobe epilepsy. *Neurology, 38*(Suppl. 1), 278.

Brown, J. W. (1980). Brain structure and language production: A dynamic view. In D. Caplan (Ed.), *Biological studies of mental processes* (pp. 287–301). Cambridge, MA: MIT Press.

Brownell, G. L., Budinger, T. F., Lauterbur, P. C., & McGeer, P. L. (1982). Positron tomography and nuclear magnetic resonance imaging. *Science, 215,* 619–626.

Brunner, R. J., Kornhuber, H. H., Seemuller, E., Suger, G., & Wallesch, C. W. (1982). Basal ganglia participation in language pathology. *Brain and Language, 16,* 281–299.

Calne, D. B., Langston, J. W., Martin, W. R., Stoessl, A. J., Ruth, T. J., Adam, M. J., Pate, B. D., & Schulzer, M. (1985). Positron emission tomography after MPTP: Observations relating to the cause of Parkinson's disease. *Nature, 317,* 246–248.

Cannito, M. P., Pool, K., Freeman, F. J., & Finitzo, T. (1985). Brain electrical activity mapping in adductor spasmodic dysphonia. *Journal of the Acoustical Society of America, 77,* S87.

Caplan, D. (1980). *Biological studies of mental processes.* Cambridge, MA: MIT Press.

Caplan, L. R., & Zervas, N. T. (1978). Speech arrest in a dextral with a right mesial frontal astrocytoma. *Archives of Neurology, 35,* 252–253.

Carpenter, M. B. (1985). *Core text of neuroanatomy.* Baltimore, MD: Williams and Wilkins.

Chiueh, C. C., Firnau, G., Burns, R. S., Hahmias, C., Chirakal, R., Kopin, I. J., & Garnett, E. S. (1987). Determination and visualization of damage to striatal dopaminergic terminals in 1-methyl-4-1, 2, 3, 6-tetrahydropyridine-induced parkinsonism by (18F)-labeled 6-fluoro-L-dopa and positron emission tomography. *Advances in Neurology, 45,* 167–169.

Crosson, B., Novack, T. A., & Trenerry, M. R. (1988). Subcortical language mechanisms: Window on a new frontier. In H. A. Whitaker (Ed.), *Phonological processes and brain mechanisms* (pp. 24–58). New York: Springer-Verlag.

Damasio, A. R., Damasio, H., Rizzo, M., Varney, N., & Gersch, F. (1982). Aphasia with nonhemorrhagic lesions in the basal ganglia and internal capsule. *Archives of Neurology, 35,* 15–20.

Damasio, A. R., & Van Hoesen, G. W. (1980). Structure and function of the supplementary motor area. *Neurology, 39,* 359.

Darby, J. K. (1985). Epidemiology of neurologic diseases that produce communication disorders. In J. K. Darby, Jr. (Ed.), *Speech and language evaluation in neurology: Adult disorders* (pp. 29–44). New York: Grune and Stratton.

Dedo, H. H., & Izdebski, K. (1983). Immediate results of 306 recurrent laryngeal nerve sections for spastic dysphonia. *Laryngoscope, 93,* 9–16.

Devous, M. D., Pool, K. D., Finitzo, T., Freeman, F. J., Schaefer, S. D., Watson, B., Kondraske, G. V., & Chapman, S. B. (1990). Evidence for cortical dysfunction in spasmodic dysphonia: Quantitative electrophysiology and regional cerebral blood flow. *Brain and Language, 39,* 331–344.

Devous, M. D., Stokely, E. M., & Bonte, F. J. (1985). Quantitative imaging of regional cerebral blood flow in man by dynamic single-photon tomography. In B. L. Holman (Ed.), *Radionuclide imaging of the brain* (pp. 135–162). London: Churchill Livington.

Duffy, F. H. (1985). The BEAM method for neurophysiological diagnosis. *Annals of the New York Academy of Sciences, 457*:19-34.

Duffy, F. H. (1986). *Topographic mapping of brain electrical activity.* Boston: Butterworth.

Duffy, F. H., Burchfiel, J. L., & Lombroso, C. T. (1979). Brain electrical activity mapping (BEAM): A method for extending the clinical utility of EEG and evoked potential data. *Annals of Neurology, 5,* 309–321.

Duffy, F. H., Denckla, M. B., Bartels, O. H., & Sandini, G. (1980). Dyslexia: Regional differences in brain electrical activity by topographic mapping. *Annals of Neurology, 7,* 412–420.

Finitzo, T., & Freeman, F. J. (1989). Spasmodic dysphonia, whether and where: Results of seven years of research. *Journal of Speech and Hearing Research, 32,* 541–555.

Finitzo, T., Pool, K. D., Freeman, F. J., Cannito, M. P., Schaefer, S., Ross, E. D., & Devous, M. D. (1987). Spasmodic dysphonia subsequent to head trauma. *Archives of Otolaryngology, 113,* 1107–1110.

Fisher, M. (1984). Putaminal hemorrhage presenting as dysarthria–clumsy hand syndrome. *Bulletin of Clinical Neuroscience, 49,* 1–3.

Flowers, K. (1978). Lack of prediction in the motor behaviour of Parkinsonism. *Brain, 101,* 35–52.

Fox, P. T., Posner, M. I., & Raichle, M. E. (1988). Localization of phonological processing in the temporoparietal cortex by PET. *Society for Neuroscience Abstracts, 14,* 217.

Freedman, M., Alexander, M. P., & Naeser, M. A. (1984). Anatomic basis of transcortical motor aphasia. *Neurology, 34,* 409–417.

Gilman, S., & Newman, S. W. (1987). *Manter and Gatz's essentials of clinical neuroanatomy and neurophysiology.* Philadelphia: F. A. Davis.

Goodglass, H., & Kaplan, E. (1983). *Assessment of aphasia and related disorders.* Philadelphia: Lea and Febiger.

Gordon, W. P. (1985). Neuropsychological assessment of aphasia. In J. K. Darby, Jr. (Ed.), *Speech and language evaluation in neurology: Adult disorders* (pp. 161–196). New York: Grune and Stratton.

Grossberg, S. (1987). *Neural networks and natural intelligence.* Cambridge, MA: MIT Press.

Groswasser, Z., Korn, C., Groswasser-Reider, I., & Solzi, P. (1988). Mutism associated with buccofacial apraxia and bihemispheric lesions. *Brain and Language, 34,* 157–168.

Helm, N. A., Butler, R. B., & Benson, D. F. (1978). Acquired stuttering. *Neurology, 28,* 1159–1165.

Herderschee, D., Stam, J., & Derex, M. M. (1987). Aphemia as a first symptom of multiple sclerosis. *Journal of Neurology, Neurosurgery and Psychiatry, 50,* 499–500.

Hirose, H., Kiritani, S., & Sawashima, M. (1980). Patterns of dysarthric movements in patients with amyotrophic lateral sclerosis and pseudobulbar palsy. *Annual Bulletin of the Research Institute of Logopedics and Phoniatrics, 14,* 231–249.

Homan, R. W., Devous, M. D., Stokely, E. M., & Bonte, F. J. (1987). Cerebellar blood flow in partial seizures. *Neurology, 37*(Suppl. 1), 327.

Horner, J., & Massey, E. W. (1983). Progressive dysfluency associated with right hemisphere disease. *Brain and Language, 18*, 71–85.

James, T. L., Chew, W. M., Giannini, D. D., Gonzalez-Mendez, R., Moseley, M. E., Pogliani, L., & Vigneron, D. (1987, August). Principles of magnetic resonance spectroscopy. *Applied Radiology*, pp. 40–52.

Kanno, I., & Lassen, N. A. (1979). Two methods for calculating regional cerebral blood flow from emission computed tomography of inert gas concentrations. *Journal of Computer Assisted Tomography, 3*, 71–76.

Kent, R. (1984). A neurobiologic view of the dysarthrias. In M. McNeil, J. Rosenbek, and A. Aronson (Eds.), *The dysarthrias* (pp. 1–36). Austin, TX: PRO-ED.

Kertesz, A., Harlock, W., & Coates, R. (1979). Computer tomographic localization, lesion size and prognosis in aphasia and nonverbal impairment. *Brain and Language, 8*, 34–50.

Kornhuber, H. H. (1977). A reconsideration of the cortical and subcortical mechanisms involved in speech and aphasia. In J. E. Desmedt (Ed.), *Progress in Clinical Neurophysiology: Vol. 3. Language and hemispheric specialization in man: Cerebral ERP's* (pp. 28–35). Basel: Karger.

Kuhl, D. E., Metter, E. J., Riege, W. H., & Markham, C. H. (1984). Patterns of cerebral glucose utilization in Parkinson's disease and Huntington's disease. *Annals of Neurology, 15*, 119–125.

Kushner, M., Reivich, M., Alavi, A., Greenberg, J., Stern, M., & Dann, R. (1987). Regional cerebral glucose metabolism in aphemia: A case report. *Brain and Language, 31*, 201–204.

Lechtenberg, R., and Gilman, S. (1978). Speech disorders in cerebellar disease. *Annals of Neurology, 3*, 285–290.

Ludlow, C. L., & Connor, N. P. (1987). Dynamic aspects of phonatory control in spasmodic dysphonia. *Journal of Speech and Hearing Research, 30*, 197–206.

Ludlow, C. L., Rosenberg, J., Salazar, A., Grafman, J., & Smutok, M. (1987). Site of penetrating brain lesions causing chronic acquired stuttering. *Annals of Neurology, 22*, 60–66.

Metter, E. J., & Hanson, W. R. (1985). Brain imaging as related to speech and language. In J. K. Darby (Ed.), *Speech and Language Evaluation in Neurology: Adult Disorders*. Orlando, FL: Grune and Stratton.

Metter, E. J., Hanson, W., Kempler, D., Jackson, C., Mazziotta, J., & Phelps, M. (1987). Left prefrontal glucose hypometabolism in aphasia. *Clinical Aphasiology, 17*, 300–313.

Metter, E. J., Hanson, W., Phelps, M., Squire, L., Wasterlain, C., & Benson, D. (1983). Comparison of metabolic rates, language and memory in subcortical aphasias. *Brain and Language, 19*, 33–47.

Metter, E. J., & Kempler, D. (1986). Cerebral glucose metabolism: Differences in Wernicke's, Broca's and conduction aphasias. *Clinical Aphasiology, 16*, 103.

Metter, E. J., Riege, W., Hanson, W., Kuhl, D., & Phelps, M. (1983). The use of (F-18)-fluorodeoxyglucose positron computed tomography in the study of aphasia. *Clinical Aphasiology, 13*, 262–276.

Metter, E. J., Wasterlain, C. G., Kuhl, D. E., Hanson, W. R., & Phelps, M. E. (1984). 18FDG positron emission computed tomography in a study of aphasia. *Annals of Neurology, 19*, 173–183.

Miller, R. H., Woodson, G. E., & Jankovic, J. (1987). Botulinum toxin injection of the vocal fold for spasmodic dysphonia: A preliminary report. *Archives of Otolaryngology, Head and Neck Surgery, 113*, 603–605.

Naeser, M. A., Alexander, M. P., Helm-Estabrooks, N., Levine, H. L., Laughlin, S. A., & Geschwind, N. (1982). Aphasia with predominately subcortical lesion sites. *Archives of Neurology, 39*, 2–14.

Naeser, M. A., Hayward, R. W., Laughlin, S. A., Becker, J. M., Jernigan, T. L., & Zatz, L. M. (1981). Quantitative CT scan studies in aphasia II: Comparison of the right and left hemispheres. *Brain and Language, 12*, 165–189.

Nagata, K., Tagawa, K., Shishido, F., & Uemura, K. (1986). Topographic EEG correlates of cerebral blood flow and oxygen consumption in patients with neuropsychological disorders. In F. Duffy (Ed.), *Brain electrical activity mapping* (pp. 357–370). Boston: Butterworth.

Nowack, W. J., & Stone, R. E. (1987). Acquired stuttering and bilateral cerebral disease. *Journal of Fluency Disorders, 12*, 141–146.

Oke, A., Keller, R., Mefford, I., & Adams, R. N. (1978). Lateralization of norepinephrine in human thalamus. *Science, 200*, 1411–1413.

Oldfield, R. C. (1971). The assessment and analysis of handedness: The Edinburgh Inventory. *Neuropsychologia, 9*, 97–113.

Ozaki, I., Baba, M., Narita, S., Matsunaga, M., & Takebe, K. (1986). Pure dysarthria due to anterior internal capsule and/or corona radiata infarction: A report of five cases. *Journal of Neurology, Neurosurgery, and Psychiatry, 49*, 1435–1437.

Peled, R., Harnes, B., Borovich, B., & Sharf, B. (1984). Speech arrest and supplementary motor area seizures. *Neurology, 34*, 110–111.

Petersen, S. E., Fox, P. T., Posner, M. I., & Raichle, M. E. (1988). Localization of phonological processing in the temporoparietal cortex by PET. *Society for Neuroscience Abstracts, 14*(1), 217.

Plum, F., & Posner, J. (1980). *The diagnosis of stupor and coma* (3rd ed.). Philadelphia: F. A. Davis.

Poeck, K., de Bleser, R., & von Keyserlingk, D. G. (1984). Neurolinguistic status and localization of lesion in aphasic patients with exclusively consonant-vowel recurring utterances. *Brain, 197*, 199–217.

Pool, K., Freeman, F. J., & Finitzo, F. (1987). Brain electrical activity mapping application to vocal motor control disorders. In H. Peters & W. Hulstijn (Eds.), *Speech motor dynamics in stuttering* (pp. 151–160). New York: Springer Press.

Posner, M. I., Petersen, S. E., Fox, P. T., & Raichle, M. E. (1988). Localization of cognitive operations in the human brain. *Science, 240*, 1627–1631.

Radda, G. K. (1986). The use of NMR spectroscopy for the understanding of disease. *Science, 223*, 640–645.

Rasmussen, T. (1974). Seizures with local onset. In P. J. Vinken & G. W. Bruyn (Eds.), *Handbook of clinical neurology* (pp. 80–81). Amsterdam: North-Holland.

Rastatter, M. P., & Harr, R. (1988). Measurements of plasma levels of adrenergic neurotransmitter and primary amino acids in five stuttering subjects: A preliminary report (biochemical aspects of stuttering). *Journal of Fluency Disorders, 13*, 127–139.

Rosenbek, J., Messert, B., Collins, M., & Wertz, R. T. (1978). Stuttering following brain damage. *Brain and Language, 6*, 314–322.

Rosenfield, D. B. (1972). Stuttering and cerebral ischemia. *New England Journal of Medicine, 287*, 991.

Rubens, A. B. (1975). Aphasia with infarction in the territory of the anterior cerebral artery. *Cortex, 11*, 239–250.

Rubens, A. B. (1976). Transcortical motor aphasia. In Whitaker & Whitaker (Eds.), *Studies in Neurolingustics* (Vol. 1, pp. 293–303). New York: Academic Press.

Ruff, R. L., & Arbit, E. (1981). Aphemia resulting from a left frontal hematoma. *Neurology, 31*, 353–356.

Schaefer, S., Freeman, F. J., Finitzo, T., Close, L., Cannito, M., Ross, E. D., Reich, J., & Maravilla, K. (1985). Magnetic resonance imaging findings and correlations in spasmodic dysphonia patients. *Annals of Otology, Rhinology and Laryngology, 94*, 595–601.

Schiff, H. B., Alexander, M. P., Naeser, M. A., & Galaburda, A. M. (1983). Aphemia. Clinical-anatomic correlations. *Archives of Neurology, 49*, 720–727.

Shaw, G. L., Silverman, D. J., & Pearson, J. C. (1985). Model of cortical organization embodying a basis for a theory of information processing and memory recall. *Proceedings of the National Academy of Science, 82*, 2364–2368.

Square, P., Darley, F. L., & Sommers, R. (1982). An analysis of the productive errors made by pure apractic speakers with differing loci of lesions. *Clinical Aphasiology, 11*, 245–250.

Starosta-Rubinstein, S., Young, A. B., Kluin, K., Hill, G., Aisen, A. M., Gabrielsen, T., & Brewer, G. J. (1987). Clinical assessment of 4 patients with Wilson's disease. Correlations with structural changes on magnetic resonance imaging. *Archives of Neurology, 44*, 365–370.

Stokely, E. M., Sveinsdotir, E., Lassen, N. A., & Rommer, P. (1980). A single photon dynamic computer assisted tomography (DCAT) for imaging brain function in multiple cross-sections. *Journal of Computer Assisted Tomography, 4*, 230–240.

Strub, R. L., & Black, F. W. (1977). *The mental status examination in neurology.* Philadelphia: F. A. Davis.

Sugishita, M., Konno, K., Kabe, S., Yunoki, K., Togashi, O., & Kawamura, M. (1987). Electropalatographic analysis of speech in a left hander and in a right hander. *Brain, 110*, 1393–1417.

Tikofsky, R. S., Collier, B. D., Hellman, R. S., Saxena, V. K., Zielonka, J. S., Krohn, L., & Gresch, A. (1985, October). *Cerebral blood flow patterns determined by SPECT I-123 iodoamphetamine (IMP) imaging and WAB AQ's in chronic aphasics: A preliminary report.* Paper presented at the meeting of the Academy of Aphasia, Pittsburgh, PA.

Van Lackner, D. (1985). Hemispheric contributions to language and communication. In J. K. Darby, Jr. (Ed.), *Speech and language evaluation in neurology: Adult disorders* (pp. 247–296). New York: Grune & Stratton.

Versteeg, D. H. G., Van der Gugten, J., DeJong, W., & Palkovts, M. (1976). Regional concentrations of noradrenaline and dopamine in rat brain. *Brain Research, 113*, 563–574.

Wagner, H. N., Jr., Burns, H. D., Dannals, R. F., Wong, D. F., Langstrom, B., & Duelfer, T. (1983). Imaging dopamine receptors in the human brain by positron tomography. *Science, 221*, 1264–1266.

Walker-Batson, D., Bonte, F. J., Devous, M. D., Ajamani, A., Nunnally, R. L., & Babcock, E. E. (1987). *31-P magnetic resonance spectroscopy in chronic aphasia; a preliminary report.* Paper presented at the annual meeting of the American Speech-Language-Hearing Association, New Orleans.

Walker-Batson, D. Devous, M. D., Bonte, J. F., & Oelschlaeger, M. (1987). Single-photon emission tomography (SPECT) in the study of aphasia: A preliminary report. *Clinical Aphasiology, 17*, 313–319.

Walker-Batson, D., Wendt, J., Barton, M. M., Devous, M. D., & Bonte, F. J. (1988). A long-term follow-up case study of crossed aphasia assessed by single-photon emission tomography (SPECT), language and neuropsychological measures. *Brain and Language, 33*: 311–322.

Walker-Batson, D., Devous, M. D., Millay, K. K., Reynolds, S., Ajamani, A. J., Grant, D. E., & Bonte, F. J. (1988). Tomographic regional cerebral blood flow (rCBF) activation during phoneme detection in normal and aphasic subjects. *Clinical Aphasiology, 18*, 75–90.

Welch, K. M. A., Chopp, M., Smith, M. B., Helpern, J. A., Walton, D., & Frinak, S., (1987). Utility of in vivo nuclear magnetic resonance spectrocopy for the study of ischemic stroke. In M. E. Raichle & W. J. Powers (Eds.), *Cerebrovascular diseases: The fifteenth Princeton conference* (pp. 210–216). New York: Raven Press.

Williamson, P.D., Spencer, D. D., Spencer, S. S., Novelly, R., & Mattson, R. H. (1985). Episodic aphemia and epileptic focus in nondominant hemisphere: Relieved by section of corpus callosum. *Neurology, 35*, 1069–1071.

ACKNOWLEDGMENTS

The authors wish to thank Drs. Michael Devous, Robert Leroy, and Donnell Johns for information on Cases 1, 2, and 3; and Jill Wilson for evaluation of Case 2. Special thanks to Texas Woman's University staff members for their contributions: Margaret McDougal, reference librarian; Era Harford, drawings; and Verda Chism, manuscript preparation. SPECT scans were made available by the Nuclear Medicine Center, The University of Texas Southwestern Medical Center, Dallas, Texas. Quantitive EEG images were provided by Cadwell Inc., Kennewick, Washington.

PART II
Generalized Movement Disorders Affecting Speech

CHAPTER 4
A Top-Down Approach to Treatment of Dysarthric Speech
Deanie Vogel and Lynda Miller

>   *Vogel and Miller describe a knowledge-driven approach that provides the cognitive scaffolding for treatment of dysarthric speech. They show how providing insight into the characteristics involved in a top-down approach to treatment for dysarthria may improve the patient's overall ability to communicate.*
>
>   1. List potential benefits of a top-down approach for treatment of dysarthric speech.
>   2. How can the concepts of primary-level and secondary-level pragmatics be used in treating the dysarthric patient?
>   3. Vogel and Miller discuss how discourse analysis can be used to counsel the dysarthric patient. How can awareness of the different types of discourse therapeutically benefit the dysarthric patient?

In their landmark papers published in 1969, Darley, Aronson, and Brown identified deviant speech dimensions and differential diagnostic patterns of dysarthric speech. These important papers revolutionized the thinking about dysarthria that was current at that time and spawned many investigations of dysarthria. A number of excellent publications followed, many of which addressed issues related to dysarthria management and treatment (Darley, Aronson, & Brown, 1975; Dworkin, 1984; Rosenbek, 1984; Wertz, 1985; Rosenbek & LaPointe, 1985; Netsell, 1986; Yorkston, Beukelman, & Bell, 1988). These publications will not be reviewed extensively here; the interested clinician is encouraged to examine these reports.

Since the publication of the work by Darley and his colleagues, several different approaches to dysarthria management have been noted. A symptomotology approach is one in which a symptom (e.g., inadequate velopharyngeal closure) is treated and the effect on a sign (e.g., hypernasality) is observed. Yorkston, Beukelman, and Bell (1988) described treatment in terms of disordered speech intelligibility, and Rosenbek and LaPointe (1985) wrote of assessment and treatment in terms of impaired respiration, phonation, resonance, articulation, and prosody. Perkins (1983) considered approaching treatment based on the underlying neuropathology of the dysarthria, but opted to organize his discussions of treatment according to the classifications described by Darley, Aronson, and Brown.

Dysarthric speakers and their clinicians should be aware that a return to normal speech probably is not a realistic goal for most dysarthric patients; compensated intelligibility as described by Rosenbek and LaPointe (1985) thus appears to be a more realistic approach, especially for dysarthric speakers who are able to use verbal communication but whose speech is not completely intelligible. Some specific techniques used to attempt to achieve compensated intelligibility involve normalizing muscle tone to increase strength and movement precision, management with a palatal lift prosthesis or laryngoplasty, engaging in phonetic drills, and attempting to control speaking rate.

Most approaches and techniques focus on the details of the patient's output signal, while seeming to neglect the wealth of knowledge available to a person with uncomplicated dysarthria. Knowledge-driven approaches, however, have been employed in the remediation of left hemisphere (Davis & Wilcox, 1985; Davis, 1986) and right hemisphere (Burns, 1985) function. These knowledge-driven approaches are top-down, whereas the peripheral signal-oriented approaches such as those traditionally used with dysarthric patients are bottom-up.

Generally dysarthria clinicians have focused on the speaker and the dysarthric speech rather than on the listener and the communication interaction. In this chapter, a top-down approach to communication will be described, involving the study of the relationships between language and the context in which language is used. The top-down process and its characteristics will be defined and contrasted with a bottom-up process in which the organization of language is largely ignored. Finally, suggestions for using a top-down approach for improving the communication of the dysarthric patient will be presented.

TOP-DOWN AND BOTTOM-UP PROCESSING

Generally, *top-down* is used to refer to the cognitive process of using available information to construct a gestalt, or whole. The whole serves as an overall form into which supporting details can be fit. The supporting details are added after the general pattern has been constructed and are used to corroborate the general pattern. As Wallach and Miller (1988) point out, "Top-down processing is analogous to deductive thinking. In deductive thinking one formulates a general hypothesis and infers specific outcomes on the basis of the general principle" (p. 20).

In contrast, *bottom-up* is employed to indicate the process of using available information to collect a group of details before constructing a general pattern. The details serve as the salient features from which a larger concept is built. Bottom-up processing can be thought of as analogous to inductive thinking in that it involves accumulating examples until a general conclusion can be reached (Wallach & Miller, 1988). Most traditional dysarthria therapies involve more bottom-up than top-down processing.

In developing knowledge of and facility with communication and language, children typically employ a learning style that is inductive or bottom-up. They hear assorted pieces of language form, various ways of encoding content, and examples of usage, which rarely suggest the organizational aspects of the language they are hearing. From these bits and pieces, children gradually construct their own methods of choosing words, forming sentences, translating them into the sound system of their language, and using them in appropriate and relevant ways.

Many language users, as they grow into adults, continue to engage in inductive learning about language and communication and may never utilize top-down thinking in considering the linguistic and nonlinguistic aspects of communicating. They may use language with facility, but have little or no insight into how it works. As bottom-up learners, they are relatively adept at choosing appropriate sound combinations, words, and sentence structures for their messages, but they remain unaware of the patterns underlying these aspects of communicating through language. For these bottom-up learners, language continues to be something that just happens; talking about it or reflecting on its myriad parts is foreign and unfamiliar, and the idea that communication patterns can be analyzed may be surprising to them.

For other language users, deciphering the general patterns and rules of language and communication from their ongoing experiences is a natural process. This group actively searches for the organizational patterns characterizing communication and language. They find the top-down characteristics salient and obvious, and they utilize them in understanding how to use both linguistic and nonlinguistic means to communicate. For these top-down learners, the general patterns stand as organizational themes from which to deduce specific examples to incorporate into their communicating. Usually by adulthood top-down learners have developed considerable ability to reflect on communication and how language and its parts function in various communicative contexts, and usually they can talk about language and its parts and understand the interactions of linguistic and nonlinguistic form, content, and use.

A third type of processing also exists, a combination of top-down and bottom-up processing. This type is referred to as interactive, and is the process language users employ when comprehending language. Language users analyze the peripheral input delivered via the input signal while consulting their central knowledge stores in order to arrive at an interpretation of the signal.

The dysarthria clinician may find it beneficial to begin treatment by attempting to discover how much a patient knows about language and communication in order to determine whether the patient is a top-down, a bottom-up, or an interactive learner. We have found that, in many cases, the question "What do you know about communication?" yields a great deal of information we can use to focus treatment. For the dysarthric patient whose knowledge of communication and language is primarily inductive or bottom-up, focusing on the deductive or top-down aspects of language and communication may constitute a significant portion of the treatment sessions, even though the patient's primary problem is disordered speech motor control rather than language impairment.

The patient who is oriented to regard the goal of dysarthria therapy as improvement in speech, rather than in overall communication, needs information about general patterns of communication and language. Top-down characteristics must be described. The patient may need assistance in discerning word patterns and sentence length. Meanings of words such as *topic* must be explained, for the patient who does not understand what a topic is will have difficulty maintaining one. Furthermore, these patients with an inductive orientation to language use may not be aware of how to get a turn in a conversation; how, either verbally or nonverbally, to signal turn-taking shifts in a conversation; or how to signal to their listeners that a humorous remark is forthcoming.

Dysarthric patients who are not bottom-up learners may benefit from a top-down orientation as well, because they have to be even better communicators than they were before becoming dysarthric. These patients have to become aware of how to use alternative strategies that may not be immediately obvious even to more top-down-oriented communicators.

The clinician's task is somewhat easier when treating the patient who, before becoming dysarthric, developed an understanding of the top-down characteristics of language. This patient may need only a reminder of those characteristics and how to manipulate them effectively.

Traditional descriptions of language focus on the patterns associated with semantic, morphological, phonological, and pragmatic components. While it is true that there are general patterns characteristic of each of these primary linguistic components, it is also true that general patterns of language exist at a secondary level of analysis. This secondary level is distinguished from the primary level by Miller (1988), who terms it the "level of higher-order language," based on the notion that a secondary level of awareness develops as a function of the acquisition of the primary level structures, forms, and uses of language. Through focusing on the general patterns of language and manipulating some of the top-down aspects of language, dysarthric persons should be able to improve the overall quality of their communication. In the following sections the top-down characteristics of both the primary and secondary levels of language processing will be described.

TOP-DOWN CHARACTERISTICS OF THE PRIMARY LEVEL OF LANGUAGE PROCESSING

Typically, the primary level of language processing is considered to consist of semantics, syntax and morphology, phonology, and pragmatics. It should be noted, however, that in this chapter some portions of the pragmatic component of language will be described as secondary-level aspects.

Semantics

The most salient semantic characteristic is that things-in-the-world are named. While this may seem obvious, what may not be so obvious is that many things have more than one name. Often alternate names or synonyms for a particular word are comprised of phonological sequences that are easier for a dysarthric patient to produce than the word the patient intended to say. Recently, a dysarthric patient attempting to tell us about his neighbor's spring planting produced several unintelligible attempts to express "rosebush." Finally, he substituted "roses" for the original word; "roses" was easier to produce. Moreover, "roses" served the same general purpose in the message as did "rosebush." The patient's word substitution was understood by his listener, communication was effective, and the conversation could continue.

Another general characteristic of the semantic component of language is that usually there is a specific word to refer to each specific thing-in-the-world. Using that specific word rather than a more general referent increases the likelihood that the word will be understood. A corollary of the specific word for a specific referent is that speakers usually maximize their intelligibility when they use a word according to the word's denotative or explicit functions rather than relying on its connotative or associative functions. This means that the literal meaning is easier to understand, and therefore to communicate, than the figurative meaning, except in certain circumstances where idiomatic or metaphoric expressions are more common. For example, the word *dog* commonly means a household pet, and most speakers of English would agree with that meaning. Another meaning, one that is less common but used among some English language users, is an undesirable person or object. The speaker who refers to a person as a dog will experience communication breakdown unless the listener understands the less common meaning of the word. We will discuss the use of figurative language and its relationship to treatment of dysarthria when we describe the characteristics of the secondary-level language components.

A third characteristic of the semantic component is that mature language users are more likely to recall overall sentence meanings than particular syntactic forms (Owens, 1988). This means that syntactic structure may not be as important as semantic meaning for the speaker with a limited ability to produce connected strings of sounds and syllables intelligibly. This is important for the clinician to consider, especially when treating the severely dysarthric patient who is using an alternative to speech. Counseling dysarthric patients to construct brief messages consisting of only nouns and verbs rather than using long, complete sentences is a common practice in dysarthria therapy. What may not be as common is making the patient aware that, for effective communication, meaning is more important than syntax.

Syntax and Morphology

The syntactical and morphological aspects of language are closely linked and are often considered to make up the same grammatical system. The most general characteristic of the grammatical component of language is that patterns underlie sentence structure and word endings. Basic sentence structures—the simple, active, declarative (John kicked the ball), the imperative (Get the ball out of the flowers), the negative (I don't want any coffee right now), and the interrogative (Is that a black tie?)—are contrasted with complex embedded sentence structures: the nonreversible passive (The book was picked up by the woman), the reversible passive (The boy was chased by the girl), the *wh* question (Why do you want to go today?), and the embedded clause (The man who came by the office yesterday is the guy I was telling you about in the park that day). To date, we know of no study comparing basic with complex embedded structures in sentences spoken by dysarthric subjects, but we hypothesize that listeners would find sentences with basic structures easier to interpret.

Patterns of word endings signal specific meanings. For example, in "the cats played in the trees," the underlined segments indicate a plural, a past tense, and another plural. These particular endings illustrate regular patterns in English, and are found in the majority of plural and past tense markers. As a general rule, regular and high-frequency irregular forms are more likely to be predicted by listeners and communicated effectively than are lower-frequency irregular markers. Many English words with irregular markers are, however, quite recognizable; the words *ate, sang, drank, hit, ought, made, children, mice, feet,* and *sheep* are examples. As in the case of underlying sentence structures, we know of no reports of systematic investigations with dysarthric subjects. We hypothesize that for dysarthric speakers, regular markers would signal meanings more effectively than would irregular morphological markers. Of course, we do recognize that forms that mark plurality by a vowel change (as in the word *women,* for example) may be easier for the dysarthric patient to produce than *s* endings, especially in words with consonant-plus-*s* combinations.

Phonology

Many primary characteristics of the phonological system are relevant to the treatment of dysarthric patients. The most apparent top-down characteristic of the phonological system is that highly visible and audible sound and sound combinations (e.g., labial and labiodental consonants, voiced and continuant consonants) are more understandable under degraded conditions than those less easily seen or heard. Deal and Darley (1972) and Darley (1984) discussed this observation within the context of apraxia of speech. The dysarthria clinician can demonstrate the differences between sounds and sound combinations that are highly visible and audible and those that are less so to make the dysarthric speaker aware of which sounds may result in the greatest amount of speech intelligibility and communicative effectiveness.

A second general characteristic of the phonological system is that shorter sequences are easier to understand than longer ones, probably because the shorter sequences place a lesser load on the working memory of the listener. The dysarthria clinician can encourage the patient to choose phonologically short phrases, underscoring the idea that both systems—phonological and grammatical—are involved in selecting a message to be communicated.

Primary-Level Pragmatics

Pragmatics involves the psychosocial uses of language and constitutes one of the most pervasive processes in communication. Pragmatic functions occur at both the primary and secondary level of language processing. At the primary level, pragmatics involves three functions: joint and mutual attending; initiating, maintaining, and shifting topics; and appropriate turn-taking.

Joint and mutual attending. It is imperative that the patient whose speech is difficult to understand use both verbal and nonverbal methods to signal joint and mutual attending. Joint attending involves sharing attention with another person during conversation. Nonverbal signals for joint attention include appropriate eye gaze (the listener watches the speaker much more frequently and closely than the speaker watches the listener), head nods, facial expression, body orientation, and other body gestures such as hand, arm, head, leg, and foot movements. The clinician can help dysarthric speakers develop a set of clear nonverbal signals to use to indicate they are engaging in joint attention.

Mutual attending occurs when conversants are engaged in observing some event, person, object, relationship, or attribute, or in participating in some event or process. Nonverbal means for mutual attending are similar to those required for joint attending, but the actual movements, expressions, orientations, and statements may be somewhat different. For instance, to indicate mutual attending conversants who are participating in some activity may need to engage in major shifts of body position, to signal to their partner, to use eye contact, or to employ specific statements to check understanding. When a speaker calls a listener's attention to an activity—for example, on the television screen or at a sports event—and that listener responds, they are participating in mutual attending. Often messages used in these situations are short: "Look here" and "Watch" are two examples.

Initiating, maintaining, and shifting topics. Topic initiation, maintenance, and shifting are critical to successful communication. To communicate a message effectively, the speaker must know how to engage a listener's attention. Listeners attend best when speakers introduce new topics in interesting and appropriate ways; when they maintain the topic through interesting, relevant, and appropriate comments; and when they shift topics appropriately. Discussing a new topic before introducing it, maintaining a topic beyond the listener's interest and attention level, and shifting topics abruptly all result in a communicative exchange that is in danger of deteriorating. The dysarthria clinician who introduces the rules of topic introduction, maintenance, and shifting can increase the chance that the patient's messages will be understood, which of course is imperative to being considered a desirable communication partner.

Turn-taking. Crucial to effective communicating is the ability to engage in appropriate turn-taking. Knowing how to get a turn, how to maintain a turn once it is obtained, and how to relinquish the turn appropriately is essential for successful communication in conversation. The ability to signal effectively is absolutely necessary for getting a turn, especially in a large conversational group. A person who wants a turn must signal this desire effectively to the person who is speaking. The signal used may be an eye gaze, a breathing pattern, a body movement, a gesture, or a verbal interjection. To be successful at getting a turn, the potential speaker often has to interject quickly, a feat that can be difficult for dysarthric patients—they may have to learn to become proficient at using nonverbal signals to get a turn in a conversation.

Maintaining a turn requires that the speaker produce relevant, interesting, and appropriate comments during a conversation. Maintenance must follow a timetable; that is, the speaker must maintain a turn for a certain amount of time, then relinquish it. Although there are no explicit guidelines, there seems to be an implicit definition of the optimum time interval for maintaining a conversation. Dysarthric speakers who are trying to increase their speech intelligibility by reducing their speaking rate may have to shorten their messages or alert their communication partners that they need a longer period of time to communicate than the partners might have anticipated.

Many a dysarthria clinician has advised many a dysarthric patient to slow down—by increasing the pause time between syllables and words—in order to increase speech intelligibility. Following this advice may create a problem for the dysarthric talker who is attempting to maintain a turn in conversation. Listeners may interpret the lengthened pause as an intention by the dysarthric talker to yield the turn in the conversation, and they may begin to speak while the dysarthric talker is pausing. The clinician can introduce nonverbal signals to use for communicating an unwillingness to relinquish a turn. Some signals that may be effective are a hand gesture that signals stop to the listener who begins to speak, or an exaggerated averting of eye gaze to indicate that the speaker is continuing to take his turn and is not yet ready to relinquish it.

Yorkston et al. (1988) offer suggestions on how to resolve a communication breakdown involving dysarthric persons. They encourage listeners to use gestures immediately to signal that the message has not been understood. This gives the dysarthric speaker a chance to decide whether to stop and repair the message or to continue with the expectation that added context will improve the communication. These authors also recommend that the patient be instructed either to repeat the misunderstood portion of the utterance, perhaps with elaboration, or to spell out the message slowly, letter by letter.

Hoskins (1987) developed an intervention program for adolescents structured around the primary-level pragmatic characteristics we have discussed. This program can be modified for use with various age groups. While a discussion of Hoskins' program is beyond the scope of this chapter, the interested clinician is encouraged to review Hoskins' work.

TOP-DOWN CHARACTERISTICS OF THE SECONDARY LEVEL OF LANGUAGE PROCESSING

There are three secondary-level processes of language: metalinguistic processing, secondary-level pragmatics, and discourse knowledge. A discussion of these language processes and their application to dysarthria therapy is provided in the next section.

Metalinguistic Processing

To be metalinguistic is to be able to reflect on language, its parts, and their functions and uses. The person with metalinguistic ability is cognizant of the various aspects of language—for example, an unfamiliar word, a humorous-sounding word, an unusual wording in a phrase, or a notable comment. Our description of the primary metalinguistic awarenesses will be from a top-down perspective, although from a metalinguistic vantage language can be considered from a top-down perspective, a bottom-up perspective, or a combination of the two.

Arbitrary relationship between words and referents. With few exceptions, words are related arbitrarily to the referents for which they stand. How things are called is largely a result of which peoples traded with each other as the language was being used. Often the names of things were determined by conquest: when a victor's language became dominant, words from the dominant language infiltrated the populace. As a result of this arbitrary relationship between words and referents, the referents have names that are understood only through convention.

Some words represent communications that are understood universally. *OK* is an example of universal agreement on a word to signify a certain meaning. Many dysarthria clinicians encourage their patients to communicate the message OK gesturally, by touching the tip of the index finger of one hand to the tip of the thumb on the same hand and pointing the remaining three fingers upward. Understanding that referents and words are separate entities allows the language user to employ synonyms and homonyms as well as verbal humor and figurative language forms.

Levels of meaning in language. Meaning exists on a variety of levels in language. For example, in every communicative interaction there is an underlying level of intent, and what is said may or may not directly signal that intent. In fact much underlying intent is communicated indirectly. In addition to the underlying level, there is a denotative, or literal, level of meaning in language, in which words stand for referents in an explicit and specific manner. Furthermore, in contrast to the denotative level, a connotative level of meaning exists through which the speaker can use a word to stand for a referent in a more associative or implied manner. Slang words typically have connotative meanings. One example, alluded to earlier in this chapter, is the word *dog*. Another example is the word *bad*, which can have either a negative connotation or a positive one, as when it is used to mean good. Also, there are figurative meanings beyond the merely connotative; examples are idioms, similes, and metaphors. To use figurative language effectively, both the speaker and the listener must know the relationship between the words used and the speaker's intended referents.

Verbal humor provides an example of how levels of meaning are used to communicate. In a riddle, for example, the listener is led into a certain set of circumstances, only to be confronted with a punch line that capitalizes on multiple meanings at the syntactic, lexical, or phonological level. For instance, in an old riddle the question is "When is a door not a door?" and the answer is "When it's ajar." The humor derived is based on the punch line, which capitalizes on the fact that, although they sound alike, the words *ajar* and *a jar* have different meanings. Another example of verbal humor is the pun. A friend, a visiting professor of anatomy from Cuba, once asked us to define the word *pun*. Knowing that he had visited the famous city in Nevada, we gave the following example:

Q. What do you get when you damage the 10th cranial nerve?
A. You get a Lost Vagus.

Our friend recognized the phonological similarities and laughed. Put another way, the verbal humor was understood by the listener because he had developed metalinguistic awareness of various levels of meaning in English. As with figurative language, users of language do not understand verbal humor unless they have developed this metalinguistic awareness of meanings.

Figurative language may carry a greater burden of inferential processing for a listener, and when it is combined with the degraded signal emitted by a dysarthric person it may well be incomprehensible. Thus the dysarthric person may do well to avoid or minimize figurative language, particularly when speaking with an unfamiliar interlocutor. Dysarthric patients should be counseled that the success or failure of their communication may depend on whether or not their listeners are familiar with various meanings of a word. This is especially important when the speaker is attempting to communicate with persons from a different background. Figure 4.1 illustrates the consequences that can occur when the listener does not know the alternative meanings of a word. The dysarthric patient who considers the listener's experience with the terminology to be used can avoid communication breakdown. We know of a dysarthric patient, a former bartender, who told his clinician that one ingredient to include when mixing a particular drink is "sparkling water." The startled clinician interpreted the message to be "talcum powder," partially because "sparkling water" was not a familiar term in the region where the conversation took place. The clinician explained this possible reason for the miscommunication to the surprised patient, who realized that his use of this unfamiliar term and its misinterpretation could have led to disastrous consequences.

Taking the listener's perspective. Although taking the listener's perspective can be considered a pragmatic function, once the speaker is conscious of the process it becomes a metalinguistic awareness. Being aware of the listener's perspective allows the speaker to manipulate language form, content, and function to accommodate the different needs of different listeners. Taking the listener's perspective allows the speaker to make good guesses about which language structures, content, and functions will result in successful communication with a particular listener. We will discuss the listener's perspective further in the section on secondary-level pragmatics.

Intervention. Metalinguistic awareness can increase communicative effectiveness. The patient who understands that words and referents are arbitrarily related may be able to choose words that the listener will understand. Furthermore, dysarthric speakers should be counseled that in situations in which they do not know their listener's education level or socioeconomic status, they should use common semantic and syntactic forms as well as phonological structures so that they can communicate with the highest degree of intelligibility. Taking the listener's perspective, the dysarthric speaker can alert the listener of the speech deficit, and ask for an agreement to violate underlying rules for com-

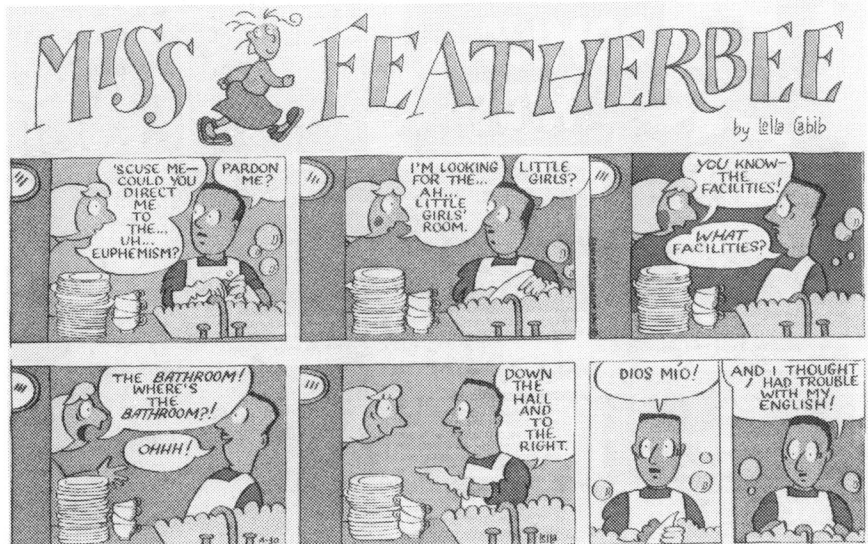

Figure 4.1 Miscommunication that can result from not knowing alternate meanings of a term.

munication such as extending speaking time in conversation. Finally, dysarthric speakers can provide cues about their communicative content; for example, they can alert their listeners when a humorous comment is forthcoming. Often these metalinguistic comments will determine whether or not a dysarthric speaker is an accepted partner in the conversation.

Dysarthria clinicians who would like additional information about intervention programs designed to develop metalinguistic knowledge are referred to the work of Wallach and Miller (1988) and the work of van Kleeck (1984a, 1984b). Much of the information reported in these publications is adaptable for use with the adult dysarthric person.

Secondary-Level Pragmatics

Most language users readily develop the primary-level pragmatic functions naturally; for most children these functions are acquired by 6 years of age. A secondary level of pragmatic functions develops throughout childhood and adolescence and is highly influenced by the social and cultural conventions of the linguistic community. As in the case of metalinguistic awareness, there are some general characteristics of secondary-level pragmatics.

Use of verbal and nonverbal behaviors to communicate intention. Part of being a successful communication partner involves the ability to use various verbal and nonverbal means to communicate underlying intention. For instance, to be clear and explicit a speaker will use semantic, syntactic, and phonological structures that state the intended message directly. The verbal message "Please close the window; I'm cold" may become clearer if accompanied by the nonverbal behaviors of shivering and rubbing the arms. An intention to tease can be communicated both verbally and nonverbally. For example, the speaker could announce:

> I'm going to tease you now. What do you mean, you can't go to the store in shorts! It's 100° in the shade and you can't go out wearing shorts because someone might see your legs.

These statements, when accompanied by exaggerated hand and body movements and an emphasis on appropriate syllables and words, will signify further that the speaker's intention is to tease.

Directness in communicating intention. Every linguistic community has indirect ways for communicating underlying intention. One indirect way of making imperative statements is using the polite form. For example, the polite request "Would you mind closing the window?" stands for "Close the window," and the polite statement "I don't mind if I do have another piece of cake" stands for "I want more cake." Idiomatic expressions provide another indirect way to communicate intention. The idiom "You're pulling my leg" to indicate that someone is teasing communicates the intended message only when the listener knows the meaning of the idiom.

Effective communication demands that speakers and listeners agree on the underlying meaning of the indirect communication. If the speaker uses an idiomatic expression that is unfamiliar to the listener, the message will not be communicated effectively unless the underlying intention is explained by the speaker. Indirect communication of intention is, by definition, more susceptible to communicative breakdown than direct communication just because it is indirect. Cultural conventions demand indirect communication of intention, however, and speakers who do not indirectly communicate underlying intention are noticed because they are not adhering to a cultural convention. There seems to be a trade-off between cultural acceptance and the probability that the communication will be effective.

Making assumptions about listeners. Speakers must make assumptions about what their listeners know in order to use the appropriate language form and content. In order to maximize the probability that a message is understood and interpreted accurately, speakers decide which words, sentence constructions, phonological sequences, and prosodic features to use, how much information to include, and how much background to provide. These decisions are based on the speaker's assumptions about such conditions and attributes of the listener as the following:

1. Listener's age, gender, and appearance (including hair color and style, clothing, and skin color)
2. Listener's speech and what it indicates (level of education and ethnicity or nationality and whether these are similar or different from those of the speaker)
3. Geographic location of the conversation
4. Speaker's perception of who functions as the authority in each communicative interaction

Adherence to and violation of community conventions for cooperating in communicating. In each linguistic community, speakers adhere to common conventions in order to communicate effectively. At the same time, speakers consistently violate the conventions in commonly agreed-upon ways, and such violation carries as much communicative information as does adherence. In fact, within each linguistic community there are institutionalized violations of the communicative conventions. Some understood rules for communicating cooperatively are: (1) tell the truth, (2) be brief, (3) be relevant, (4) be unambiguous, (5) ask only for information you want, and (6) give only information you believe is wanted.

One of the maxims associated with cooperativeness is to be informative. One way we express that information is new or important is through prosody. We use prosody to mark sarcasm, for example. If we say "You really look *terrific*" when we mean "You really look *terrible*," we are using prosody to mark and communicate meaning. Dysarthric persons who are also dysprosodic lose this ability, and this may be a reason for counseling patients to use alternative strategies for marking and conveying meaning.

Another aspect of prosody for expressing salient or new information is the use of intonation. Again, dysprosody might impede this function. If a listener does not know what part of a word to focus on, a message will be more difficult to interpret than it would be if the listener were aware of this important information. For a more complete discussion of how prosody can be utilized in the treatment of disordered speech motor control, see Chapter 9.

Many indirect means of communicating intentions also violate communicative conventions. For instance, the intention underlying the question "How are you?" spoken to a colleague at work on a Monday morning usually is to extend a simple greeting, not to obtain a comprehensive account of the state of the colleague's health. The question itself, then, violates the rule to ask only for information you want.

Intervention. Focusing on the secondary level of pragmatic functions may constitute a crucial part of clinical intervention. Knowledge of ways to manipulate language functions can increase the dysarthric patient's communicative ability. The dysarthria clinician can aid the patient in discriminating between direct statements of intent and indirect means of communicating, and in constructing examples of each. Rather than making assumptions about what listeners know, dysarthric speakers can practice asking communication partners for explicit information; with this information they can tailor their own remarks to be direct and explicit. The clinician can advise patients to reduce or eliminate low-frequency idiomatic expressions and metaphoric forms and to concentrate instead on direct, literal terms or frequently used idioms and metaphors that are understood by most speakers.

For a discussion of intervention for higher-level pragmatics with school-age children, see Wallach and Miller (1988). Also, Hoskins (1987) describes a general program that includes both primary- and secondary-level pragmatics that may be of interest to clinicians who are treating dysarthric patients.

Discourse Knowledge

Communication takes place in a variety of situations and contexts. Speakers and listeners have varying levels of familiarity and topics range from everyday to esoteric. The study of discourse processes and knowledge focuses on how speakers and listeners organize their communication in various types of conversations. These conversations differ with the context in which they take place. The type of discourse used in a coffee shop between good friends is different from the discourse used between teacher and students, and both are different from the type of discourse used in a corporate office between a middle-level manager and an upper-level executive. Not only does each of these conversations employ different types of discourse, but each type carries with it a separate set of rules and conventions for participating. We will discuss everyday and job-related discourses and their relevance to therapy of dysarthria.

Everyday discourse. Everyday discourse is the most frequent and familiar type of conversational form. Most people engage in everyday conversations without thinking about the rules and conventions underlying the utterances. Even though it is the most familiar conversational form for most people, however, everyday discourse is characterized by a variety of features that, if omitted or altered, significantly influence the understandability of a conversation. The primary characteristics of everyday conversations are the following:

1. Informal language and conversational style are familiar to participants, for example, "Hey, how's it going?" or "Wow, it was a super experience, you know?"
2. Participants share assumptions about experiences and knowledge upon which to base language content and context; therefore, there is no need to provide background.
3. Meaning is conveyed in the immediate, nonverbal context; therefore, there is no need for participants to explain terms or to use descriptors extensively to convey meaning.
4. Language use is specific to the immediate context. For example, "Hand it to me" or "Bring it here" can be understood easily because the desired object can be seen by both the listener and the speaker.
5. Turn-taking is relatively equal among participants according to cultural conventions.
6. There are frequent, ongoing checks for at-the-moment understanding; that is, participants frequently ask for confirmation that their messages were understood. Often the speaker accomplishes this by asking the listener questions such as "Do you understand?" or "Is that clear?"
7. Typically language structures are short and concise, for example, "I want one" or "Is it there?"

Job-related discourse. Conversing in a job setting may be a relatively formal and unfamiliar process for a new employee. The person must learn the vocabulary, topics, and context that form the bases for conversation in the work setting. Usually, once the new employee has become familiar with both the co-workers and the context within which conversations will occur, the employee can begin to engage in everyday conversations at work. Eventually beginning workers learn the new vocabulary, topics, and contexts well enough to participate in everyday discourse. Of course there can be situations in a job setting in which information must be conveyed in a more formal style. Or, depending on the employee's position, the employee may be required to use everyday discourse in combination with job-related discourse.

Intervention. Everyday conversation may be the easiest type of discourse for the dysarthric talker to engage in because of its familiarity, informality, and characteristically short structures. The clinician can inform the patient that it is easier to converse with partners who share the speaker's own experiences and knowledge than to talk with partners who do not share the same background. It is well known that communication is more effective when the dysarthric speaker's message can be anticipated, whether the message is delivered by speech, gesture, or an augmentative communicative device. The patient should be made aware that the success of the communication is, in a large measure, dependent upon the listener's ability to anticipate the patient's message, which, in turn, is dependent upon how much the listener knows about the patient. The patient should also be made aware that redundancy or providing background information also improves communication.

Dysarthric speakers who are planning to return to their previous work settings have probably already made the transition into everyday discourse in their job settings. It is likely that for them job-related discourse will be as familiar as everyday discourse. The dysarthric patient who must enter a new job situation, however, will be confronted with the conversational requirements of the new job. The clinician can make the patient aware of different types of discourse so that the patient will be better prepared to communicate in the new setting.

Determining familiarity. Clinicians can assist dysarthric patients in assessing familiarity with partners, topics, and contexts. Determining familiarity will enable the dysarthric speakers to predict if participating in a conversation would cause frustration. Dysarthric patients who have learned to judge familiarity can then concentrate on deciding the length and complexity of the linguistic structures necessary for participating in the conversation. In situations where it appears likely that their speech will not be intelligible enough for effective verbal communication, the patients can inform their conversation partners that they will be writing, typing, drawing, using a communication board, or communicating in whatever ways are most effective for them. Attending to the top-down characteristics of the discourse type in progress may enable the patients to avoid the frustration that can accompany unsuccessful attempts at communication in conversation. Dysarthric patients who are able to prevent frustration or failure in conversation have a level of control over the communicative interchange that they would not have achieved if they were unaware of how discourse functions. This control is especially important because patients who are able to exert some control in their communicative interactions can reduce much of the anxiety and stress that occurs when dysarthria interferes with their ability to produce intelligible speech.

CASE STUDY

The case study that follows illustrates how a top-down approach to dysarthria therapy was utilized. D. M., a 40-year-old bilingual Spanish- and English-speaking male, was admitted to the rehabilitation unit of a hospital in San Antonio, Texas. Eleven years prior to his admission, he had sustained a gunshot wound to the temporal-parietal lobe of his right cortex. Subsequently D. M. underwent a complicated course that included hematoma evacuation, tracheostomy placement, and multiple episodes of grand mal seizures.

D. M. was unemployed. For approximately 10 of his posttrauma years, he had lived in a nursing home. He was pleasant and cooperative, and he followed complex commands without flaw. Cranial nerve deficits included a mild central VIIth and an absent gag reflex. His gait was ataxic and he had a left hemiparesis. Oral mechanism exam revealed facial flaccidity, reduced range and mobility of the lips, severe lip weakness, reduced speed and mobility of the tongue, and chronic deviation of the tongue to the right with the tongue tip lodged in the right cheek. He did not move his tongue voluntarily.

The patient's speech was severely dysarthric. Disturbances in speech alternate motion rate (production and timing of the syllables /pa/, /ta/, and /ka/) were observed. Speech intelligibility as measured by the *Computerized Assessment of the Intelligibility of Dysarthric Speech* (CAIDS) (Yorkston, Beukelman, & Traynor, 1984) was judged to be an average of 0.9% (2 words out of a possible 220 words transcribed correctly by two judges). A disturbance in rhythm and stress was noted; often he produced two words as if they were one. For example, when repeating the sentence "Tie my shoe" he said, "Tiemy shoe" and when instructed to count to five he said, "Onetwo, threefour, five."

As noted previously, D. M.'s comprehension of verbal instructions was good. Reading comprehension of single words was within normal limits; however, his writing was not intelligible enough for consistent, clear communication.

To improve overall communication, we attempted rhythmic cuing using an alphabet board supplementation technique as described by Beukelman and Yorkston (1977), a metronome as described by Dworkin, Abkarian, and Johns (1988), and a pacing board as described by Helm (1979). None was effective. Instructing him to mark on a page, one stroke per spoken syllable, or to swing his arm from side to side while producing a syllable or a word with each swing was also ineffective. We tried many techniques to improve his speech, but the techniques we tried did not work. D. M.'s speech remained too unintelligible for effective communication.

D. M. could type using one finger of his right hand. He could write two-word sentences legibly enough to communicate the message. He could answer questions by indicating yes or no with appropriate head gestures, and often his verbalizations "yeah" or "no" were interpretable. Occasionally, when asked a question and given a choice of two words, he produced a response that could be understood by his listener.

With D. M.'s help we constructed a communication board consisting of printed words and symbols for communicating in everyday conversation. Among these words were "excuse me," "thank you," "nurse," "doctor," "more," "less," "A.M.," "P.M."

In order to expand his communication capabilities still further, we introduced drawing for communication as outlined by Lyon and Helm-Estabrooks (1987) for use with nonfluent aphasic patients. Figure 4.2 is an example of how, by drawing, he communicated about his favorite spectator sport.

We asked D. M. what he knew about communication and he wrote, "Many ways." It was then that we decided to try a top-down approach to dysarthria treatment.

We introduced D. M. to the idea of alerting his communication partners before beginning a conversation. Because he was bilingual—he communicated frequently in both English and Spanish—we suggested that D. M. alert his listeners as to which language he would be using. He could do so either by writing "English" or "Spanish" or by pointing to the appropriate word on his communication board. We also suggested that before he begin he inform his communication partners of the method he would be using for communicating, that is, whether he would be speaking, drawing, writing, using a communication board, or using a combination of methods. The words *drawing, speaking, writing, board,* and *all* were written on a card and he practiced pointing to the appropriate words before beginning a conversation.

D. M. demonstrated how he could use gestures for alerting his conversation partners that he wanted a turn in conversation. For example, at one time he raised his left hand and at another he used finger snapping.

We suggested that D. M. shorten his written messages, writing the name of an object or action rather than attempting sentences longer than two words. He found that when he did so he was able to communicate more effectively.

After 11 years of relative inactivity, D. M. was ready to return to work. Prior to his accident, he had worked in a tax preparation office and he was interested in returning to employment related to accounting. After being introduced to the concept of job-related discourse, he spent some time reviewing the terminology he had used in his previous work setting, thinking about how he would communicate those terms most effectively should he work in tax preparation again.

At the time of this writing, D. M. uses an electronic pocket computer on which he types short messages. During our first meeting after receiving the computer, he directed our attention to the LED display and typed, "I talk, again." D. M. is motivated to communicate as effectively as he can, and he has demonstrated that he can access a knowledge-driven

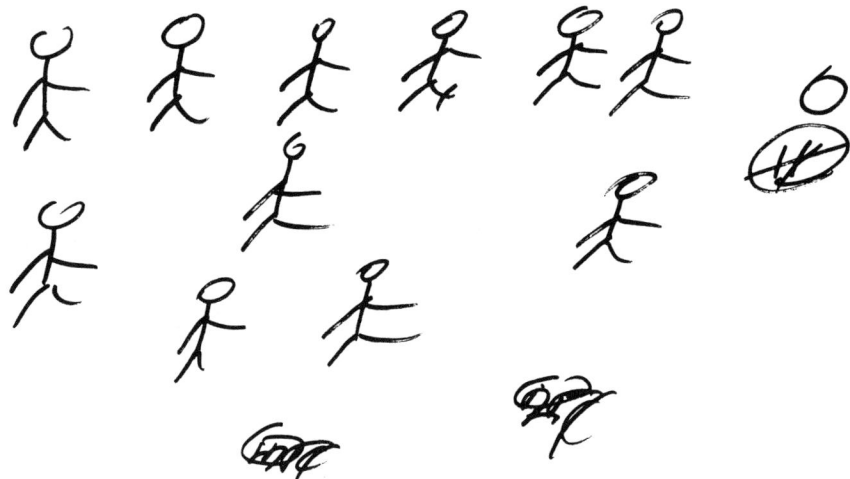

Figure 4.2 D. M.'s drawing to communicate his favorite spectator sport.

top-down approach to improve his communication. He is severely dysarthric and his speech may never be more intelligible than it is today, but we believe that his ability to communicate has improved as a result of his becoming aware of some of the characteristics of a top-down approach to treatment of dysarthria.

CONCLUSION

In this chapter we have taken the position that for optimum communicative effectiveness, it is essential to make the dysarthric patient aware of how language is communicated. That is not to say that we are discounting the importance of bottom-up learning in dysarthria therapy, of instrumental procedures, palatal lift fitting, bite-block construction and use, and additional behavioral therapies. Certainly we recognize that many techniques are basic to treatment of the dysarthric patient. Also, we acknowledge that at present our observations have not been substantiated by results of systematic investigation. On the other hand, we have observed that a top-down approach to treatment of dysarthric speech has therapeutic value and that it can provide the cognitive scaffolding for an effective communication experience for the dysarthric patient. We urge the dysarthria clinician to consider this approach with patients who demonstrate they can understand the characteristics and can use the approach effectively. Furthermore, we believe that a combination of bottom-up and top-down processing is analogous to normal interactive processing in which top-down and bottom-up information sources interact in ongoing communication, and therefore that this combination should be used to attempt to improve communication for the dysarthric patient.

We recognize also that the success of the dysarthric patient's ability to use top-down information may be compromised as a result of aging, dementia, and left hemisphere (aphasia) and right hemisphere dysfunction. To the extent that dysarthria is complicated by these co-occuring deficits, top-down approaches may be contraindicated or may require specific types of modification for certain patients. As research in this area has been neglected, we can offer no answers based on the results of systematic investigations, and can only hypothesize that compromising conditions, such as those listed above, will affect a patient's ability to benefit from a top-down approach. Our conclusions will have to await the results of studies of dysarthric patients in which the success of simultaneous verbal, gestural, and written communication is investigated.

REFERENCES

Beukelman, D. R., & Yorkston, K. M. (1977). A communication system for the severely dysarthric speaker with an intact language system. *Journal of Speech and Hearing Disorders, 42*, 265–270.

Burns, M. (1985). *Clinical management of right hemisphere dysfunction.* Gaithersburg, MD: Aspen Publishers.

Darley. F. L. (1984). Apraxia of speech: A neurogenic articulation disorder. In H. Winitz (Ed.), *For clinicians by clinicians: Vol. 1. Treating articulation disorders* (pp. 289–305). Austin, TX: PRO-ED.

Darley, F. L., Aronson, A. E., & Brown, J. R. (1969a). Differential diagnostic patterns of dysarthria. *Journal of Speech and Hearing Research, 12*, 246–269.

Darley, F. L., Aronson, A. E., & Brown, J. R. (1969b). Clusters of deviant speech dimensions in the dysarthrias. *Journal of Speech and Hearing Research, 12*, 462–469.

Darley, F. L., Aronson, A. E., & Brown, J. R. (1975). *Motor speech disorders.* Philadelphia: Saunders.

Davis, G. A. (1986). Pragmatics and treatment. In R. Chapey (Ed.), *Language intervention strategies in adult aphasia* (pp. 251–265). Baltimore, MD: Williams and Wilkins.

Davis, G. A., & Wilcox, M. J. (1985). *Adult aphasia rehabilitation.* Austin, TX: PRO-ED.

Deal, J. L., & Darley, F. L. (1972). The influence of linguistic and situational variables on phoneme accuracy in apraxia of speech. *Journal of Speech and Hearing Disorders, 15*, 639–653.

Dworkin, J. P. (1984). Specific characteristics and treatments of the dysarthrias. In H. Winitz (Ed.), *For clinicians by clinicians: Vol. 1. Treating articulation disorders* (pp. 263–288). Austin, TX: PRO-ED.

Dworkin, J. P. (1989, May). *Motor-speech disorders.* Paper presented at a workshop at Baylor College of Medicine, Houston.

Dworkin, J. P., Abkarian, G. G., & Johns, D. F. (1988). Apraxia of speech: The effectiveness of a treatment regimen. *Journal of Speech and Hearing Disorders, 53,* 280–294.

Helm, N. A. (1979). Management of palilalia with a pacing board. *Journal of Speech and Hearing Disorders, 44,* 350–353.

Hoskins, B. (1987). *Conversations.* Allen, TX: Developmental Learning Materials.

Lyon, J., & Helm-Estabrooks, N. A. (1987). Drawing: Its communicative significance for expressively restricted aphasic adults. *Topics in Language Disorders, 8*(1), 61–71.

Miller, L. (1988). *Components of language processing: An intervention model for academic success.* Paper presented at the annual meeting of the American Speech-Language-Hearing Association, Boston.

Netsell, R. A. (1986). *A neurobiologic view of speech production and the dysarthrias.* Austin, TX: PRO-ED.

Owens, R. E., Jr. (1988). *Language development: An introduction* (2nd ed.). Columbus, OH: Merrill Publishing.

Perkins, W. H. (1983). *Dysarthria and apraxia: Current therapy of communication disorders.* New York: Thieme-Stratton.

Rosenbek, J. C. (1984). Alternatives for the dysarthric adult: In H. Winitz (Ed.), *For clinicians by clinicians: Vol. 1. Treating articulation disorders* (pp. 249–262). Austin, TX: PRO-ED.

Rosenbek, J., & LaPointe, L. L. (1985). The dysarthrias. Description, diagnosis and treatment. In D. F. Johns (Ed.), *Clinical management of neurogenic communicative disorders* (pp. 97–152). Austin, TX: PRO-ED.

van Kleeck, A. (1984a). Metalinguistic skills: Cutting across spoken and written language and problem-solving abilities. In C. P. Wallach & K. G. Butler (Eds.), *Language learning disabilities in school-age children* (pp. 128–153). Baltimore, MD: Williams and Wilkins.

van Kleeck, A. (1984b). Assessment and intervention: Does "meta" matter? In G. P. Wallach & K. G. Butler (Eds.), *Language learning disabilities in school-age children* (pp. 179–198). Baltimore, MD: Williams and Wilkins.

Wallach, G. P., & Miller, L. (1988). *Language intervention and academic success.* Austin, TX: PRO-ED.

Wertz, R T. (1985). Neuropathologies of speech and language: An introduction to patient management. In D. F. Johns (Ed.), *Clinical management of neurogenic communicative disorders.* Austin, TX: PRO-ED.

Yorkston, K. M., Beukelman, D. R., & Bell, K. R. (1988). *Clinical management of dysarthric speakers.* Austin, TX: PRO-ED.

Yorkston, K. M., Beukelman, D. R., & Traynor, C. D. (1984). *Computerized assessment of intelligibility of dysarthric speech.* Austin, TX: PRO-ED.

CHAPTER 5

Pharmacologic Approaches to Speech Motor Disorders

David B. Rosenfield

> *Rosenfield discusses principles of pharmacologic therapeutics, basic aspects of pharmacology, and particular neurologic diseases that can compromise speech. He discusses various medications used to treat these disturbances, as well as their possible side effects.*

1. *List the major movement disorders discussed by Rosenfield and the drugs that can be used to treat these disorders. Name the side effects of each of these drugs. If some symptoms are reduced with the administration of a particular drug but other symptoms increase, what factors are important in deciding whether or not that medication should be continued?*
2. *Is it probable that a drug will be discovered that will cure stuttering? Discuss the different parts of the brain involved in speech production that might be involved in stuttering. Is the etiology of stuttering different for different people?*
3. *What are some of the diseases associated with spasmodic dysphonia? What pharmacologic therapies are efficacious for treatment of this disorder? Review arguments for and against the use of recurrent laryngeal nerve sectioning and botulinum toxin injections as treatment possibilities.*

It would be foolhardy to undertake a discussion of pharmacologic therapies of speech motor disturbances without first dispelling some misconceptions about this subject. First, there is the assumption that since these therapies exist, cures are available. Furthermore, there is the idea that speech motor disturbances have an underlying locus of breakdown that can be medicinally "fixed." Finally, there is the supposition that disturbances of nervous system motor output can themselves be fixed. None of these assumptions is true.

It is this conundrum of implausibilities that underlies this chapter. Add to this an awareness that speech-language pathologists do not prescribe medicine and that most graduate programs in speech-language pathology do not require students to learn pharmacology and the question becomes "Why include a chapter on neuropharmacology in a book for the speech-language clinician?" There are several answers.

First, many patients with movement disorders affecting speech are treated routinely with pharmacologic agents. Understanding the effects of such medications should enhance the speech-language pathologist's interaction with both patient and neurologist. Second, the fact that patients tend to see their speech-language pathologists more often than they see their physicians suggests that the informed clinician may participate more effectively in the monitoring of symptomatic changes or side effects that may be related to a particular pharmacologic regimen. Finally, there is growing interest in experimentation with pharmacologic trials for patients with "ideopathic" speech disorders such as spasmodic dysphonia or stuttering. Typically such patients are seen by speech-language pathologists but might not routinely be referred to a neurologist. It seems prudent to suggest that the practicing speech clinicians have a realistic appreciation of the current status of pharmacotherapies for these disorders and their limitations.

The employment of medication in treating a particular symptom is not simple. Different drugs can have different effects in different patients. Too often a patient may have a symptom that worsens with time. The physician may not know whether the symptom is worsening from the disease or from side effects of the drug that is being employed to treat the underlying ailment.

It is my personal experience that attentive speech-language pathologists can be of considerable assistance in providing health care. Doctors welcome personnel with the types of skills that they have. These skills come from experience, from being attuned to a particular presentation of symptoms, from knowledge pertaining to medications, and from a knowledge of pharmacology. The remainder of this chapter provides information in three broad categories. The first is a survey of fundamental concepts pertinent to an understanding of pharmacology in general. These concepts include principles of therapeutics, sources of drug information, and information regarding neurotransmitters. Second, the disorders of movement are treated somewhat extensively, including discussions of etiology, symptomatology, and the positive and negative effects of medication. These disorders characteristically involve neurochemical systems and frequently are managed by pharmacologic means. Collectively, movement-disordered patients comprise the largest population for whom pharmacologic approaches to speech motor control may be of interest. The final topic area involves pharmacologic issues relevant to other speech disturbances and includes discussions of normal speech motor control, stuttering, and spasmodic dysphonia. Throughout this chapter, frequent reference will be made to a variety of neuroanatomical structures. For a review of basic neuroanatomy, the reader is referred to Chapter 3.

FUNDAMENTAL CONCEPTS

Principles of Therapeutics

Well-designed and well-executed clinical trials exemplify the application of the scientific method to experimental therapeutics. Clinical trials form the basis for physicians' therapeutic decisions. In excellent summaries of the scientific requirements for clinical trials (Hill, 1960, 1962), it is agreed that the sine qua non of any clinical trial is its controls. There are many different types of controls, and one should understand that a controlled trial is not the same as a randomized double-blind trial. Although the randomized double-blind controlled trial is the most effective design for distributing variables between treatment and control groups, it is not always optimal or ethical. It is not always possible to employ this design to study disorders that are rare, or to study populations of patients that cannot, due to regulation or ethics or both, be studied, or to study treatment of patients with a uniformly fatal disorder (Hill, 1960, 1962).

Results of clinical trials of therapeutic agents may not generalize to use with all patients. This is because often patients selected for experimental drug trials do not have coexisting diseases, and usually such trials assess the efficacy of only one or two drugs rather than the many drugs that may be taken by a patient who is not in the study. Clinical trials usually are conducted over small periods of time and usually involve small numbers of patients. Compliance may be better controlled for patients participating in experimental trials than for those who are not. These factors lead to the following conclusions.

1. Even if the findings of a well-executed clinical trial of a drug are understood, a physician only can hypothesize about what effects that

drug will have on a particular patient. One cannot assume that what occurred in patients participating in the drug trial will also occur in other patients. Thus a physician uses the results of earlier clinical trials to establish an experiment for each patient. The physician must detect side effects and also must determine whether these effects truly are a result of the drug administered. Approximately one-half or more of both the useful and adverse effects of drugs that have not been recognized in initial formal trials are subsequently discovered and reported by practicing physicians (Ingelfinger, Mosteller, Thibodeau, & Ware, 1983).

2. If a drug does not produce its anticipated effect in one patient, it cannot be assumed that the effect cannot occur in that patient or in another patient. Many factors may contribute to a drug's lack of efficacy in an individual patient. Some of these factors are misdiagnosis, poor compliance by the patient with the regimen, improper dosage or dosage intervals, simultaneous development of another disease, use of other agents that interact with the primary drug to nullify or to alter its effects, undetected genetic or environmental variables that modify the disease or the pharmacological actions of the drug, and unknown therapy by another physician who is caring for the same patient. Even if the medication appears to be efficacious and without harm, a physician must not attribute uncritically all improvement to the therapeutic regimen chosen. Nor can a physician assume that a deteriorating condition reflects only the natural course of the disease.

3. Rational drug therapies are based upon critical observations. A physician, in effect, employs as scientific an approach in treating each individual patient as do researchers when formally investigating drugs.

Therapy itself is a science. All treatments of all patients should focus upon each patient as an individual. Individual patients can demonstrate wide variability of response to the same drug. The basic concepts that underlie these sources of variability include the prescribed dose, the administered dose, and the concentration of the medication at the locus of action. These three factors alter the intensity of the effect (Koch-Weser, 1972).

Patient noncompliance as well as possible medication errors can result in the prescribed dose differing from the actual dose taken by the patient. The administered dose will have varying effect upon the concentration of the medication at the intended locus of action. The amount of medication delivered to this locus of action depends upon the rate and degree of the drug's absorption, the patient's body size and composition, the distribution of the medicine in body fluids, the degree of chemical binding of the drug in plasma and tissues, and the rate of elimination from the body. The relationship between the concentration of the medicine at the locus of action to its intensity of effect upon the patient is altered by drug-receptor interactions, the overall functional state of the patient, and any placebo effects.

The relationship between the administered dose and the concentration of medication at the locus of action, as well as the relationship between the concentration of the medication at the locus of action to the intensity of the effect, is further acted upon by physiological variables, pathological factors, genetic factors, interaction with other drugs, and development of drug tolerance by the patient. Nothing mandates that any particular patient will have any particular response to any particular drug. There are multiple variables within each individual patient (Balashke, Nies, & Mamelok, 1985).

Sources of Drug Information

Textbooks on pharmacology and therapeutics, leading medical journals, drug compendia, professional seminars, meetings, and advertisements are all sources of drug information. *Goodman and Gillman's "The pharmacological basis of therapeutics"* (Gillman, Goodman, Rall, & Murad, 1985) is a good source of information on pharmacology and, although it may be intimidating due to its size, it is highly readable and extremely informative. Other sources of pharmacologic information are listed in the review by Balashke et al. (1985).

Another good source of information is an industry survey, the *Physician's Desk Reference (PDR)*. Brand-name manufacturers list various medications. There are no comparative data on product efficacy, safety, or cost. Descriptions of pharmacologic actions of medication are terse and highly technical. The information is virtually identical to that contained in drug package inserts. The *PDR* is not intended as a pharmacology text; rather, its primary value lies in its information concerning what indications for use of a drug have been approved by the Food and Drug Administration.

One problem with the *PDR* is that almost all possible side effects are listed. Thus when a patient has a particular symptom or sign and it is important to know whether a prescribed drug is causing it, the PDR often does not provide as much help as one would hope. If the complaint is not listed in the *PDR*, the likelihood is remote that the symptom or sign is due to the drug. However, if it is listed in the *PDR*, there is no guarantee that the clinical findings are attributable to the drug. I have found that the *PDR* often unintentionally frightens patients because of the myriad of side effects it lists. Some patients have been reluctant to take a much-needed medication after reading the *PDR*.

One useful aspect of the *PDR* is the picture section. The photographs of major drugs help patients to identify the drugs they are taking. It is for this reason that I recommend owning a copy of the *PDR*.

Another possible source of confusion when interpreting a patient's prescription is the dosage interval. These tend to be reported as abbreviations that may not be obvious. Some abbreviations and their definitions are provided in Table 5.1.

Neurotransmitters

It is the brain that underlies the neuromotor control system of speech, which involves respiratory movements, laryngeal neuromotor dynamics, and articulatory muscles. Medications aimed at treating particular diseases that affect this system affect alleged "chemical inequities." Certain chemicals called neurotransmitters are involved in translation of the neural impulse from the brain to the end organ, whether that end organ be respiratory muscle, laryngeal muscle, articulatory muscle, or other tissue. The complex role of neurotransmitters in the transmission of nerve impulses is elaborated in the next sections.

Cholinergic and adrenergic nerves. Peripheral nerves consist of motor (efferent) nerves that terminate in skeletal muscle (e.g., muscles in limbs). Motor fibers interact with muscles through the neuromuscular junction. These motor nerves are under voluntary control.

The nervous system can be divided into voluntary and nonvoluntary components. The nonvoluntary portion includes the autonomic nervous system which, in turn, includes the sympathetic and the parasympathetic nervous system.

TABLE 5.1
Abbreviations of Terms Associated with Dosages

Abbreviation	Term
ac (a.c.)	Before meals
Ad lib	As needed; as desired
alt. hor.	Every other hour
h.s.	At bedtime
NKA	No known allergies
NPO	Nothing by mouth
pc (p.c.)	After meals
Po, po	By mouth
PRN	As necessary
q.d.	Every day
q. (4) h.	Every 4 hours (number specified)
q.i.d.	Four times per day
q.o.d.	Every other day
t.i.d.	Three times per day

The terms *adrenergic* and *cholinergic* reflect the concept that chemicals transmit nerve impulses across the microscopic gap between nerve fibers and the structures they innervate. Epinephrine (adrenaline) and a closely related compound called norepinephrine (noradrenalin) are important neurotransmitters at peripheral (nonbrain, non–spinal cord) sympathetic, or adrenergic, terminations. Acetylcholine is generally associated with parasympathetic, or cholinergic, effects. However, acetylcholine is also an important neurotransmitter at some synapses in both sympathetic and parasympathetic pathways.

Impulses conducted by sympathetic, or adrenergic, nerve fibers usually elicit an active reaction in the effector structure, such as smooth (nonstriated) muscle (e.g., the muscle in the bowel) or glands. This is the reverse of parasympathetic, or cholinergic, fibers, which diminish these activities. Thus, stimulating sympathetic cardiac nerves increases heart rate whereas stimulation of parasympathetic cardiac nerves decreases heart rate. These effects, however, are not universal: adrenergic nerves slow gastric and intestinal movement motility whereas cholinergic nerves accelerate these movements. Likewise, sympathetic nerves cause the bladder wall to relax whereas the parasympathetic nerves cause bladder contraction.

In Table 5.2 the basic pharmacology of the autonomic nervous system is reviewed.

Activities of the agonists and antagonists are shown in Table 5.2. It should be understood that there is a finely tuned sympathetic and parasympathetic nervous system and that different receptors and end organs and nerve pathways serve different functions. A drug acting on one set of receptors may have effects on others. The system overall is in a fine balance.

Acetylcholine. Acetylcholine (ACh) is a chemical synthesized by a chemical reaction; that is, it is catalyzed by the enzyme choline acetyltransferase. This process is described by the following reaction:

$$\text{AcetylCoA} + \text{choline} \xrightleftharpoons{\text{enzyme}} \text{ACh} + \text{CoA}$$

As this reaction indicates, ACh is produced by certain chemicals that interact with one another. ACh can also be degraded back into those chemicals. Acetylcholine is found in parts of the autonomic nervous system, the brain (especially the basal ganglia), and the neuromuscular junction (Cooper, Bloom, & Roth, 1986).

The neuromuscular junction (motor end plate) is a specialized connection between an axon of a motor neuron and a somatic (striated) muscle fiber. The structure of the neuromuscular junction is such that an action potential (or neural impulse) in the motor axon produces

TABLE 5.2
Pharmacology of Autonomic Nervous System

	Sympathetic		Parasympathetic
	α-adrenergic Receptors	β-adrenergic Receptors	Muscarinic Cholinergic Receptors
Natural agonists			
Norepinephrine (released by sympathetic nerve endings)	+++	+	—
Epinephrine (released by adrenal medulla)	+	+++	—
Acetylcholine (released by parasympathetic nerve endings)	—	—	+++
Other (artificial) agonists	Methoxamine Phenylephrine	Isoproterenol Methoxyphenamine	Muscarine Pilocarpine Carbachol
Direct effects of agonists on:			
Heart	—	Increased rate and force of contraction	Decreased rate and force of contraction
Blood vessels	Vasoconstriction	Vasodilatation	Vasodilatation
Intestines	Decreased motility	Decreased motility	Increased motility
Antagonists (blocking agents)	Phentolamine Phenoxybenzamine Ergot alkaloids	Propranolol	Atropine Scopolamine

TABLE 5.2. Continued

	Sympathetic		Parasympathetic
	α-adrenergic Receptors	β-adrenergic Receptors	Muscarinic Cholinergic Receptors
Agents that block enzymatic degradation of transmitter	Monoamine Oxidase (MAO) inhibitors Catechol-O-Methyltransferase (COMT) inhibitors		Anticholinesterase

Note. Adapted from *The CIBA collection of medical illustrations:* Vol. 1. *Nervous System:* Part 1. Anatomy and Physiology (p. 90) by F. H. Netter, 1983, West Caldwell, NJ: CIBA Pharmaceutical Co. Copyright 1983 by CIBA-Geigy Corp. Adapted by permission.

synaptic depolarization of the muscle fiber, thus triggering a muscle action potential and, in turn, making the muscle contract (Cooper et al., 1986; Gillman, Goodman, Rall, & Murad, 1985).

Reviewing the pharmacology of the neuromuscular junction offers an example of certain basic concepts. The point to observe is not to note every chemical that alters acetylcholine activity. Rather, observe that there is a dynamic process involved in the synthesis, metabolism, release, and reuptake of this neurotransmitter. Different drugs affect this process and, as a result, can alter particular actions of the nervous system. All neurotransmitters—ACh and others—are synthesized and degraded, although each has its own independent chemical processes.

Pharmacological agents can affect transmission at the neuromuscular junction in three major ways. They can (1) alter the amount of ACh that the nerve impulse releases; (2) alter the response of the muscle cell membrane itself to the ACh that has been released; and (3) act upon the enzymes that degrade the ACh after it has been released. Some drugs have only one action, but many have more than one effect.

Five classes of drugs are described in Table 5.3. The choline uptake inhibitors decrease production of ACh in the nerve terminal by blocking the uptake of the choline molecules that are required in its synthesis. This results in decreased ACh synthesis, causing a reduction in the number of ACh molecules reaching the muscle. The net effect is a decrease in the number of muscle fibers activated per nerve impulse, resulting in a lessened strength of muscle contraction.

The ACh release blockers act on the motor nerve terminal by blocking the process through which a nerve impulse liberates ACh into the space between the nerve and muscle. The amount of ACh released may decrease to an amount insufficient to produce an electrical potential in the muscle fibers, thus causing severe weakness.

The ACh antagonists block the electrical depolarizing effect of the acetylcholine on the membrane. Drugs in this class are sometimes referred to as nicotinic antagonists, differentiating them from those blocking the action of ACh at autonomic endings (nicotine mimics the action of acetylcholine at the neuromuscular junction but not at autonomic endings). Many of these antagonists also have a weak depolarizing action on the muscle cells, but their major effect is blocking muscle activation by ACh, thus producing paralysis.

Cholinomimetics mimic the action of ACh, producing a strong, long-lasting muscle cell depolarization, making these cells less sensitive to the ACh subsequently released at the nerve terminal. This process is referred to as desensitization. Accommodation of the muscle cell membrane to the central depolarization eventually blocks muscle action potentials completely, causing paralysis.

Cholinesterase inhibitors decrease the chemical breakdown of ACh, normally achieved by enzymes called cholinesterases. ACh released by nerve impulse acts for a longer time on the muscle membrane, producing a larger end plate potential that results in muscle contraction.

Catecholamines. Catecholamines generically refer to a particular type of chemical, one containing a catechol nucleus (a benzine ring with two adjacent hytroxyl substituents) and an amine group. In practice, catecholamines usually imply dihydroxyphenylethylamine (dopamine, DA) and its metabolic products, norepinephrine (NE) and epinephrine (E).

Tyrosine, as are many other (aromatic) amino acids, is actively taken up into the central nervous system and converted to dihydroxyphenylalanine (dopa). This is the most important (rate-limiting) step in this biosynthetic pathway. Dopa is subsequently converted to dopamine (DA) which, in some nerve terminals, is converted to NE.

Dopamine is found in many areas in the brain. The major dopamine pathways are the nigrostriatal, mesolimbic, mesocortical, tuberoinfundibular, and hypothalamic pathways. There is a rich interconnection between cortex, subcortex, and brainstem cells, interacting through dopamine as well as other neurotransmitters. One of the most important pathways of dopamine, apparently involved in Parkinson's disease, is the projection from an area known as the substantia nigra, through the nigral striatal pathway, into the caudate and putamen (Cooper et al., 1986).

The central noradrenergic system (i.e., the noradrenergic system in the central nervous system, thereby excluding the peripheral nervous system) contains two major clusterings of norepinephrine cell bodies from which axons arise that will innervate targets throughout the entire neuraxis. This is the locus ceruleus, a compact cell group in the bottom part of the pons, and the lateral tegmental noradrenergic neurons, a more loosely scattered group of cells lying outside of the locus ceruleus (Cooper et al., 1986).

The central dopamine-containing systems are more complex in their organization than are the noradrenergic systems. There are many more dopamine cells. The number of dopamine cells in the midbrain alone has been estimated to be between 15,000 and 20,000 on each side, whereas the number of noradrenergic neurons in the entire brainstem is thought to be about 5,000 in each side. There are also several major dopamine-containing cells as well as specialized dopamine neurons that make extremely localized connections within the retina and olfactory bulb. Dopamine, too, has multiple connections throughout the neuraxis (Cooper et al., 1986).

Serotonin. Since the mid-19th century, scientists have been aware that a substance found in the serum of patients can cause powerful contrac-

TABLE 5.3
Pharmacology of Neuromuscular Junction

Drug	Effect on Supply of Acetylcholine in Terminal	Effect on Amount of Acetylcholine Released in Terminal by Action Potential	Effect of Amplitude on End Plate Potential	Effect of Muscle Response to Application of Acetylcholine	Direct Effect of Muscle Membrane Resting Potential	Clinical Effect
Choline uptake inhibitors						
Hemicholinium Triethylcholine	Decreased	Decreased (smaller quanta)	Decreased	—	—	Weakness
Acetylcholine release blockers						
Botulinum toxin Low CA^{++} or high Mg^{++}	—	Decreased (fewer quanta)	Decreased			Paralysis (low Ca^{++} concentration may also produce tetany by direct action on nerves)
Acetylcholine (nicotinic) antagonists						
D-tubocurarine (curare)	—	—	Decreased	Decreased	Depolarized (in high dosage)	Paralysis
Cholinomimetics						
Nicotine Carbamylcholine Succinylcholine	—	—	Decreased (by desensitization)	Decreased (by desensitization)	Strongly depolarized	Paralysis

TABLE 5.3. Continued

Drug	Effect on Supply of Acetylcholine in Terminal	Effect on Amount of Acetylcholine Released in Terminal by Action Potential	Effect of Amplitude on End Plate Potential	Effect of Muscle Response to Application of Acetylcholine	Direct Effect of Muscle Membrane Resting Potential	Clinical Effect
Cholinesterase inhibitors						
Physostigmine	—	—			Depolarized slightly in high doses	Muscle power and duration of contraction increased
Neostigmine						
Edrophonium						
Organophosphorous compounds (nerve gases)	—	—	Increased; prolonged	Increased; prolonged	No change	Convulsions

Note. Adapted from The CIBA collection of medical illustrations: Vol. 1. Nervous System: Part 1. Anatomy and Physiology (p. 219) by F. H. Netter, 1983, West Caldwell, NJ: CIBA Pharmaceutical Co. Copyright 1983 by CIBA-Geigy Corp. Adapted by permission.

tion of smooth muscle organs. This substance, serotonin (5-hydroxytryptamine, 5-HT), has a basic chemical structure underlying it known as an indole. The indole nature of serotonin bears much resemblance to the psychedelic drug LSD, as well as to many other agents that alter mentation. Many of the serotonin pathways originate in the brainstem, primarily in midline nuclei. They go to the cortex and subcortical tissue, and have other brainstem connections as well. Serotonin is very important in behavior as well as in other brain functions.

In summary, the brain is a conundrum of different pathways and so-called centers, many of these pathways and centers having particular activities but none acting alone without influence from other centers and other pathways. Together, they enable the brain to program movement as well as other functions. As already noted, medications that allegedly affect one area of the brain sometimes (intentionally or unintentionally) affect other areas. For the reader who is interested in pursuing pharmacology further, and who requires more information about major and minor pathways, an excellent source is Cooper, Bloom, and Roth (1986).

DISORDERS OF MOVEMENT

Extrapyramidal diseases are a group of motor disorders associated with disease in the basal ganglia. From a clinical standpoint, these diseases consist of one or a combination of the following signs: (*a*) abnormal involuntary movements, (*b*) altered skeletal muscle tone, (*c*) a decrease or increase in movement, and (*d*) alteration of automatic associated movements.

The involuntary movements seen in extrapyramidal diseases are without purpose. They can be patterned or nonpatterned, predictable or unpredictable, and repetitive or nonrepetitive. The most frequently encountered clinical entities are Parkinson's disease, chorea, dystonia, athetosis, and hemiballismus. Although there are terms that designate these various clinical entities, a thorough understanding of the etiology of these disorders does not exist. Any one of these disorders may result from a wide variety of different types of central nervous system pathology.

Anatomy of the Extrapyramidal Motor System

The extrapyramidal system usually refers to gray matter structures lying deep within the cerebral hemispheres, although other areas also may be involved. Its function is predominantly motor in nature. The extrapyramidal structures are very richly interconnected, and include the basal ganglia. The basal ganglia consist of the caudate nucleus, putamen, globus pallidus, and several brainstem structures, including the subthalamic nucleus, the substantia nigra, and portions of the reticular formation. The caudate and putamen together are referred to as the corpus striatum (or neostriatum). The putamen and globus pallidus together are known as the lenticular (lenslike) nucleus (Gilman & Winans, 1982).

Extrapyramidal disorders are characterized either by too much (hyperkinetic) movement or too little (hypokinetic) movement.

Hyperkinesia

Hyperkinesias include tremor, chorea, ballismus, dystonia, and athetosis. Tremor is the nonpurposeful, rhythmic, patterned to-and-fro oscillation produced by contractions of antagonistic and agonistic muscles. There are many types of regular tremors: physiologic, metabolic (enhanced physiologic), tremor at rest, benign essential tremor, intention (cerebellar) tremor, and rubral tremor (Koller 1984; McDowell & Cedarbaum, 1988).

Tremor may be classified further as to whether it occurs at rest (resting tremor), during sustained posture of an extremity (postural tremor), or during intentional acts (action or intention tremor). The "pill rolling" tremor of Parkinson's disease is the prototype of resting tremor, usually decreasing substantially with voluntary activity of the affected limb. Essential, intention, and rubral tremors are exacerbated by and occur only during movement.

Physiologic tremor is fast (8–12 cycles per second compared to Parkinson tremor, which is 3–7 cycles per second) and has a low amplitude. It is usually observed in circumstances of fatigue, fear, or emotional stress. Physiologic tremor is often prominent in the extremities, is induced by sustained posture, is a natural phenomenon, and has little pathologic significance.

Hyperthyroidism, emotional stress, and certain medications—steroids and beta-adrenergic agonist medications—can increase the amplitude of physiologic tremor. Hyperthyroidism can cause a fine, rapid tremor (10–20 cycles per second), especially in the hands. This tremor often is confused with physiologic tremor.

A slower and coarser tremor is observed in patients with a metabolic disturbance such as electrolyte imbalance, withdrawal from alcohol, withdrawal from various drugs, or liver, kidney, or lung disease. Intention tremor, present upon intentional activity, is often seen in cerebellar disease. It is especially prominent when many joints are involved in movements, such as pointing a fully extended arm to an object. Patients with extrapyramidal diseases often have tremor at rest, but the tremor may also have an intentional component. Intentional tremor may be hereditary and familial.

Rubral tremor is a rotatory tremor of the upper portions of the extremities due to a disturbed outflow of impulses from the cerebellum. This tremor usually involves the superior cerebellar peduncle, known as the brachium conjunctivum, usually in an area of the midbrain near the red nucleus.

Tics. Tics are rapid, stereotyped, repetitive involuntary movements resembling fragments of normal motor acts. As opposed to chorea, tics seldom interfere with ongoing movement and can be suppressed by the patient for variable periods of time (McDowell & Cedarbaum, 1988).

Chorea. Chorea (Greek for "dance") varies greatly, depending upon the severity, the site, and the distribution of the underlying brain disturbance. Variability is the cardinal rule; a particular movement is rarely repeated. Choreic movement may be generally distributed all over the body or may be confined to a restricted part of the body. Usually, however, chorea is observed in the face or in outstretched hands. The movements last from approximately 1/10 to 1 second. Those movements involving larger joints appear to be more rapid than those in the fingers and toes. Although dependent upon the severity, voluntary action is often compromised because of the incoordination of the afflicted muscles. When requested to protrude the tongue, the patient with chorea may properly carry out all anticipatory movements but may be very slow in thrusting the tongue forward and may have difficulty maintaining protrusion. Rapid successive movements and intentional acts are impaired (McDowell & Cedarbaum, 1988).

Ballismus. *Ballismus* comes from the Greek word meaning "jumping about," and refers to violent flinging, flailing, or flipping limb movements. *Hemiballismus* refers to ballismus in one-half of the body. Usually ballismus resembles chorea and is sometimes classified as an extremely violent chorea (McDowell & Cedarbaum, 1988).

Dystonia. Dystonic movements are characterized by slow, long, sustained, powerful, nonpatterned contorting movements of the axial (trunk, neck) and appendicular (hand, foot) muscles as well as slow, sustained contractions in the platysma (superficial neck muscles), shoulder, and pectoral (chest) muscles. The muscles of the neck, trunk, and upper portions of the extremities are involved most commonly. Involvement may be generalized (dystonia musculorum deformans) or confined to a restricted region such as the neck, face, or tongue (Fahn, 1984).

Athetosis. Athetotic movements appear phenomenologically as a mixture of chorea and dystonia. In fact, some authorities deny the existence of athetosis as a separate entity.

Athetotic movements are irregular, nonpatterned, and slow. They are frequently described as writhing, cramplike, and spasmodic, and often consist of single movements lacking prompt initiation, smooth continuity of excursion, and smooth termination. Athetotic movements occur when antagonistic muscles contract simultaneously; the resultant movement is caused by differences in the power of the various opposing muscles (McDowell & Cedarbaum, 1988).

Hypokinesia

Akinesia refers to the absence of, and hypokinesia (bradykinesia) refers to a decrease in, the initiation, implementation, and ease of execution of automatic and volitional movement. When muscle is at rest, it has a particular tone that represents activity provided by the brain, the spinal cord, and the nerves. Too little tone usually means damage to the neurons or the nerves that are supplying the muscle. Two types of increased muscle tone encountered clinically are rigidity and spasticity. Rigidity involves simultaneous agonist and antagonist muscle activity; spasticity involves only one. If an extremity is rigid, passive movement encounters resistance in flexion as well as in extension. In contrast, resistance to passive movement in a spastic extremity is encountered only in the direction opposite the pull of the muscles with the increased tone. Spastic resistance is not uniform throughout the range of motion; there is increasing opposition up to a point, at which time the resistance suddenly gives, resulting in what is referred to as the "clasped-knife" phenomenon (Gilman & Winans, 1982; McDowell & Cedarbaum, 1988).

Rigidity of the upper extremity usually involves flexors and extensors (i.e., the pro-gravity and the antigravity muscles), whereas spasticity usually involves only the leg extensors and arm flexors. Increased stretch reflexes (hyperreflexia) accompany spasticity but are not observed with rigidity. Basal ganglia diseases and extrapyramidal disorders frequently cause rigidity. In most patients, bradykinesia, or hypokinesia, is a result of rigidity, although sometimes spasticity plays a role (McDowell & Cedarbaum, 1988; Gilman & Winans, 1982).

Bradykinesia can impair voluntary activity, causing the patient to initiate movements slowly. The patient may freeze upon initiating voluntary acts. This becomes especially evident during walking. Despite good strength, normal fist closure lacks the synergic dorsiflexion of the hand and impairs overall function. In writing, the patient begins well but makes the letters increasingly smaller and often freezes and stops. There is usually limitation of quick successive movements such as rapid skilled finger and foot movements (McDowell & Cedarbaum, 1988).

Hyperkinetic Movement Disorders

Dystonia. Dystonia can occur by itself or in association with other complex involuntary movements, and can be classified according to whether an etiology for the disorder is known, as well as according to hereditary pattern, age of onset, and region of the body afflicted. Usually, in the primary dystonias no underlying pathology or radiologic changes are found. In secondary or symptomatic dystonias, there is a variety of central nervous system disorders. These disorders include trauma (perinatal brain injury, head trauma), focal intracranial pathology (stroke, tumor, or arteriovenous malformation), infection, and metabolic disturbance (Wilson's disease, Hallervorden-Spatz syndrome, hexosaminidase deficiency, lipidoses, gangliosidoses). Other causes of secondary dystonia include toxins such as manganese and various medications (McDowell & Cedarbaum, 1988; Fahn, 1984; Fahn, 1988; Fahn, Marsden, & Calne, 1988; Marsden, 1988; Calne & Lang, 1988).

Focal dystonias appear to represent only a fragment of the dystonic process. They usually begin during adulthood. The most common forms of focal dystonias include torticollis (wry neck), writer's cramp, typist's cramp, musician's cramp, and Meige's syndrome. Meige's syndrome refers to oromandibular dystonias with blepharospasm (involuntary eye closure). This disorder may begin with blepharospasm or spasms and contractions of the muscles of the mouth, jaw, pharynx, and tongue (oromandibular dystonia). Meige's syndrome usually begins between the fourth and the eighth decade, most often in the sixth decade of life. Symptoms are often triggered by bright light, stress, or attempts to read. Some patients wear dark glasses to reduce photic stimulation. As the disorder progresses, eye closure becomes more prolonged and many patients become functionally blind. Spasmodic dysphonia or grunting noises can appear often in this syndrome (Fahn, 1984; McDowell & Cedarbaum, 1988).

Dystonias probably represent a combination of dopaminergic and cholinergic overactivity within the basal ganglia. Their therapy, unfortunately often unrewarding, employs dopamine receptor antagonists and anticholinergic drugs; these drugs will be discussed later.

Chorea. Table 5.4 provides the classification of chorea. Degenerative (Huntington's) chorea is inherited as an autosomal dominant disease with complete penetrance. This means there is a 50% chance that each offspring of a person with Huntington's will inherit the disease. Huntington's disease has different clinical characteristics and different ages of onset, depending upon the sex of the transmitting parent. Brains of patients who have died from Huntington's disease reveal a significant change in the levels of some neurotransmitters. The most striking change is the reduction in the level of gamma-aminobutyric acid and

TABLE 5.4
Classification of Chorea

Degenerative
　Huntington's chorea
　Senile chorea

Metabolic
　Hepatolenticular degeneration (Wilson's disease)
　Choreoacanthocytosis

Acute infectious
　Rheumatic (Sydenham's chorea)
　Diphtheria
　Rubella
　Pertussis
　Encephalitis

Vascular
　Systemic lupus erythematosus, Henoch-Schönlein purpura, basal ganglia infarction (caudate nucleus or subthalamic nucleus)

Endocrine
　Thyrotoxicosis, chorea gravidarum

Drug-induced chorea
　Neuroleptics, anticonvulsants (phenytoin, carbamazepine), oral contraceptives, levodopa and other dopamine agonists, antiemetics (promethazine, metoclopramide)

Paroxysmal
　Paroxysmal dystonic choreoathetosis

Miscellaneous
　Basal ganglia neoplasms
　Subdural hematoma

Note. Adapted from "The Extrapyramidal System and Disorders of Movement" by Fletcher H. McDowell and Jesse M. Cedarbaum, 1988, in *Clinical Neurology*, Vol. 3 (p. 50), edited by Robert J. Joynt, Philadelphia; J. B. Lippincott. Copyright 1988 by J. B. Lippincott. Adapted by permission.

its synthesizing enzyme, glutamic acid decarboxylase (McDowell & Cedarbaum, 1988).

The clinical onset of degenerative chorea is insidious. Some patients complain of abnormal movements whereas others complain of emotional disturbances. Still others complain of intellectual compromise. Often there is a combination of these manifestations. There may be a history of an insidious onset of restlessness, progressive clumsiness, and general diminution of motor proficiency. The patient or the patient's family may notice involuntary facial grimaces, twitching of the fingers, or movements of the arms. Dysarthria can be an early symptom. Speech may become severely impaired by the choreoathetotic movements of the tongue, lips, larynx, palate, pharynx, diaphragm, and chest. Facial expression may be contorted and there may be continuous sucking, grimacing, and lip-smacking movements. Examination reveals abnormal choreic movements that may often be demonstrated by asking the patient to hold hands or feet outstretched.

There is no specific treatment for Huntington's disease. Choreic movements can be reduced with reserpine, haloperidol, or tetrabenazine. Reserpine also has a calming effect on the aggressive behavior of some Huntington's patients, but it usually has less effect than haloperidol. Haloperidol in doses of 1 mg to 10 mg per day lessens the choreic movements. The dosage is gradually increased from a minimal amount (1 mg per day) until symptoms are relieved. Tetrabenazine is still an experimental drug in the United States; most physicians do not have access to it. Sometimes baclofen is used because of its GABA-like action in inhibiting glutamate. Any of these medications may reduce chorea-induced dysarthria, but their effect is often minimal (McDowell & Cedarbaum, 1988).

Drug-induced chorea. Limb chorea in combination with athetoid movements of the head, face, mouth, and neck may be the result of long-term administration of phenothiazines, butyrophenones, and other medications. Choreiform movements are most likely to occur with the use of phenothiazines such as prochlorperazine, perphenazine, fluphenazine, and triflupromazine. Phenothiazine-induced choreiform movements are most common in young people receiving high doses of these drugs for acute schizophrenia and in elderly females. In 25% of the patients who have developed choreiform movements while taking phenothiazines, these movements have become permanent and may be labeled tardive dyskinesia (McDowell & Cedarbaum, 1988).

Choreiform movements have been noted in many patients with Parkinson's disease who have been treated with levodopa. The occurrence of these movements is dose-related. The dose at which the movements appear varies widely, but tends to be low in patients with a longer duration of disease. In most instances reported, these movements have stopped with lower doses or on discontinuation of the medication (McDowell & Cedarbaum, 1988).

Tic disorders. As already noted, tics are repetitive, stereotyped involuntary motor acts that resemble normal patterns of muscle movement. They usually do not interfere with voluntary skilled motor performance. They are often volitionally suppressible for long periods of time. They should not be confused with the lightninglike jerks of a single muscle or group of muscles occurring as myoclonus, or from the distal twitch-like movement of chorea (McDowell & Cedarbaum, 1988).

The most notorious of all tic disorders is Gilles de la Tourette syndrome. This is a chronic but fluctuating disorder that begins early in life. Onset in adult life is rare. The major symptoms of this disorder are multiple motor and vocal tics. Tourette syndrome begins between ages 2 and 15 years, the median age of onset being 7 years. Ninety-three percent of the patients are symptomatic by age 11. This syndrome is often misdiagnosed, a median 10-year interval being present between onset of symptoms and establishment of diagnosis. Unlike acute simple tics of childhood, there is a male-to-female ratio of 3:1. In 37% of the patients, tics begin in the head and face. In 8%, the disorder begins with vocal tics. Seventy-five percent of the patients have vocal tics characterized by grunting or barking noises; 62% by squeaks or shrieks; 59% by sniffing or snorting; and 22% by repetitive dysfluencies. Coprolalia, or involuntary swearing, occurs in 60% of the patients. In addition to simple tics, 73% of the patients have complicated movements, consisting of touching, hitting, jumping, skipping, squatting, or echopraxia (McDowell & Cedarbaum, 1988).

The tics in Tourette's syndrome, as in other movement disorders, decrease during distraction, disappear during sleep, and increase with tension or anxiety. Unlike other involuntary movements, patients can voluntarily suppress their tics for variable periods of time (Butler, 1984).

Haloperidol is frequently used to treat Tourette's syndrome. Other dopamine antagonist drugs have also been employed. The major side effects of haloperidol include bradykinesia, restlessness, and sedation. Tardive dyskinesia has rarely been reported in patients receiving neuroleptics for treatment of Tourette's syndrome. Clonidine has been reported to be useful. However, some studies have not been able to corroborate its effectiveness. Recently, the more highly specific dopamine antagonist pimozide has been used (McDowell & Cedarbaum, 1988).

Tremor. Essential tremor is characterized by involuntary rhythmic movements of the head, face, jaw, tongue, arms, hands, and, rarely, the legs. It can also involve laryngeal muscles. It can begin at any time but usually begins in adult life, commonly around the age of 50. It is a gradually progressive disorder, but remissions for long periods of time have been reported. Many patients note that alcohol reduces their tremor (McDowell & Cedarbaum, 1988; Rosenfield, 1988c).

Propranolol, 10 mg 3 to 4 times a day, increasing up to 320 mg per day in divided doses, is usually effective for decreasing tremor. The dose should be increased from a small starting dose until tremor or adverse effects, such as bradycardia (slowed heart rate, less than 60 beats per minute), hypotension, dizziness, or fatigue supervene. Propranolol should not be given to patients with known congestive heart failure, bronchospasm, or diabetes. Sometimes propranolol causes sedation, depression, and delirium, so that patients may prefer not to use it. Other effective medications include primidone (Mysoline), beginning at 50 mg 3 times per day and then gradually increasing the dose until the tremor is reduced or disappears (Koller, 1984; McDowell & Cedarbaum, 1988).

Hyperkinetic drug-induced movement disorders. Many pharmacologic agents can produce extrapyramidal symptoms resembling naturally occurring movement disorders. These symptoms may result from the effects of blocking some of the brain's dopamine receptors, but this is not certain. Drug-induced hyperkinetic syndromes (tardive dyskinesias) as well as hypokinetic syndromes have been described.

The most common drug-induced movement disorder is parkinsonism, which will be more fully discussed in the next section. Paradoxically, drugs that cause parkinsonism, a hypokinetic movement disorder, can also cause hyperkinetic disorders. Drug-induced hyperkinesias can present as dystonia or chorea. Treatment is difficult and, unfortunately, often unsuccessful.

Acute dystonic reactions may occur within minutes after patients receive a dopamine-blocking agent. Many of the antipsychotic drugs have dopamine-blocking capabilities. Movements may consist of forced upward ocular deviation or other orofacial dystonias. Anticholinergic therapy or antihistamines may be effective.

Tardive dyskinesia is an increasing problem. These involuntary movements consist of orobuccolingual masticatory movements, with tongue thrusting, grimacing, chewing, and blepharospasm the most common. These oral movements may be associated with choreiform movements of the hands and feet, as well as dystonic postures or laryngeal-pharyngeal dystonic spasms. Tardive dyskinesia occurs in 25% of patients treated with neuroleptic medications. The disorder usually begins several weeks to months after treatment with the offending medication. Fifty percent of the patients are asymptomatic within 6 months after discontinuing the offending drug. The incidence of remission decreases with increasing patient age. Whether the combination of anticholinergic and neuroleptic medications increases the predisposition toward development of tardive dyskinesia has been questioned. It is postulated that tardive dyskinesia results from supersensitivity of postsynaptic dopamine receptors in the striatum or from overactivity of presynaptic dopamine neurons induced by a dopamine receptor antagonist (Goetz & Klawans, 1984; McDowell & Cedarbaum, 1988).

It is not known why this condition persists after medication has been discontinued. All known dopamine-receptor blocking agents, including antiemitics, prochlorperazine, and metoclopromide, can cause tardive dyskinesia. Many drugs not known to affect dopamine transmission or dopaminergic receptors can produce choreiform dyskinesias, which usually remit after the medication is stopped. These agents include phenytoin (Dilantin), carbamazepine (Tegretol), and, rarely, anticholinergic medications (Goetz & Klawans, 1984; McDowell & Cedarbaum, 1988).

The initial treatment for tardive dyskinesia is to reduce or to eliminate the offending agent. Often this is not possible because of the severity of the underlying psychiatric condition. When dyskinetic symptoms persist or when continuing the offending medication is necessary, treatment of the movement disorder is usually very difficult. Increasing the dose of the neuroleptic drug often masks the symptoms, but this usually exacerbates the underlying pathologic factor. Treatment with presynaptic dopamine-depleting agents (e.g., reserpine) is beneficial in approximately 65% of the patients. Depression is a side effect sometimes. Baclofen and amantadine have been employed also (Goetz & Klawans, 1984; McDowell & Cedarbaum, 1988).

Hypokinetic Movement Disorders

Parkinson's disease. Parkinson's disease—sometimes known as parkinsonism or Parkinson's syndrome—consists of tremor, rigidity, postural changes, and a decrease in spontaneous movement. This syndrome can be associated with several pathologic processes that can damage the extrapyramidal system (Table 5.5).

Parkinson's disease usually develops insidiously and progresses slowly. Usually patients cannot tell exactly when the symptoms began. Bradykinesia and rigidity may not occur in the limbs and trunk only, but can appear in speech also. Patients complain that their voices lack volume and force and that they "run out of steam" when they talk for long periods. Some speak in whispers. Articulation may be impaired. Speech is often monotonous with rapid staccato quality. It is as though patients' speech, handwriting, and other motor activities are affected by the same phenomenon that causes the freezing of their gait.

Frequently, early symptoms of Parkinson's disease are unilateral tremor and alteration in facial expression. In early Parkinson's disease, patients may have only a mild unilateral tremor that decreases with activity and decreased arm swing on the same side as the tremor. The tongue may not be weak, but it may have a rapid tremor.

Treatment: Anticholinergics. The earliest effective treatment for parkinsonism was a tincture of belladonna, discovered by Charcot. Belladonna and its derivatives have anticholinergic activity. A variety of related anticholinergic compounds since have been synthesized and employed in treating parkinsonism. The exact mechanism of action in these compounds in relieving the symptoms of parkinsonism is not known. Researchers question whether dopamine inhibits and acetylcho-

TABLE 5.5
Classification of Parkinsonism

Primary	Secondary	Pseudoparkinsonism
Idiopathic	Metabolic	"Arteriosclerotic"
Parkinsonism plus	Wilson's disease	"Normal-pressure" hydrocephalus
Olivopontocerebellar degeneration	Chronic nonwilsonian hepato-cerebral degeneration	Mass lesions (tumor, subdural hematoma)
Shy-Drager syndrome	Hallervoorden-Spatz syndrome	Tremor syndromes
Striatonigral degeneration	Infectious	
Guamanian parkinsonism-ALS-dementia complex	Acute, postencephalitic	
Azorian motor system degeneration	Toxic	
Progressive supranuclear palsy	Irreversible	
	Carbon monoxide	
	Carbon disulfide	
	Manganese	
	Meperidine analogs (MPTP)	
	Reversible	
	Reserpine	
	Phenothiazine	
	Butyrophenone	
	Neuroleptics	
	Antiemetics	
	Metoclopramide	
	Alpha-methyldopa	

Note. Adapted from "The Extrapyramidal System and Disorders of Movement" by Fletcher H. McDowell and Jesse M. Cedarbaum, 1988, in *Clinical Neurology*, Vol. 3 (p. 18), edited by Robert J. Joynt, Philadelphia: J. B. Lippincott. Copyright 1988 by J. B. Lippincott. Adapted by permission.

line excites the individual cells in the neostriatum (McDowell & Cedarbaum, 1988).

Diminished dopamine activity in Parkinson's disease renders the excitatory effects of acetylcholine more prominent. Before levodopa, anticholinergic agents were often employed alone for therapy in Parkinson's disease. These agents are still useful in some patients, especially when tremor occurs.

Anticholinergic agents rarely produce more than 20% improvement. Despite continued use of these drugs, the symptoms and signs of parkinsonism progress. Sudden discontinuation of them can cause a marked increase in symptoms. The side effects of anticholinergic agents include dry mouth, aggravation of glaucoma, blurred vision, constipation, urinary retention, and psychiatric side effects (delirium, impaired memory, disorientation, anxiety, agitation, and hallucinations).

The most commonly used anticholinergic medications are trihexyphenidyl hydrochloride (Artane), benztropine mesylate (Cogentin), and ethopropazine (Parsidol). The usual starting doses are as indicated in Table 5.6, but patients can have a wide variation of response. Dosages, initially small, are increased until improvement occurs or side effects prevent further increase (see Table 5.6).

Certain antihistamines, such as diphenhydramine (Benadryl), have anticholinergic side effects and are sometimes helpful if patients cannot tolerate more potent anticholinergics. Antihistamines may cause sedation.

Anticholinergic drugs may help patients who are taking levodopa. Some patients deteriorate markedly if anticholinergics are withdrawn suddenly. Thus, if discontinued, the dose should be reduced gradually.

Treatment: Levodopa and Decarboxylase Inhibitors. Following the discovery of striatal dopamine depletion in patients with parkinsonism, many investigators began treating patients with dihydroxyphenylalanine (dopa) in an effort to replace brain dopamine. Dihydroxyphenylalanine was used instead of dopamine because dopamine does not cross the blood-brain barrier. Only a particular form of dopa, the levorotatory isomer (L-dopa on levodopa) is effective.

L-dopa greatly decreases hypokinesia and bradykinesia. Postural instability may resist improvement. Some patients become more alert and mental functioning improves after beginning levodopa.

Levodopa treatment is initiated with a small dose that is gradually increased until maximum benefit is achieved or until intolerable side effects occur. These side effects include dyskinesias, loss of efficacy, fluctuations in response, confusion, hallucinations, and drop in blood pressure upon standing (orthostasis hypotension).

Eighty percent of the patients develop dyskinesia at some time during levodopa treatment. These abnormal movements are dose-related

TABLE 5.6
Dosages and Side Effects of Commonly Used Drugs

Drug	Dose Range	Major Side Effects
Acetazolamide (Diamox)	215–1,000 mg/day	Numbness of extremities, appetite loss, frequent urination, drowsiness, confusion
Amantadine (Symmetrel)	100–200 mg/day	Depression, hallucinations, ankle swelling, skin lesions
Anticholinergics		Dry mouth, constipation, urinary retention, aggravation of glaucoma, impaired memory, hallucinations, confusion
Trihexyphenidyl (Artane)	2–20 mg/day	
Procyclidine (Kemadrin)	5–40 mg/day	
Benztropine mesylate (Cogentin)	0.5–7 mg/day	
Biperiden (Akineton)	2–6 mg/day	
Ethopropazine (Parsidol)	50–400 mg/day	
Antidepressants		Dry mouth, blurred vision, sleepiness
Amitriptyline (Elavil, Endep)	25–150 mg/day	
Imipramine (Tofranil)	25–150 mg/day	
Antihistamines		Dry mouth, constipation, urinary retention, aggravation of glaucoma, impaired memory, hallucinations, confusion
Diphenhydramine (Benadryl)	50–150 mg/day	
Orphenadrine (Disipal)	50–300 mg/day	
Carbamazepine (Tegretol)	200–1,200 mg/day	Dizziness, drowsiness, blurred vision, nausea, skin rashes, disturbances in bone marrow production
Clonazepam (Klonopin)	1.5–20 mg/day	Drowsiness, clumsiness, behavior changes, tremor, hair loss, hairiness, appetite loss

TABLE 5.6. Continued

Drug	Dose Range	Major Side Effects
Diphenylhydantoin (Dilantin)	300–500 mg/day	Clumsiness, insomnia, motor twitching, nausea, rash, gum overgrowth, hairiness
Dopamine agonists Bromocriptine (Parlodel)	2.5–100 mg/day	Mental disturbances, nightmares, agitation, hallucinations, paranoid delusions, angina, impotence, skin changes, spasm of arteries
Dopamine precursors Levodopa Levodopa/carbidopa (Sinemet)	2,000–6,000 mg/day 75/300 mg–250/2,500 mg/day	Dyskinesias, dystonias, unpleasant dreams, hallucinations, mental confusion
Ethosuximide (Zarontin)	500 mg–1.5 g/day	Appetite loss, nausea, drowsiness, headache, dizziness
Haloperidol (Haldol)	Varies considerably	Restlessness, tremor, bradykinesia, sedation, dry mouth
Phenobarbital	60–240 mg/day	Drowsiness, irritability, hyperactivity
Primidone (Mysoline)	250–1,000 mg/day	Clumsiness, vertigo, loss of appetite, fatigue, irritability
Propranolol (Inderal)	40–320 mg/day	Slow heart rate, confusion, fatigue, low blood pressure, dizziness
Valproate (Depakene)	1,750–3,000 mg/day	Upset stomach, altered bleeding time, liver toxicity

side effects and can be relieved by decreasing the dose, but the movements may reappear. Often some dyskinetic movement has to be accepted by the patient as the price of levodopa's therapeutic effect.

Reduced blood pressure (orhtostatic hypotension) can occur in 25% of the patients early in the course of treatment with levodopa alone. It is rarely symptomatic and usually disappears as treatment continues. Palpitations and cardiac arrhythmias occur in approximately 10% of the patients.

Abnormal behavior appears in approximately one-fifth of the patients early in treatment. This is more common in older patients, those with severe Parkinson's disease, and those with dementia. The most prominent of these abnormalities is delirium with episodes of confusion, agitation, disorientation, and visual hallucination. The episodes are often related to excessive intake of the antiparkinsonian medication, as well as other prescribed drugs such as sedatives, antidepressants, anticholinergic agents, and tranquilizers. Delirium can be precipitated by infection, fever, dehydration, electrolyte imbalance, and frequently by exposing the patient to a new or strange environment. Episodes of delirium seldom occur in nondemented patients. Visual hallucinations are common in patients receiving levodopa but are not threatening to the patient. These mental abnormalities are usually reversed by lowering the dose of levodopa or by eliminating concomitant medications, especially anticholinergics and sedatives (McDowell & Cedarbaum, 1988).

If a Parkinson's patient develops impaired mental status, it is important to determine whether this is due to medication side effects. All medications used to treat the Parkinson's disease can compromise cognition, but the ones most likely to do this are the anticholinergic agents. These medications should be decreased or discontinued in patients with altered mental status and patients should be observed for difficulty in their thinking (McDowell & Cedarbaum, 1988).

Hallucinations are a common problem for patients who are becoming demented. Dopa, dopamine agonists, and anticholinergic medications can all cause hallucinations, and each should be reduced systematically to determine which contributes to the symptom. Some patients continue to hallucinate while off the medication. Families usually prefer an immobile clearheaded member to one who is mobile but grossly confused.

Loss of intellectual function increases with time and is not recovered until levodopa is discontinued. Effective daily doses of levodopa average 4 gm per day, but some patients require as much as 16 gm. Currently, levodopa alone rarely is used for treatment of Parkinson's disease except in the case of an unusual patient who develops an allergic reaction to carbidopa-levodopa tablets or who suffers severe dyskinesia or orthostatic hypotension when using the drugs in combination.

Inhibiting the extracerebral metabolism of levodopa to dopamine is important in the treatment of Parkinson's disease. Drugs accomplish this by inhibiting dopa-decarboxylase, the enzyme that metabolizes levodopa into dopamine. These drugs do not pass the blood-brain barrier. The net effect is a larger amount of unmetabolized levodopa available for transport into the brain, where conversion to dopamine occurs. Thus the total dose of dopa required is lowered and peripheral side effects, due to increased dopamine outside the brain, are markedly reduced. Some adverse effects of levodopa (dyskinesia, agitated confusion, hallucinations) may be more prevalent and more serious when decarboxylase inhibitors are used, because these side effects are directly related to the amount of dopa entering the brain. The dopa-decarboxylase inhibitor used in the United States is alpha-methyldopa hydrazine (carbidopa).

Carbidopa combined in a tablet with levodopa (Sinemet) is marketed in three strengths: 10/100 mg, 25/100 mg, and 25/250 mg. Initial dosage is usually one-half to one 25/100 tablet 3 times per day. The dose is slowly increased until maximum benefit is obtained, which usually requires a minimum total dose of 75 mg to 100 mg of carbidopa and 750 mg to 1,000 mg of levodopa.

Patients initially placed on levodopa and then switched to decarboxylase inhibitors with dopa often feel better and have improved appetites. Changing from regular dopa to combinations of levodopa with decarboxylase inhibitors is accomplished by reducing the overall levodopa dose by 75% and by giving the remaining amount in divided doses with carbidopa (McDowell & Cedarbaum, 1988).

The side effects of decarboxylase inhibitors with levodopa are identical to those of levodopa alone. No specific ill effects have been attributed solely to these or decarboxylase inhibitors.

Improvement using dopa alone usually begins to appear at a dosage of 1.5 gm to 2.5 gm per day or with 100 mg to 400 mg of levodopa with the decarboxylase inhibitor. Improvement is manifested first as a subjective increase in liveliness or ease of movement. Maximal improvement may not occur until the patient has taken a steady dose of levodopa or the levodopa-decarboxylase inhibitor for several weeks.

With few exceptions, levodopa and levodopa with decarboxylase inhibitors can be taken concomitantly with drugs used to treat other illnesses. The combination of levodopa with monoamine oxidase inhibitors (used in treating depression) can cause hypertension. Phenothiazines and reserpine tend to counteract the effect of levodopa. Pyridoxine, found in most vitamin preparations, can interfere with the action of levodopa, but large supplements have to be ingested to produce this action. Vitamin preparations containing large amounts of pyridoxine should be avoided. Since decarboxylase inhibitors act by blocking the binding of pyridoxal phosphate (related to pyridoxine) to decarboxylase enzymes, patients taking the combination need not avoid pyridoxine.

The pharmacokinetics of levodopa are complex and may be altered by its chronic use. There are on-off signs as well as wearing-off signs. Some patients have sudden fluctuations between mobility and immobility; this is known as the on-off phenomenon. Patients who have marked fluctuations, or even mild fluctuations, should report this to their physicians. Levodopa is most effective in the first 2 to 5 years of treatment. Later, as the disease progresses, the benefits provided lessen. This is known as the wearing-off effect.

Treatment: Amantadine. Amantadine (Symmetrel) is an antiviral agent that also helps relieve symptoms of parkinsonism. The mechanism of action is unknown, but it appears to act by releasing dopamine from striatal neurons. Most of the drug is not metabolized; 90% of it passes from the body into the urine. Thus the drug should be used cautiously in patients with kidney disease. Amantadine is recommended for Parkinson patients with mild disease who have not received levodopa.

A dose of 100 mg 2 to 3 times daily produces rapid benefit, usually within a day, but efficacy diminishes in some patients after several weeks. Amantadine is effective in approximately 60% of the patients and partially relieves rigidity, akinesia, and to a lesser extent tremor. Side effects, which are seldom troublesome, include nervousness, insomnia, confusion, hallucinations, dry mouth, nausea, ankle edema, and skin lesions.

Some patients may not respond to amantadine, but the drug should be taken for 10–14 days before assuming that it is ineffective. Amantadine and anticholinergics, when used at the same time, can adversely affect mental function (McDowell & Cedarbaum, 1988).

Treatment: Bromocriptine. Bromocriptine (Parlodel) mimics the action of dopamine. It can relieve akinesia, rigidity, and tremor in many Parkinson patients. It has less antiparkinsonism effect than levodopa used alone, but may cause less abnormal involuntary movement. It also has a longer duration of action. Nausea and orthostatic hypotension may occur early in treatment, but this is usually avoided by increasing the dosage slowly.

Major disadvantages of bromocriptine, especially in high doses (more than 30 mg a day), are mental disturbance, nightmares, agitation, hallucinations, and paranoid delusions. The latter are more common in older patients. Angina pectoris (chest pain due to lack of appropriate blood supply to the heart), sexual impotence, swelling and redness of the lower extremities, and arterial spasm in the hands and feet causing pain and weakness are rare but have been reported.

The best results of bromocriptine occur early in the treatment, when the drug is used with Sinemet. Low doses of bromocriptine (less than 30 mg a day) combined with Sinemet can ameliorate the wearing-off and on-off effects that sometimes results from prolonged use of levodopa. When bromocriptine is given concurrently, levodopa can be given in lower doses (less than 1,000 mg per day), thus causing fewer dyskinesias and dystonias. However, the toxicity of levodopa and bromocriptine may be additive. This is especially true of their adverse mental effects.

Adjunctive drugs in Parkinson's disease. Depression often accompanies Parkinson's disease. Tricyclic antidepressants such as trazodone (Desyrel) or fluoxetine (Prozac) may be useful. Monoamine oxidase inhibitors used for depression can cause marked swings in blood pressure in patients taking levodopa. Propranolol (Inderal) and other similar medications (known as beta-adrenergic blockers) are useful for decreasing action tremor that may accompany the resting tremor of Parkinson's disease.

Parkinsonism-plus syndromes. Parkinsonian symptoms are sometimes the presenting features of parkinsonism-plus syndromes. These neurologic conditions are distinguished clinically from idiopathic Parkinson's disease by the presence of associated signs and symptoms that occur together in various combinations. These signs and symptoms include impaired eye movements; spinocerebellar, corticospinal, and autonomic nervous system dysfunction; motor neuronal degeneration; peripheral neuropathy; and dementia.

The most common of these syndromes is progressive supranuclear palsy (PSP), also known as Steele-Richardson-Olszewski syndrome. Usually the patient's first complaint is difficulty with posture. Gait is slow. There may be axial rigidity and extension of head and neck. Disturbed eye motility usually is present; loss of downward gaze is common, followed by loss of upward gaze. Levodopa may be effective for some patients. Occasionally bromocriptine is helpful (McDowell & Cedarbaum, 1988).

The family of multiple systems degeneration constitutes another group of parkinsonism-plus syndromes. Multiple systems degenerations have three major subgroups: those with predominant cerebellar features (olivopontocerebellar degeneration), those with predominant autonomic features (Shy-Drager's syndrome) such as orthostatic hypotension without associated rise in pulse, and those in which drug-resistant parkinsonism is the major clinical finding.

Other parkinsonian syndromes. The symptoms and signs of postencephalitic parkinsonism are similar to the idiopathic form, but the former usually have more autonomic dysfunction and may have more seborrhea (oily skin), sialorrhea (salivation), and hyperhidrosis (increased perspiration). Blepharospasm (frequent and tight closing of the eyelids) may be prominent.

Many pharmacological agents can cause movement disorders. The disorders appear to result from the actions these drugs have on dopamine receptors, but this is not certain. Hyperkinetic as well as hypokinetic syndromes can occur.

The most common drug-induced movement disorder is parkinsonism. Parkinsonism can be produced by drugs that deplete the brain of dopamine, interfere with its synthesis and release, block dopamine receptors, or destroy dopaminergic neurons. Reserpine and tetrabenazine deplete the brain of biogenic amines including dopamine. Phenothiazine (e.g., Thorazine), thiothixene (e.g., Navane), and butyrophenone (e.g., Haldol) neuroleptics owe their therapeutic efficacy to the blocking of dopamine receptors. Further, antiemetic (antinausea) preparations such as prochlorperazine (Compazine) and metoclopramide (Reglan) may cause parkinsonism.

The clinical syndrome of drug-induced parkinsonism is similar to that of the idiopathic form of the disease, but postural reflexes are less likely to be disturbed in drug-induced parkinsonism and tremor is often prominent. This syndrome is usually reversible upon withdrawal of the offending medication.

The "treatment" for drug-induced parkinsonism is prevention. Rest, using as small a dose as possible of the potentially offending medication, and avoiding use of the stronger parkinsonism-producing agents—especially in the elderly who may have limited dopaminergic reserve—is best. If drug-induced parkinsonism cannot be avoided, small doses of anticholinergic medication such as trihexyphenidyl (2 mg to 6 mg per day) or benztropine (0.5 mg to 2 mg per day) or amantadine (100 mg to 200 mg per day) are useful (Goetz & Klawans, 1984; McDowell & Cedarbaum, 1988).

Any disturbance that causes an increased movement of respiratory muscles, laryngeal muscles, or supralaryngeal articulators can interfere with speech (Darley, Aronson, & Brown, 1975; Hartman & Abbs, 1988). Likewise, any medication that decreases the movement of these muscles can compromise speech. Any of the movement disorders can cause speech compromise. The data pertaining to this realm are continually increasing, as an increasing number of physicians and speech-language pathologists investigate speech motor disturbances.

When a patient presents with speech symptoms or other disturbances, medications are directed at treating the underlying disease state. Thus a patient who has a known, diagnosed essential tremor, for example, might be prescribed a beta blocker, whereas a Parkinson's patient might be prescribed a parkinsonian medication. The drug therapy will address the underlying disease state and hopefully will decrease or eliminate the symptoms. Problems arise when there are a presenting speech symptom and associated nonspeech signs and the symptoms are not recognized. In my experience, this frequently is the case of patients with spasmodic dysphonia. Many of these patients have focal dystonia or essential tremor (Rosenfield, 1988b).

An example of speech problems without nonspeech signs or symptoms is dysfunction of the neuromuscular junction. Patients with myasthenia gravis have weak muscles because an appropriate amount of acetylcholine does not reach the muscle receptors at the neuromuscular junction. There are different classifications of myasthenia gravis. Some individuals have only double vision or droopy eyelids, while others are so weak that they cannot breathe. Often myasthenic patients— whatever their symptoms—improve with rest, which may be as short as 2 to 3 minutes (Rosenfield & Barroso, 1989). The characteristics of speech disturbance due to myasthenia gravis may be poor volume, slurred speech, and hypernasality. As patients continue to talk, they may become short of breath and increasingly hypernasal.

The diagnosis of myasthenia gravis is not always simple—it involves multiple medical and electrical tests. When myasthenia gravis is suspected, the physician should be consulted as soon as possible, especially if the patient complains of shortness of breath. Anticholinesterase medication, such as pyridostigmine bromide (Mestinon), provides an increased amount of acetylicholine at the neuromuscular junction. Worsening of speech can result if the patient is either on too little or too much medication. Patients with myasthenia gravis should be followed carefully and should be treated by a physician who has experience with this disease.

SPEECH MOTOR CONTROL

Normal Speech Motor Output

As previously stated, when a patient takes a drug the drug does not go only to one particular spot in the brain. Rather, the drug can affect various cerebral sites as well as areas outside the brain, causing behaviors that may or may not be anticipated. Many of these cerebral sites can be involved in production of speech. If one is to discuss the realm of speech motor dysfunction further, however, one needs to understand how it is that speech is produced. Our understanding is far from complete. The ensuing discussion pertains only to speech motor output, not aphasia (an acquired disturbance of language).

Mammalian vocalization involves appropriate coordination between respiration, laryngeal activity, and articulatory movements. The lower motor neurons that control the respiratory movements reside in the anterior portion of the cervical, thoracic, and upper lumbar spinal cord. Motor neurons controlling laryngeal closure reside in the nucleus ambiguous, located in the lower part of the brainstem. Neurons directly responsible for articulatory control are the trigeminal motor nucleus, facial nucleus, rostral portion of the nucleus ambiguous, hypoglossal nucleus, and the anterior horn cells of the rostral portion of the cervical spinal cord. This wide array of neural tissue extends from the pons to the lower part of the spinal cord (Jürgens & Ploog, 1981).

Considerable evidence supports the thesis that there is bilateral cortical bulbar input to the periaqueductal gray, an area located in the middle part of the midbrain (the midbrain is the upper part of the brainstem, located above the pons which, in turn, is above the medulla). There is also major input from the limbic system, a part of the brain that has a strong role in emotions. It is important to note that there are multiple inputs to the lower motor neurons involved with speech motor output. Thus, compromising cortex, subcortex, basal ganglia, thalamus, and multiple areas of the brainstem can independently alter speech. The above-noted compromise can result from lesions (e.g., tumor, stroke, or infection), but can also result from medications affecting these areas (Jürgens & Ploog, 1981; Rosenfield & Barroso, 1991).

Stuttering

There are very cogent arguments that stutterers have a neurophysiologic predisposition toward stuttering, resulting in speech motor dynamic disturbance. No singular psychiatric theory can explain the fact that the prevalence of stuttering has not decreased (Porfert & Rosenfield, 1978); stuttered dysfluencies are not random; there are genetically determined patterns of inheritance for stuttering; and particular fluency-evoking maneuvers (e.g., singing, speaking with loud broad-band noise, speaking during inhalation) eliminate stuttering behaviors. Further, there is no evidence that stuttering has ever been cured by psychiatric intervention (Rosenfield, 1984; Rosenfield & Boller, 1985; Rosenfield & Nudelman, 1987).

Stutterers do talk. Stutterers have some fluent output, just as fluent speakers have some dysfluent output. Stress alters the degree and frequency of dysfluent output, as it alters the motor output of all individuals with underlying motor control disturbances. This affect-sensitivity reminds us that speech output is a highly delicate motor coordinative task. Just as emotional stress can exacerbate a parkinsonian tremor or an underlying dystonic disturbance, so can it alter stuttered dysfluencies.

It is in this context that the pharmacotherapy of stuttering is discussed. The degree of emotional stress sometimes can be curtailed through psychotherapy, biofeedback, or pharmacotherapy. Phamacotherapies that might be effective in treating stuttering are alprazolam (Xanax) and other tranquilizers. Xanax might be most effective for reducing speech anxiety in that it can decrease some of the autonomic nervous system responses, such as increased heart rate. For example, if a student who stutters has to give a book report in class and has a rapid heartbeat, that heartbeat itself might cause the student to be more dysfluent. Xanax might lessen some of the student's anxiety. It should be stated, however, that no control studies have been conducted with results that support this thesis. There could be a strong placebo effect.

The usual dosage of Xanax is 0.75 mg to 1.5 mg daily, taken orally. The drug is one of the benzodiazepine derivatives. Other benzodiazepines include chlordiazepoxide (Librium), oxazepam (Serax), diazepam (Valium), and clorazepate (Tranxene). In general, the clinical toxicity of these drugs is low, although they can cause drowsiness and unsteadiness, and there can be physical dependence and withdrawal symptoms.

There have been several investigations pertaining to pharmacotherapies for stuttering. Bloodstein (1987) reviews many of these, but none of the drugs studied has proved unequivocally effective. Several years ago, some schizophrenics who stuttered were treated with the antidopamine medication haloperidol. While taking this medication, they stuttered less. This observation led to multiple studies in which stutterers were given dopamine-blocking agents such as haloperidol to determine whether dysfluencies decreased. The results were inconclusive. It may be that the patients on haloperidol who had fewer dysfluencies following medication were somewhat somnolent or slightly fatigued while on the medication, in effect causing them to speak more slowly. Slowed speech is a well-known therapy technique that decreases dysfluencies independently of pharmacologic agents (Rosenberger, Wheelden, & Kalotkin, 1976; Rosenberger, 1980; Bloodstein, 1987).

To explore further the possible relationship of haloperidol and stuttering, Rosenfield, Freeman, and Jankovic (1983) reasoned that if haloperidol truly reduces stuttering, the effect presumably results from the blocking by haloperidol of CNS dopamine receptors. They questioned whether stutterers who had lost dopamine might actually become more fluent. That is, they reasoned that if stutterers developed Parkinson's disease—which is associated with dopamine depletion in parts of the brain—perhaps their speech would improve.

Rosenfield and colleagues reviewed a large series of stutterers who subsequent to stuttering developed Parkinson's disease. They could not ascertain whether or not their speech improved. In some instances, when speech did improve, it may have been because slowing of speech resulted from the Parkinson's disease itself. It is well known that many Parkinson's patients develop dysfluencies as a result of the disease and that these dysfluencies are different from those of developmental stutterers (Canter, 1971; Deal & Cannito, this volume). Regardless, they were not able to document any improvement in stuttering behavior during the course of treatment for Parkinson's disease.

Personally, I have prescribed different pharmacologic agents for stuttering, thinking that these drugs might be effective in controlling stuttering. These were not prescribed as part of double-blind controlled studies. The stutterers could have had a marked placebo overlay, and all patients were told that there was no guarantee that the medication would control their stuttering, although a pharmacologic rationale for administering the drug did exist. In this context, each of the following drugs was prescribed for five stuttering patients: carbamazepine (Tegretol), diphenylhydantoin (Dilantin), clonidine (Catapres), and propranolol (Inderal). In a noncontrolled environment with an admittedly high placebo predisposition, none of these patients reported any improvement in answering the telephone, addressing large audiences, introducing themselves, or doing anything else of speech-related importance. Finally, to this author's knowledge, there have been no substantiated reports of Dilantin curing stuttering. There have been some reports of improved speech output under Dilantin, but these have never been substantiated (Bloodstein, 1987).

Hays (1987) wrote a letter stating that bethanechol may help stuttering. Another letter (Goldstein, 1987) contended that carbamazepine helps stutterers. A subsequent letter by Rosenfield (1988a) discussed the efficacy of this drug for stuttering.

Stuttering is so variable that it is difficult to be certain whether a stutterer is better one day or the next, one week or the next, and so on. In this setting, double-blind studies with qualified people evaluating the speech output become imperative.

At the present time, there is no indication for pharmacologic therapy in stuttering. In all likelihood, no singular curative drug will be found, since many individuals stutter for different reasons and possibly each one stutters for different reasons at different times. However, there may be a subclass of stutterers who could benefit from the appropriate medications.

Spasmodic Dysphonia

Spasmodic dysphonia (SD) is a chronic phonatory disorder of unknown etiology that usually appears in adulthood. The speech of SD patients is characterized by choppy breaks in phonation, staccatolike catches, a strained-strangled voice quality, and monopitch. Phonation in SD patients is often accompanied by effortful, jerky strained sounds that are frequently associated with pain in the laryngeal area.

Interruptions of phonatory airflow in SD presumably result from the intermittent hyperadduction of the vocal folds. Endoscopy usually fails to reveal evidence of nerve or muscle disease. No singular cause of SD has been identified, and there is great argument regarding the possibility of psychogenic disturbance in these individuals.

The nature of the referral base determines the type of SD patients that an individual clinician may see. Neurologists typically see those SD patients who have been seen by multiple speech-language pathologists and several ear, nose, and throat physicians. The majority of patients in our clinic have been seen by several professionals over a long period of time. Neurologic disturbance is evident in two-thirds of these patients. Of those patients who have neurologic disturbance, the majority have evidence of dystonia elsewhere (usually face, eyes, head, or neck) or tremor elsewhere (seen in finger-to-nose testing or head movements at rest). Usually these individuals' voices improve with pharmacotherapy, though the symptoms persist. The symptoms that are most distressing are tightness in the larynx and neck and the presence of glottal stops (Rosenfield, 1988b, 1988c).

Patients with spasmodic dysphonia as a result of underlying phonatory tremor often report that their speech improves when they drink alcohol. This is because alcohol affects the tremor, not because it makes the patient more relaxed. Individuals who have phonatory tremor, and especially those who improve with alcohol, can be treated with a beta blocker such as propranolol (Inderal). If this fails, sometimes a regimen of a low dose of Mysoline or Tegretol is efficacious. In my experience, I have found that the majority of patients respond to propranolol. The symptom that improves the most is glottal stopping. The patients also frequently report a diminished sensation of straining and pain (Rosenfield, 1988b, 1988c).

Patients with evidence of dystonia—frequently associated with Meige syndrome (oromandibular dystonia associated with blepharospasm)—often respond to a regimen of baclofen (Lioresal). If they fail to respond to this, a combination of trihexyphenidyl (Artane) and lithium may be effective.

Individuals who have no evidence of disease elsewhere may nevertheless be initiated on a regimen of Lioresal, which may reduce the feeling of tightness in their vocal folds. If this fails to help, a regimen of alprazolam (Xanax) may decrease muscle tension as well as tranquilize the patient.

I believe that all SD patients should be seen by a speech-language pathologist. Sometimes, but not often, patients respond better to speech therapy when they are on medication. If patients do respond to the above medications, they do so in the first 1 or 2 weeks. When patients fail to respond to a medical regimen, local anesthetic blocking of a recurrent laryngeal nerve may be considered, with evaluation for later possible nerve section. Unilateral sectioning of the recurrent laryngeal nerve produces ipsilateral vocal cord paralysis, placing the vocal fold in an abducted position. This abduction curtails the degree of bilateral laryngeal closure during phonation. The procedure frequently ameliorates symptoms for several months, but symptoms often return after 1 to 3 years. Recurrent laryngeal nerve sectioning appears to help some patients for longer periods, but such outcomes remain as yet impossible to predict. Because so many of our patients respond well enough to speech therapy and medication, they do not even wish to consider a local anesthetic injection into the recurrent laryngeal nerve.

Another form of therapy suggested for SD patients is intralaryngeal muscle botulinum toxin injection. Botulinum toxin, as already noted, blocks the release of acetylcholine, a most important neurotransmitter at the neuromuscular junction. Blocking the release of acetylcholine causes the muscle to be weak and thus decreases laryngeal muscle activity. Information regarding distribution of vocal fold neuromuscular junctions is important in deciding where to inject the toxin, although the chemical appears to diffuse fairly well. Certainly it diffuses well enough to produce side effects in peripheral muscles. If transient vocal cord paralysis produced by local anesthetic injection fails to improve voice output, blocking the vocal cord at the level of the neuromuscular junction with botulinum toxin will probably be no more effective. One of the arguments in favor of botulinum toxin injection is that blocking the recurrent laryngeal nerve compromises abductors as well as adductors of the vocal folds, although the net result of the nerve blockage causes abduction. Even if the botulinum toxin is injected only into the adductors, there might be more abduction of the vocal fold as well. One of the concerns I have about botulinum toxin is whether or not antibodies to the botulinum toxin will cause harmful effects in the years to come and whether vocal atrophy might occur, resulting in an altered mucosal wave. This outcome could result in further vocal strain. Considerable research is being conducted on botulinum toxin injection, which in the next few years should reveal its efficacy and which patients it will help. I do not believe that botulinum toxin should be employed if the patient fails to improve following local anesthetic block of the recurrent laryngeal nerve. This nerve block, resulting in temporary ipsilateral vocal cord abduction, enables a clinician to observe whether speech improves during the temporary unilateral vocal cord paralysis. If speech does improve following this maneuver, there is no guarantee that the recurrent laryngeal nerve sectioning will provide long-term efficacy, but failure to respond to the local anesthetic suggests that neither nerve sectioning nor botulinum toxin injection is likely to be beneficial (DeBito, Malmgren, & Gacek, 1985; Jankovic, 1988; Jankovic & Tolosa, 1988;

Rosenfield, 1988b, 1988c). For a case study of a spasmodic dysphonic patient treated using combined pharmacotherapy and speech therapy, the reader is referred to Chapter 10.

CONCLUSION

The fact that a speech deficit such as stuttering or spasmodic dysphonia worsens under emotional stress does not prove that the disturbance is purely psychogenic (Rosenfield, 1982). Although it is tempting to look to neuropharmacology for a potential mode of treatment, there are many speech motor disturbances that have no real definitive cures. Few clinicians cure stuttering (in adults), spasmodic dysphonia, or speech tremor. However, many excellent therapists can make people considerably better. What is important is to be certain that underlying disease processes have been ruled out and that any medications which might be effective have been tried.

I have discussed some major disease processes as well as basic pharmacology and medication. If a patient has a neurologic disease that is causing speech symptoms, and if the symptoms that are not related to speech respond to medication, then often the speech symptoms will also respond. However, sometimes there is a trade-off in that patients have worsening speech while otherwise improving. Individuals on anticholinergic medication may have improvement in their Parkinson's disease but also a dry mouth. A simple, effective truism is that any drug can do just about anything to anyone. If a patient is on a medication and after a few weeks develops a speech symptom, question whether that drug has caused the symptom. If a speech-language pathologist who is seeing a patient has questions about a prescribed medication, the pathologist should insist that the patient speak to the referring physician.

Speech-language pathologists, physicians, and other health care personnel have one primary goal: that the patient do well. A working knowledge of pharmacology and its basic mechanisms can help speech clinicians move toward that goal. Taking care of sick patients is not easy, and the more input physicians have from health care personnel who interact with the patients, the more effective medical care they can provide. It is hoped that the information presented in this chapter will contribute to that end.

REFERENCES

Balashke, T. F., Nies, A. S., & Mamelok, R. D. (1985). Principles of therapeutics. In A. G. Gillman, L. S. Goodman, T. W. Rall, & F. Murad (Eds.), *Goodman and Gillman's "The pharmacological basis of therapeutics."* New York: Macmillan.

Bloodstein, O. (1987). *The handbook of stuttering.* Chicago: National Easter Seal Society.
Butler, I. J. (1984). Tourette's syndrome: Some new concepts. In J. Jankovic (Ed.), *Neurologic clinics—Movement disorders.* Philadelphia: W. B. Saunders.
Calne, D. B., & Lang, A. E. (1988). Secondary dystonia. In S. Fahn, C. D. Marsden, & D. B. Calne (Eds.), *Advances in neurology: Vol. 50. Dystonia 2* (pp. 9–33). New York: Raven Press.
Canter, G. J. (1971). Observations on neurogenic stuttering: A contribution to differential diagnosis. *British Journal of Disorders of Communication, 6,* 139–143.
Cooper, J. R., Bloom, F. E., & Roth, R. H. (1986). *The biochemical basis of neuropharmacology.* New York: Oxford University Press.
Darley, F. L., Aronson, A. E., & Brown, J. R. (1975). *Motor speech disorders.* Philadelphia: W. B. Saunders.
DeBito, M. A., Malmgren, L. T., & Gacek, P. R. (1985). Three-dimensional distribution of neuromuscular junction in human cricothyroid. *Archives of Otolaryngology, 111,* 110–113.
Fahn, S. (1984). The varied clinical expressions of dystonia. In J. Jankovic (Ed.), *Neurologic clinics—Movement disorders* (pp. 541–555). Philadelphia: W. B. Saunders.
Fahn, S. (1988). Concept and classification of dystonia. In S. Fahn, C. D. Marsden, & D. B. Calne (Eds.), *Advances in neurology: Vol. 50, Dystonia 2* (pp. 1–8). New York: Raven Press.
Fahn, S., Marsden, C. D., & Calne, D. B. (Eds.). (1988). *Advances in neurology: Vol. 50. Dystonia 2.* New York: Raven Press.
Gillman, A. G., Goodman, L. S., Rall, T. W., & Murad, F. (1985). *Goodman and Gillman's "The pharmacological basis of therapeutics."* New York: Macmillan.
Gilman, S., & Winans, S. S. (1982). *Manter and Gatz's "Essentials of clinical neuroanatomy and neurophysiology."* Philadelphia: F. A. Davis.
Goetz, C. J., & Klawans, H. L. (1984). Tardive dyskinesia. In J. Jankovic (Ed.), *Neurologic clinics—Movement disorders* (pp. 605–614). Philadelphia: W. B. Saunders.
Goldstein, J. A. (1987). Carbamazepine treatment for stuttering. *Journal of Clinical Psychology, 48,* 39.
Hartman, D. E., & Abbs, J. H. (1988). Dysarthrias of movement disorders. In J. Jankovic & E. Tolosa (Eds.), *Advances in neurology: Vol. 49. Facial dyskinesias* (pp. 289–306). New York: Raven Press.
Hays, P. (1987). Bethanechol chloride in the treatment of stuttering. *Lancet, 1,* 271.
Hill, A. B. (1960). *Controlled clinical trials: Conference of Council for International Organization of Medical Sciences.* Oxford: Blackwell Scientific Publications.
Hill, A. B. (1962). *Statistical methods in clinical and preventative medicine.* New York: Oxford University Press.
Ingelfinger, J. A., Mosteller, F., Thibodeau, I. A., & Ware, J. H. (1983). *Biostatistics in clinical medicine.* New York: Macmillan.
Jankovic, J. (1988). Blepharospasm and oromandibular-laryngeal-cervical dystonia: A controlled trial of botulinum A toxin therapy. In S. Fahn, C. D. Marsden, & D. B. Calne (Eds.), *Advances in neurology: Vol. 50. Dystonia 2* (pp. 583–591). New York: Raven Press.

Jankovic, J., & Tolosa, E. (Eds.). (1988). *Advances in neurology: Vol. 49. Facial dyskinesias*. New York: Raven Press.

Jürgens, U., & Ploog, D. (1981). On the neural control of mammalian vocalization. *Trends in Neuroscience, 4,* 135–137.

Koch-Weser, J. (1972). Serum drug concentrations as therapeutic guides. *New England Journal of Medicine, 287,* 227–231.

Koller, W. C. (1984). Diagnosis and treatment of tremors. In J. Jankovic (Ed.), *Neurologic clinics—Movement disorders* (pp. 499–514). Philadelphia: W. B. Saunders.

Marsden, C. D. (1988). The investigation of dystonia. In S. Fahn, C. D. Marsden, & D. B. Calne (Eds.), *Advances in neurology: Vol. 50. Dystonia 2* (pp. 35–44). New York: Raven Press.

McDowell, F. H., & Cedarbaum, J. M. (1988). The extrapyramidal system and disorders of movement. In Robert J. Joynt (Ed.), *Clinical neurology* (Vol. 3, Chap. 38) (rev. ed.). Philadelphia: J. B. Lippincott.

Netter, F. H. (1983). *The CIBA collection of medical illustrations: Vol. 1. Nervous System: Part 1. Anatomy and Physiology*. West Caldwell, NJ: CIBA Pharmaceutical.

Porfert, A. R., & Rosenfield, D. B. (1978). Prevalence of stuttering. *Journal of Neurology, Neurosurgery and Psychiatry, 41,* 954–956.

Rosenberger, P. B. (1980). Dopaminergic systems and speech fluency. *Journal of Fluency Disorders, 5,* 255–267.

Rosenberger, P. B., Wheelden, L. A., & Kalotkin, M. (1976). The effect of haloperidol on stuttering. *American Journal of Psychiatry, 133,* 331–333.

Rosenfield, D. B. (1982). A comment on stuttering. *Journal of Fluency Disorders, 7,* 79–80.

Rosenfield, D. B. (1984). Scientific approaches to stuttering. *Critical Reviews in Clinical Neurobiology, 1,* 117–139.

Rosenfield, D. B. (1988a). Carbamazepine treatment for stuttering. *Journal of Clinical Psychology, 49,* 38.

Rosenfield, D. B. (1988b). Spasmodic dysphonia. In J. Jankovic & E. Tolosa (Eds.), *Advances in neurology: Vol. 49. Facial dyskinesias*. New York: Raven Press.

Rosenfield, D. B. (1988c). Spasmodic dysphonia. In S. Fahn, C. D. Marsden, & D. B. Calne (Eds.), *Advances in neurology: Vol. 50. Dystonia 2* (pp. 537–545). New York: Raven Press.

Rosenfield, D. B., & Barroso, A. B. (1991). Dysarthria, dysfluency and dysphagia. In W. G. Bradley, R. B. Daroff, G. M. Fenichel, & C. D. Marsden (Eds.), *Neurology in clinical practice: Vol. 1. Principles of diagnosis and management* (pp. 129–141). Stoneham, MA: Butterworth-Heinemann.

Rosenfield, D. B., & Boller, F. (1985). Stuttering. In P. J. Binken, G. W. Bruyn, & H. L. Klawans (Eds.), *Handbook of clinical neurology* (Vol. 2, No. 46).

Rosenfield, D. B., Freeman, F., & Jankovic, J. (1983, April). *Stuttering and the dopamine system*. Paper presented at the 35th annual meeting of the American Academy of Neurology, San Diego, CA.

Rosenfield, D. B., & Nudelman, H. B. (1987). Neuropsychological models of dysfluency. In L. Rustin, H. Purser, & D. Rowley (Eds.), *Progress in the treatment of fluency disorders*. London: Taylor and Francis.

ACKNOWLEDGMENTS

This work was supported by the M. R. Bauer Foundation and the Ariel-Benjamin-Jeremiah-Gideon-Abigail Maida Lowin Medical Research Foundation.

CHAPTER 6
Dysarthria: A Breakdown in Interpersonal Communication
Rosemary Lubinski

> *Lubinski writes of dysarthria as a breakdown in the patient's social system, focusing on the effect of the speech disorder on the patient, the family, and the clinician.*
>
> 1. What are the psychological, social, and emotional impacts of progressive deterioration in speech intelligibility on an adult with dysarthria?
> 2. What is the role of the speech-language pathologist in identifying and remediating psychological, social, and emotional problems of an adult with dysarthria?
> 3. How does dysarthria affect the daily lives of family members of dysarthric individuals?
> 4. How does institutionalization affect a dysarthric individual's motivation for speech therapy?
> 5. What for speech pathologists are the personal and professional consequences of working with severely dysarthric adults over long periods of time?

Although the multifaceted nature of dysarthria has become better understood in recent years than in years past, more attention has been directed toward investigating respiratory, laryngeal, and supralaryngeal structures and functions than to the psychosocial impact of reduced intelligibility on dysarthric individuals, their caregivers, and their families. This chapter focuses on dysarthria acquired in adulthood, which is usually associated with progressive neurological disease, trauma, or stroke. Specifically, the chapter explores dysarthria as a breakdown in the individual's social system and communication opportunities. It is divided into four main sections, all of which stress diagnostic and therapeutic implications for the speech-language pathologist providing service to dysarthric individuals and their significant others. The first part focuses on the individual with dysarthria and hence on the psychosocial impact on interpersonal functioning and communication. The second section explores how dysarthria may affect the individual in a family context. The next part describes the impact of institutionalization on the dysarthric person. The final section discusses the stress that the speech-language pathologist may incur in working with dysarthric individuals, particularly those with progressive degenerative disorders. The theme inherent throughout this chapter is that dysarthria should be considered from a broad psychosocial perspective if quality speech-language pathology services are to be meaningful to the individuals served.

IMPACT OF DYSARTHRIA ON THE INDIVIDUAL

The ability to communicate effectively is a skill that many adults take for granted on a daily basis. While we may desire a richer vocabulary or more sophisticated social communication skills, we assume that we will be able to produce the sounds of our language clearly. The mastery over our phonological system is a developmental skill accomplished early and relatively easily in our lives with little conscious attention to individual sounds or how these sounds are produced physiologically. It is not until adults encounter a chronic illness, trauma, or stroke that affects the motor-speech system that it is realized how complex the mechanism is that produces sounds and how devastating the psychosocial effects of the impairment are for the individual.

Phonology and Social Development

While unintelligibility may be tolerated in young children, mastery over the sound system is encouraged and eventually expected. The reciprocal nature of conversation is difficult until the young child's sound system at least minimally matches that of the linguistic environment. Before this match occurs, parents and others anticipate what the child may be trying to say; they guess, look for cues in the environment, say something encouraging, and sometimes eventually give up trying to converse with the child. As the child's sound system concurs with the environment, more opportunities for social interaction and social role development arise, more stimulation is given, vocabulary and syntax develop, and the child gains communicative competence. While the cognitive and sensory abilities of the child are contributors to this competence, mastery over the sound system to an acceptable level is crucial for others to perceive the child as a viable communication partner. The sound system becomes the building blocks for further communication skill learning and refinement.

The phonological system and its mastery is a part of the foundation for social development not only in childhood but throughout the life span. It is unusual for adults to experience difficulty with their phonological system—that is, failure in their ability to produce intelligible speech—and so when the phonological system becomes impaired individuals may experience some degree of breakdown in their emotional well-being and social system. At a time when communication may be integral to maintaining a positive self-concept, receiving optimum medical care, and providing feedback to caregivers, reduction or loss of speech intelligibility may cause tremendous frustration and anger.

Psychosocial Impact of Dysarthria

The literature reveals little research regarding the psychological, social, and emotional consequences of dysarthria. However, it is easy to extrapolate from research on the impact of chronic illness, aphasia, and other long-term disabilities on the psychosocial functioning of adults. Caplan and Schecter (1987) state that individuals with chronic illnesses may exhibit confusion, emotional numbing, depression, grief, anxiety, paranoia, and denial. Goodstein (1983) adds such emotional feelings as fear surrounding loss of control, independence, and affection, and the fear of recurrence of illness or death itself. In addition, changes in cognitive functioning may impair judgment, critical thinking ability, and appropriate pragmatic skills.

Dysarthric individuals, as any persons with a disability, may display a wide range of coping styles and mechanisms. Henderson and Bryan (1984) state that persons with disabilities are "more vulnerable to stress than persons without disabilities . . . and react more intensively" (p. 125). These authors describe three major coping or defense mechanisms that are likely to be used by the disabled person: (1) deception such as repression, projection, and displacement; (2) substitution devices such as compensation and reaction formation; and (3) avoidance devices including fantasy and regression. Safilios-Rothchild (1970) provides another source of discussion about the effects of disability by examining the sociology and social psychology of disability at the personality, societal, and cultural levels.

Furthermore, for those persons experiencing progressive disorders, uncertainty about increasing incapacity and fear of reduction in speech intelligibility complicate the emotional turmoil. These factors may contribute to gradual or precipitous withdrawal from social, occupational, leisure, and other activities. Patients may experience a sense of loss over behaviors that were once easily executed and taken for granted and are now irretrievable. Part of their fear may be attributable to the uncertainty of not knowing how and to what degree their communication will deteriorate. Progressive phonological incompetence combined with other physical or psychological deterioration can be devastating to the individual regardless of the person's original level of motivation and positive self-esteem.

Soon after becoming dysarthric, the individual perceives that our society values communicative competence, a characteristic that the patient now lacks. Thus, previous social roles are difficult to maintain or reassume. The person with dysarthria has become part of a minority group of disabled adults and may incur some or all of the negative reactions and stereotyping ascribed to the handicapped in our society. Sussman (1977) describes these handicapped individuals as "marginal." Certainly those adults who cannot express themselves clearly and easily are marginal members of our society inasmuch as they do not fit our society's definition of effective adult communicators.

When dysarthria occurs in a person age 65 or older, the individual is placed in double jeopardy. This individual faces the negative attitudes directed toward the aged plus those directed toward the handicapped. The older dysarthric individual presents unique and perhaps even more difficult diagnostic and rehabilitative dilemmas because of this double handicap. The older dysarthric person is likely to have one or more chronic illnesses, is likely to be dependent on others for assistance in activities of daily living, and is likely to face a variety of personal and social changes or losses including those that occur with retirement, death of spouse, and relocation.

Furthermore, communication partners may not know how to interact with a physically disabled adult, especially one with decreased speech intelligibility. Researchers have documented the negative attitudes toward the disabled stemming from such factors as ignorance of the problem, anxiety, fear of embarrassment, and stereotypes of handicapped individuals (Dunn, 1987). These attitudes are reflected in the reduction of communicative opportunity for the dysarthric individual. Dunn (1987) states that individuals who are not handicapped do not know the "rules" for interacting with the handicapped. This fact can be extended to the area of communication with the dysarthric individual who may have sustained both physical and communication handicaps. In fact, the dysarthric person may pose a dual threat for communication partners in that the possible presence of a visible physical handicap coupled with the speech disorder may heighten communication anxiety and discourage interaction. Many dysarthric persons are physically handicapped from stroke or progressive neurological disease and require assistance with ambulation and activities of daily living. The more visible and debilitating the handicap, the less likely that others will want to encourage interaction. Conversation with the communicatively handicapped individual may be terminated as quickly as possible.

Communication partners may not have a repertoire of strategies to help decode unintelligible messages and therefore maintain a conversation with the dysarthric individual. If the dysarthric person fails to speak clearly, the communication partner may feel failure for not interpreting the dysarthric person's speech accurately, and may minimize communication contact to prevent further failure and frustration.

Dysarthria as Stress

Dysarthria appears to create a source of communicative stress for the patient and for the communication partners. Stress is defined as the "physical, mental or emotional reaction resulting from an individual's response to environmental tensions, conflicts and pressures" (Greenberg & Valletutti, 1980). Stress may occur during the actual or even in the anticipated interaction with a dysarthric individual. This stress may arise from the frustration created by an unsuccessful attempt at sending or receiving a message. It may stem from the conflict between wanting to express oneself successfully and the fear of failure to do so. Or it may originate from the internal and societal expectations that articulatory proficiency equals communicative competence. Dysarthria—particularly severe dysarthria—by its very nature may create chronic stress that will be evident over long periods of time. For those dysarthric individuals with progressive disease, the awareness that the present level of intelligibility may be difficult to maintain is sure to add to the stress already perceived.

The speech-language pathologist treating a dysarthric individual should consider the potential psychological, social, and emotional impacts of the speech disorder. Traditionally speech-language pathologists have focused on identifying the speech process components of the problem, designing remedial programs to improve the specific areas of the disorder or recommending assistive communicative devices. It is not axiomatic that improving communication skills will result in an immediate resolution of the entire communication problem. Despite improved communication skills, individuals may continue to perceive themselves as handicapped and subsequently may withdraw from communication opportunities. It is difficult to shed a coat of disability once it has been worn. Further, improved skills may not result in perfect intelligibility, regardless of how much effort has been expended by the clinician and the client. The dysarthric individual may insist on obtaining the goal of producing 100% intelligible speech, a goal that is unrealistic for the patient. Or the individual may continue to react to other physical and mental disabilities that do not improve. Communication partners may have withdrawn so much opportunity for interaction that the social bonds which instigate communication are weakened. People cannot always pick up relationships or activities where they left off months or even years ago.

Compliance to Therapy

Speech-language pathologists may wonder why some dysarthric clients are not highly motivated to improve their speech intelligibility. They wonder why a person whose communication world is limited would not take every possible opportunity to learn how to speak clearly or to learn how to use an assistive device. They wonder why the reinforcement of being able to communicate more effectively does not seem to motivate the patient to work diligently to attain that goal. Basically the speech-language pathologist is asking, "Why doesn't every dysarthric patient follow my advice?" This is called compliance and has been an area of great interest in the medical arena for years (Gerber & Nekemkis, 1986).

Dysarthric clients vary in the amount of commitment to speech therapy despite its golden goals. Commitment is dependent on a person's positive and negative experiences with a task and on the bond between these two factors (Lemkau, Bryant, & Brickman, 1982). Some individuals come to the therapy situation with a compliant, committed personal attitude. Others may be cautious of accepting help from a stranger. Some individuals expect the clinician to accept all the responsibility for improvement, while others enter the therapy situation certain that nothing can be done to improve their speech. Hopefully, few are noncompliant because they do not understand the nature of the speech problem or the procedures being used to treat it. Previous positive and negative experiences with speech therapy can also affect commitment to therapy. Unfortunately, little is known about the nature of dysarthric individuals' commitment to speech therapy or the factors that contribute to an unsuccessful experience and noncompliance. Understanding these factors could lead to obtaining a stronger commitment from the patient to achieve therapy goals.

Probe Questions

The set of questions in Table 6.1 is designed to help the speech-language pathologist explore and understand the psychological, social, and emotional impacts of dysarthria on the individual during the therapy process. The questions are probe questions that can be followed later with more in-depth queries appropriate for a given client. The questions are not designed for scoring or to compare the client with other clients. These questions can be repeated during the course of therapy to examine the impact of therapy and to determine continued psychosocial needs.

TABLE 6.1
Probe Questions for the Client

Definition of the Problem
1. What concerns you about your speech?
2. What kinds of sounds or words give you the most difficulty?
3. In what situations do you feel you have the most difficulty talking?

Impact of the Problem
1. How do you feel when you have difficulty being understood?
2. How do others react when you have difficulty being understood?
3. Do you ever avoid a situation or a person because of your speech problem? If yes,
   a. What is this situation (person)?
   b. Why do you think this happens?
4. How has your speech problem affected your interaction with your family?
5. How has your speech problem affected your social life (employment, etc.)?
6. Do you think you have less opportunity to talk now than previously? If yes,
   a. Why?
   b. How can you change this?

Motivation to Improve
1. Why would you like to improve your speech?
2. What would you like to improve?
3. What have you done on your own to improve your speech?
4. What techniques did you find helped you talk better?
5. Have you attended speech therapy sessions before this? If so,
   a. Where were they held?
   b. What were your goals?
   c. What were the results?
6. How will your family work to help you improve your speech?
7. How will we know when speech therapy has been successful?
8. What do you think is my role in the speech therapy situation?

EXPLORING THE PSYCHOSOCIAL IMPACT OF DYSARTHRIA: THE FAMILY

Although the stroke, trauma, or progressive neurological disease that results in dysarthria is incurred by an individual, in actuality the family acquires the problem. The family equilibrium is disrupted at several levels. At one level the family must face the problem of a severe physical disability and/or progressive chronic illness. Bray (1987) provided a schema for understanding the reaction of family members to chronic illness. He cautions that families vary in their reactions to chronic illness, and observes that numerous, often amorphous, factors complicate their feelings. The major courses of reactions exhibited by families include fear, denial, bargaining, depression, mourning, and rapprochement.

Bray (1987) describes fear as the first response of the family. Family members often are shocked by the occurrence or identification of the chronic illness. They may coalesce into some type of unified group to fight the problem. This may manifest itself through criticizing, as family members attack or unreasonably question care or rehabilitation efforts. Another natural response is to flee. Although few family members would outrightly deny care to a chronically ill person, some may more insidiously withdraw emotional support and interaction from the affected individual. Another fear is based on not understanding the course of a chronic illness; family members may automatically assume the worst possible consequences. There is also an egocentric type of fear in which family members may project the same chronic illness on themselves sometime in the future.

Denial is a second response exhibited by some or all family members. Bray (1987) describes this as a defensive posture. While denial may at first help to cushion the impact of the disorder on the family, eventually it can result in providing less than optimal care and rehabilitation possibilities (Power, 1985).

A third response by a family is bargaining. Bray states that some families attempt to trade their "compliance and oversolicitness" for the patient's recovery. Bargaining can be summed up as an "if we, then you" situation. Although family involvement, concern, and commitment are necessary and important factors in meaningful rehabilitation of the dysarthric individual, no guarantees can be made. Speech identical to that produced before the stroke, trauma, or disease occurred is an unreasonable expectation in spite of the efforts expended by the clinician, patient, and family.

Depression constitutes the fourth possible reaction by the family. Depression may result in a lack of affect by the family members, a sense of giving up, and a pervasive sadness that invades all aspects of their lives. The depression felt by the dysarthric individual or by the family members may spread to persons outside the family. A vicious cycle can occur: others limit or cut off interaction opportunities with the dysarthric individual or the family and thus reduce the social interaction needed for achieving an environment free of depression.

Mourning is defined as the quiescent phase (Bray, 1987). During this stage the family begins to accept the actual disability and feels sorrow at the loss that has occurred or—in the case of progressive disease—will occur eventually. This letting-go may result in withdrawal from the dysarthric individual, as a new family system is being created.

The final stage in reaction to chronic illness as described by Bray is rapprochement. This stage usually occurs after rehabilitation efforts have been completed. The family now establishes its new equilibrium, often with family members accepting new roles and with the chronically ill person either being reintegrated into former roles, or assuming a role commensurate with abilities and desires. At this point the chronically impaired person may become a marginal member of the family.

The family equilibrium also is broken at a more fundamental, personal level. Each time the dysarthric individual tries to communicate and experiences difficulty, the reciprocal nature of communication is compromised. Like society at large, most family members lack experience in communicating with persons who have sustained speech or language impairment. They may exhibit the same negative attitudes that society holds toward the disabled, and in fact may be more intolerant, embarrassed, and frustrated than others outside the family unit as they attempt to interact with someone who is difficult to understand. Family members may let down their social guard and exhibit their frustration in more open—if not hostile—ways than persons outside the family, particularly in the confines of the home and other familiar places. Some may be overly solicitous and anticipate what the dysarthric individual may want to say, thereby denying the dysarthric person opportunities to use remaining or improving speech and language skills. Other family members may place an unrealistic burden for improvement on the dysarthric speaker. Still others may feel that communication rehabilitation will result in return to normal speech if only the dysarthric individual and the clinician work hard enough. Finally, some family members may fluctuate in their interactions with the dysarthric person. At times they may demonstrate overexpectations and at other times underexpectations; at still other times they may provide few opportunities for any interactions at all.

Thus, the family is a complex factor in the life of the dysarthric individual, and hence in the rehabilitation process. Nevertheless, speech-language clinicians should consider Luterman's (1984) advice when he says we must "come to realize that the people we deal with are part of a system and that we cannot treat one element [the person with the communication disorder] without some attention to the entire system [the family]" (p. 160).

Family as a System

The concept that a family is a system has become well accepted in the family theory and counseling areas (Satir, 1981). The components of the system include individuals, marital dyads, parental relationships, sibling relationships, and relationships with other significant family members. Jones (1988) states that the family can be viewed as an interdependent, interacting system of roles in a state of dynamic equilibrium. Family roles are developed through verbal and nonverbal communication over time. Each member of the family brings individual characteristics, expectations, resources, and limitations to any family situation. Individuals and the family itself influence each other and in turn are influenced by societal rules and expectations. Thus the family cannot be understood without any of its parts, yet the parts individually do not constitute the family. It is the interaction of family members and their evolution over time that create a system.

Therefore, we can see that when the individual incurs a communication problem such as dysarthria, there must be an impact on the family system. Initially the stroke, trauma, or progressive neurological disease creates a crisis for the individual and the family, and eventually the resulting dysarthria comprises a chronic stress for the family system. Hill (1949) proposed a model for understanding family systems under stress and called this paradigm the ABCX model. The A variable constitutes the stressor event and the demands placed on the family system. The B variable describes the resources brought to the stressful situation by the individual family members. The family's definition of the problem is the C variable. The interaction of the A, B, and C variables creates the X variable, or the actual crisis.

This model has been expanded upon by McCubbin, Boss, Wilson, and Lester (1980) in the Double ABCX model. The revised model, which is shown in Figure 6.1, provides a way of understanding how a family reacts to multiple stressors over a period of time, not just at the time of the crisis.

The primary crisis—having the stroke, incurring trauma, or identification of a progressive neurological disorder—is not static in time within the family. The family comes to that crisis with other demands on it (A variable). For example, there may be any variety and combination of preexisting demands on the family prior to the dysarthria-causing crisis. These may include social, occupational, and financial problems within the family itself or between members of the family and groups

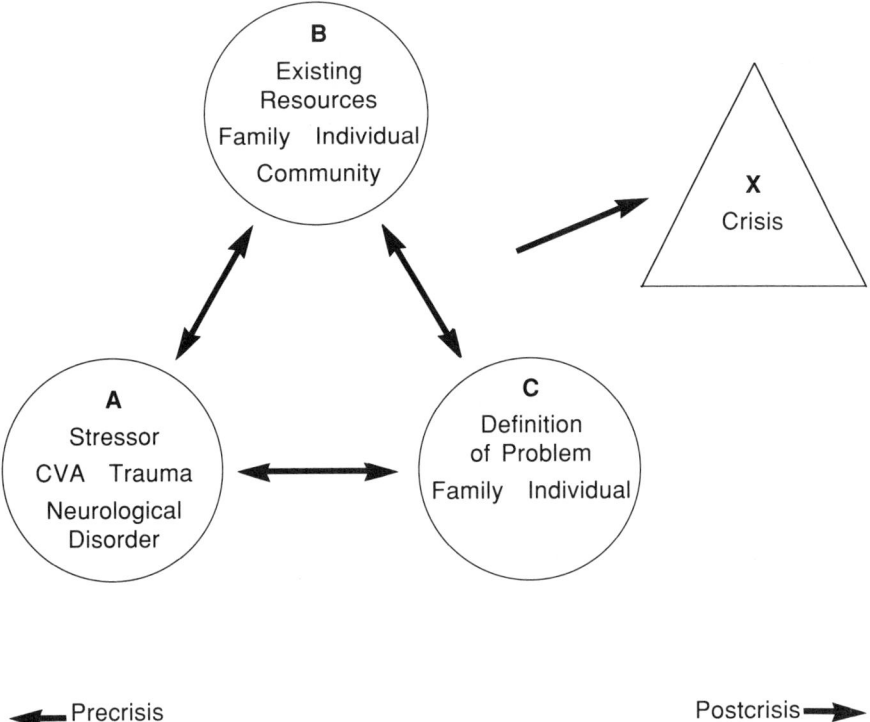

Figure 6.1 ABCX model of family stress adapted from Hill (1949) and McCubbin and Patterson (1983).

outside the family. These demands do not disappear when the individual becomes dysarthric. The family with previous financial concerns may find that problem exacerbated and contributing to the present crisis. Thus clinicians working with dysarthric individuals and their families must explore demands on the family that existed before the dysarthria and that affect the present condition.

The family brings not only a history of other small and large demands, but also a cadre of resources (B variable) that have helped them cope with previous stresses and problems. Some families have positive, functional styles that help them cope well with both everyday and major problems. Friedman (1986) states that a family most likely to use its resources is one that has a broad repertoire of resources. Similarly, Imber-Black (1986) describes families as perpetual problem-solving mechanisms. Families may not even be aware of the resources or strengths they are bringing to a problem situation.

Imber-Black (1986) describes the resources families may bring to any problem. One set includes religious, cultural, and racial identify. These three factors have helped shape the family in particular ways over a long period of time. A second source of strength is the family's "inner language." Family members have special and idiosyncratic ways of communicating with each other that help to define them as a family. A third source of strength is individual and family commitment, loyalties, and sense of connection. Individuals within a family and the family as a whole may be dedicated to its members and to the survival of the family system in different ways. The final resource factor that Imber-Black postulates is the family's capacity to interact with the outside world. This factor describes how family members and the family as a whole interface with groups or systems outside themselves. Some families are inner-directed in that they seldom if ever seek assistance from anyone outside the family. This type of family is seen as a free-standing entity capable of providing its own sustenance. Other families, in contrast, are open in that they seek outside stimulation and assistance as needed. Many families probably fall between the closed, self-sufficient family and the open, society-integrating family on this continuum. A family that hesitates to interface with groups outside its own family unit may be more hesitant to accept rehabilitative and counseling efforts than a family that interacts easily outside its own unit.

To this list of resources might be added the family's adaptability. Baird and Doherty (1986) define adaptability as "flexibility in responding to demands imposed by stressors" (p. 371). A crucial element in a family's adaptability is its ability to shift family roles easily. The family's natural response to the crisis facing it is to maintain relative homeostasis; therefore individual family members may need to assume different roles even though this may add extra demands.

Cohesion is a strength that a family may bring to a problem situation. Similar to Imber-Black's concept of commitment, loyalty, and sense of connection and inner language, cohesion emanates from the family's "tightly woven communication" (Baird & Doherty, 1986, p. 372). Cohesive families have clear roles, exhibit open communication, and provide support when needed.

Resources may also stem from outside the family. Informal family support systems include the extended family, friends, and community and religious groups. Social agencies and self-help groups offer support outside the familiar family system. As stated previously, some families may be more open than others to using the resources generated by these groups.

How families define the actual stressor is the third variable in Hill's ABCX model. Individuals may perceive the dysarthria-causing event and the resulting dysarthria in different ways. The definition of stress partly emanates from our societal definition of what is identified as a problem. It also originates from individual perceptions. Such factors as the suddenness of onset, the degree of severity, the length of adjustment to the problem, the impact on other individuals, and the solvability of the problem all contribute to individuals' definition of the problem (Jones, 1988). One family member may view the dysarthria as an inevitable problem associated with advancing age, another may see it as a problem during each interaction, and still another may perceive it as remedial with time and therapy. Speech-language pathologists need to explore how both family members and the dysarthric individual describe and view the problem. This exploration needs to take place over time, since the definition of the problem may change as the dysarthric patient becomes more intelligible or family members gain more experience in communicating with the dysarthric person.

Probe Questions for Family Members

The set of questions in Table 6.2 is based on Hill's ABCX Model. The first set of questions explores the demands created by the dysarthria, the second searches for resources that the family may be able to bring to the situation, and the third focuses on how the family defines the problem itself. All three components combined should indicate the stress the family may be experiencing and consequently the loci of counseling needs.

INSTITUTIONALIZATION OF THE DYSARTHRIC INDIVIDUAL

The decision to institutionalize a family member is a difficult one to make. Contrary to what we might expect, most persons are not callously dumped in this setting (Committee on Aging, 1974). The decision often comes after a crisis or a burdensome, unsuccessful period of trying to care for the individual at home. An older spouse may not be able to meet the physical needs of a neurologically impaired person. Some dysarthric individuals may need maximum assistance with activities of daily living that an older, perhaps frail, spouse cannot provide. Some dysarthric individuals may not have a spouse or family member to care for them at home. In-home services may be considered too expensive or intrusive or may not be easily and consistently available.

In other cases the lifestyle of adult children may preclude providing full-time care for a parent. Adult daughters tend to be the primary caregivers for their parents, and their move into the work force complicates the issue (Bernard & Thompson, 1970). Basically, the person who resides in a nursing home cannot live independently and needs maxi-

TABLE 6.2
Probe Questions for Family Members

Demands
1. What significant events were occurring in your family prior to the onset of your (dad's, mom's, husband's, wife's, etc.) chronic illness or communication difficulties?
2. How have these events changed since the onset of the physical and communication problems?
3. Who has primary care or responsibility for your (dad's, etc.) physical needs?
4. How does this care affect (you, her, him, them)?
5. How has the chronic illness or communication difficulty affected your (dad's, etc.) social life?
6. How has the chronic illness or communication difficulty affected the primary caregiver's social life?
7. What physical stress or strains does the primary caregiver have because of the physical problem?
8. What financial problems is your family incurring related to the physical or communication problem?
9. How has the primary caregiver's daily life changed since the onset of the problem?
10. What physical or psychological changes have you noted in the primary caregiver since the inception of the problem?
11. How did the family change immediately at the onset of the problem? How has it changed over time?

Resources
1. How would you describe your family's strengths?
2. What other problems did your family have in the past and how did they solve them?
3. How successful do you think your family is in solving difficult problems?
4. How willing is your (dad, etc.) to seek help from friends? counselors? religious institutions? social service? others?
5. During difficult times, will your family call a family conference and discuss problems? Who is likely to be the leader or take-charge person in these situations?
6. Who will be the primary communication partner of your (dad, etc.)? Will this individual be available to come to therapy sessions on occasion?

Definition of the Problem
1. What do you perceive as the major problem facing your family at the present time?
2. Why is this problem so paramount?
3. What do you think can be done about this problem?
4. Should the communication problem not be mentioned, then ask the following: How does your (dad's, etc.) communication problem compare to this problem you have just defined?
5. Do other members of your family define the impact of your (dad's, etc.) problem in the same way as you have just done? How is their definition different from yours?

mum assistance in daily living (Rauth, 1968). How the loss of intelligibility contributes to the decision to institutionalize a dysarthric person is an unknown factor.

In 1980 there were 23,065 nursing homes in the United States serving 1.4 million elderly and chronically ill individuals. In addition, there were over 1,100 nursing and extended care facilities attached to acute care hospitals (Advancedata, 1983). While it is usually estimated that only about 5% of the elderly are institutionalized (Kastenbaum & Candy, 1973), many more will spend some time in a long-term care setting. In general the nursing home patient population consists of very old white females. The average nursing home patient is 82 years old, has at least four chronic disabilities, and will reside there at least one year. Most of these individuals will die in this setting (Committee on Aging, 1974). The number of dysarthric individuals in nursing homes is unclear due to the variety of conditions that cause dysarthria. It does appear that the number is likely to be significant since dysarthria is associated with aphasia following stroke, progressive neurological disease, and head trauma and can coexist with dementia (Hudson, 1981).

Effects of Institutionalization

An individual who enters a nursing home undergoes a drastic change in lifestyle. Goffman (1961) and Bennett (1963) describe the totality of this context. The individual must adhere to a regimented lifestyle in which there are few opportunities for self-determination and choice. Kleemeier (1961) described this regimentation as a dimension of institutional control. In most nursing homes the physical environment is designed for the efficient functioning of staff in the provision of long-term custodial care. The staff of the nursing home generally controls or manages the daily life and possessions of the patient. The social environment is also limited, particularly in the number and type of social roles the individual may assume. The primary social role for the dysarthric individual in this setting is that of patient, one who receives care. Frequently there is little regard for the person's privacy and personal possessions. The right to self-actualization and self-determination is limited as are opportunities to be independent (Ainsworth, 1977).

Many patients react to this depersonalization and dehumanization with feelings of fear, hostility, rejection, despair, loss, anxiety, dependency, and isolation (Ainsworth, 1977; Committee on Aging, 1974; Kahana, 1973; Lieberman, 1969). Some of them react negatively to their caregivers and become verbally and physically abusive; others withdraw from available social activities and passively receive care; still others attempt to instill guilt in family members who come to visit. Other individuals accept institutional life and interact positively with other patients, staff, and family. They feel that their institutionalization is necessary and expected by family members and thus reconcile themselves to their new lifestyle. For them there appears to be little alternative to institutionalization. In general, most people adapt to institutional life at some level though few regard this as a positive living experience.

Communication Impaired Environment

Nursing homes have been described by Lubinski (1981, 1988, 1991) and by Lubinski, Morrison, and Rigrodski (1981) as an example of a communication-impaired or -deprived environment. This concept adds another dimension to Goffman's and Bennett's concepts of institutional totality. According to Lubinski (1981), the nursing home is a setting where there are (1) few reasons to talk, (2) few people of choice with whom to talk, (3) few things to talk about which emanate from stimulating activities, (4) few private places to communicate, and (5) a variety of rules that restrict communication opportunities. In addition, staff members state that they do not have enough time to communicate with patients.

Koury and Lubinski (1991) found that nursing assistants had a limited knowledge of the communication problems of the elderly, and furthermore, they could generate few strategies for communicating with communicatively impaired older persons. Thus, when confronted with an individual with reduced speech intelligibility, nursing assistants often lack the skills for facilitating communication. As a result they may avoid interaction with the dysarthric person. Communication therefore becomes a by-product of daily life in this setting rather than a priority of care.

In addition to the restrictive physical and psychosocial environment of this setting, the patients themselves contribute to the impoverished communication atmosphere of long-term care settings. Patients make few efforts to get to know each other, perceive others as incapable of communication, and are highly selective about whom they choose as communication partners. In an interview study of communication in a nursing home, elderly patients stated that they did not talk to "aphasic" patients because they perceived such patients as being incapable of communication (Lubinski, 1981). It is not known how amenable nursing home patients are to communicating with dysarthric patients who may be difficult to understand or who may use an assistive communication device. It can be hypothesized, however, that the dysarthric individual is likely to be rejected as a communication partner along with other severely communicatively impaired persons. This in turn places more burden on staff and family to be available as communication partners for dysarthric individuals in long-term care settings.

Positive Communication Environment

Despite the bleak portrayal of nursing home life, it is likely that improvements can be made that would result in a better quality of life for the patients and in greater job satisfaction for staff members. Major improvements would entail a drastic conceptual change in the design and management of nursing homes as well as in their everyday interaction. Ideally, nursing homes would mirror independent life in the community as nearly as possible. Maxwell Jones (1976) describes this ideal institutional setting as a "therapeutic community." In a therapeutic milieu, patients and staff work cooperatively and share responsibility for daily life. Social interaction between patients and staff and among the patients themselves is viewed as the means of promoting self-actualization and self-determination. This concept emanates from the principle that people, even the institutionalized elderly, can and should be active participants in their own care and not simply passive respondents. Excellent reviews of the concept of the therapeutic community are contained in Rosenstock, Goldman, and Rothenberg (1969), Rossi and Filstead (1973), and Gottesman (1973).

Full implementation of a therapeutic milieu in all nursing homes may be unrealistic. Although there is increased governmental pressure to improve nursing homes, much of the emphasis is on factors such as cleanliness, dietary considerations, nursing care, and availability of rehabilitation and leisure activities. While these are important aspects of nursing home life, they do not address the socialization that occurs between patients and staff and among patients. Opportunities for choice and self-actualization are amorphous and difficult to evaluate. Thus nursing homes are usually not evaluated on the amount of socialization that occurs nor on the quality of the communication that exists.

Staff, families, and patients may be unaware of what a nursing home could be and what the alternatives to the present conditions could be. During the institutionalization process, families are likely to focus on the apparent cleanliness and nursing care of the setting. Staff, accustomed to the usual scheme of interaction in the nursing home, are likely to maintain the status quo. Patients are even less likely to make any major changes. So much time in the nursing home is spent on meeting the physical demands of the patients and documenting caregiving that the cycle of dehumanization and depersonalization becomes entrenched and is considered the norm for that setting.

The communication disorders specialist can become involved in creating a more positive communication environment in nursing homes. This should benefit all patients but especially those with communication difficulties such as dysarthria.

A positive communication environment is one in which patients and staff have maximum opportunity to interact with each other in a variety of meaningful activities. It is based on the following premises: (1) elderly and chronically ill patients want to talk and feel that is important to their well-being to communicate; (2) members of the staff are the primary communication partners of the patients and thus play a crucial role in the patients' communication life; (3) it is possible to change the physical environment to make it more conducive to communication; and (4) people need to be able to engage in activities that foster communication and to be allowed access to their choice of communication partners in order for optimum communication to occur.

The first step in creating this positive communication environment is to help administrators and staff understand the vital importance of communication to the daily lives and functioning of their patients. Communication should be as high a priority of care as a clean environment and adequate nursing. Staff, in particular the nursing assistants, should receive inservice training focusing on skills for initiating and facilitating conversations with patients and emphasizing their important role in communicating with the patients (Koury & Lubinski, 1991). Nursing assistants need to know how assistive devices work and how valuable these devices can be to dysarthric patients. Also, they need to know how to manage the physical environment to promote visual and auditory aspects of communication. Finally, and most important, they need to become sensitive to their role in communicating with patients. Many staff persons are not aware of how vital their role is in communicating with patients or of how their own verbal and nonverbal communication is received and interpreted by patients. Communication occurs between people who perceive themselves as similar, who have similar interests, and who work interdependently. Chipping away at what Goffman (1961) calls the staff-inmate split could be one of the most valuable ways to enhance communication in the nursing home environment.

Communication disorders specialists can work with the staff to identify the physical aspects of the environment that can be made more conducive to communication. Proper management of lighting and sound control can be incorporated easily by most nursing homes. For example, adding more light so that patients can see one another and turning down the volume on a television set so that the patients can hear one another are management procedures that can be accomplished easily. Also, providing physical access to the activities that are available for patients in the institution can stimulate communication. Speech-language pathologists should work with activities directors in nursing homes to aid them in designing activities and programs that are both meaningful and stimulating to the age and physical abilities of the residents. For further information, the reader is referred to Lubinski (1981,

1988, 1991), who in a series of articles and book chapters has outlined the concept of a positive communication environment as well as identification and intervention strategies.

STRESS OF DYSARTHRIA THERAPY

The major focus of this chapter thus far has been on the impact of dysarthria on the individual and the significant others in the dysarthric person's environment. There is an additional person to be considered: the speech-language pathologist. For many dysarthric clients, the speech-language pathologist will become the primary helper. The thrust of dysarthria therapy is to help the individual regain as much communicative competence as possible. Therapy if successful can result in the client's overall improved quality of life. When this is possible, both client and clinician feel successful. The joy of seeing a client communicate effectively can be an immense reward for the speech-language pathologist even if the client does not directly express gratitude. Positive comments from family, caregivers, and other professionals can be an added incentive for both client and clinician.

Therapy progress with dysarthric clients is likely to be slow, limited, and prolonged. For those clients with degenerative diseases, the progressive loss of intelligibility, along with the loss of physical and mental abilities that can accompany the disease, may cause strain for client and clinician. Clients may expect progress even when it is not realistic, may reject assistive communicative devices, or may exert less than optimum effort to use the communication skills that remain. The speech-language pathologist may be frustrated, if not angry, at a client's lack of compliance with therapy procedures and with the client's minimal motivation. Further, families and significant others in the environment may pay little attention to therapy, reduce communicative opportunities for the dysarthric individual, and even sabotage therapy efforts in subtle ways. For example, placing a communication board out of the reach of a client may extinguish the client's motivation to use it.

Indeed, the help offered by the speech-language pathologist may be simultaneously intense, complicated, demanding, and tedious for the patient. The speech-language pathologist who has a caseload of individuals who need this type of therapy may incur stress and eventually burn out.

It is only recently that our profession has become aware that speech-language pathologists may react physically and emotionally to the work that they do. Miller and Potter (1982) and Potter and Rudensey (1984) were among the first to describe the personal impact of our professional work. Miller and Potter (1982) found that 43% of speech-language pathologists were experiencing moderate to severe burnout. Although their work does not focus specifically on the speech-language pathologist working with the dysarthric client, many implications can be derived from the existing theories and empirical research on stress and the helping professions.

Helping Relationship

Speech-language therapy, in which one individual helps another to communicate, is one of the most intimate forms of helping relationships. The relationship between the client and clinician is a complex one. The clinician brings to the situation clinical knowledge, competency, and experience combined with a variety of important personal qualities. Numerous authors have delineated the following characteristics of a helping relationship: empathy, warmth, genuineness, concreteness, immediacy, self-understanding, and open communication (e.g., Rogers, 1951; Murgatroyd, 1985). The client, in turn, also brings certain factors to the relationship: (1) a personal history, (2) the communication handicap, (3) the need and motivation to improve, (4) other complicating physical and mental problems, and (5) a social environment, which can be supportive or not. The client may be in the therapy situation by choice or because others have deemed it necessary. In addition, the client and clinician will form a working relationship over time, making their relationship dynamic rather than static.

The helping relationship in dysarthria therapy focuses on assisting the individual to improve or maintain speaking abilities or to use compensatory strategies to communicate. Therapy also may focus on motivating the client and working with significant others to improve their strategies for communicating with the dysarthric individual. Thus the helping relationship incorporates a series of decisions: judgments involving the diagnostic process and techniques, therapy strategies, how to motivate the client and family, and counseling.

Stress

This process of dysarthria therapy may be a stressful one for the speech-language pathologist. Stress is a person's "physical, mental, or emotional reaction to tension, conflict, and pressure" (Greenberg & Valletutti, 1980, p. 2). The sources of stress may arise from the clinician's personal outlook, the client, significant others, and the work environment (Farmer, Monahan, & Hekeler, 1984). These factors are intertwined as they impact on the clinician.

The very nature of the helping relationship may be a source of stress for the clinician working with a dysarthric individual. Clinicians who are idealistic or perfectionistic may find this type of therapy stressful.

Normal speech may not be attainable. Regression may occur. Therapy gains can evaporate even after months of success. Clinicians may expect the dysarthric client to maintain high levels of motivation and involvement in the therapy even though the client is facing multiple other problems. The clinician may experience role overload, wherein the clinician has too many tasks to perform often without enough preparation time (Greenberg & Valletutti, 1980). Clinicians also bring to the therapy situation their own constellation of personal problems from other parts of their lives.

Stress may arise from the client or from significant others in the client's life. Clients may lack motivation, be noncompliant, fluctuate in their motivation and performance, become ill, and impose unrealistic expectations on the therapy process. Further, their own personal problems may hamper the helping process and indirectly cause stress for the clinician.

Stress can also stem from the work environment. Greenberg and Vallettuti (1980) describe such sources of stress as role ambiguity, role conflict, inequities in pay, and inadequate job status. Maslach (1982) adds conflict between co-workers, poor relationships with supervisors, and even the goals of the work setting. The agency's definition of success in therapy may be contrary to what clinician or client determines. It may be very difficult for a clinician to continue therapy for a dysarthric client when third-party insurers expect continued documented progress. While a client may need therapy to maintain existing skills, many governmental and private sources of therapy funding do not support maintenance therapy.

Burnout

The result of chronic stress incurred in a helping relationship is burnout. Maslach (1982) defines burnout as a "syndrome of emotional exhaustion, depersonalization, and reduced personal accomplishment that occurs among individuals who do 'people work'" (p. 3). She states that burnout is a unique form of stress because it stems from the "social interaction between helper and recipient" (p. 3). Corey (1982) lists nine causes of helper burnout: repetition of therapy tasks, minimal reward for maximal expenditure of energy, unrealistic expectations, minimal evident progress, lack of collegial support, conflict between organization administration and clinician, few opportunities for independent decision making, few opportunities for self-improvement, and unresolved personal problems. A speech-language pathologist providing dysarthria therapy is likely to incur some if not all of these causes of burnout.

The results of burnout also are numerous. The effects of burnout include "physical depletion and chronic fatigue, feelings of hopelessness and helplessness, and development of a negative self-concept and negative attitudes toward work, life, and other people" (Pines, 1982, p. 455). One of the most devastating effects of burnout is that the clinician stops caring about the client, provides only the most basic, nonchallenging therapy, and views the client and significant others in a cynical fashion. Eventually the clinician internalizes a negative concept about the helping relationship and broadcasts this attitude to other clients, caregivers, and families.

Coping with Stress and Burnout

The first step in coping with stress and burnout is identification. A variety of tools is available for clinicians to use to help identify and measure their burnout, including those developed by Pines (1982) and Maslach and Jackson (1982). These tools stress identifying the sources of stress within the individual, the client-clinician relationship, and the work environment. They also focus on identification of stress effects and behaviors. For example, the physical effects of stress can include headaches, colds, gastrointestinal problems, hypertension, and numerous other physical problems. Emotional stress effects can include feelings of hopelessness, frustration, powerlessness, and loneliness. Finally, the identification tools can help clinicians under stress to delineate specific stress behaviors in their lives. These may include eating and sleeping disorders, withdrawing, engaging in medication and alcohol abuse, and other negative activities.

A number of positive actions can be taken to prevent or ameliorate stress and burnout among helping professionals. These include reducing the staff-client ratio, making client selection more flexible, changing job tasks, and taking time out (Pines, 1982). Maslach (1982) states that a critical factor in helping to deal with burnout is the formal or informal support given by colleagues. She states that peers can provide help, insight, a basis for personal comparison, recognition, and a means of escape. She adds that the colleagues can help ease the burden through positive humor. Other techniques that help reduce burnout include improving communication skills with colleagues, administrators, clients, and significant others.

Finally, for some clinicians a period of time out will be crucial. This can be done through taking planned vacations, changing client types, and refocusing job tasks. Some clinicians may be helped by assuming a new role within the organization, participating in a research project, or attending a professional workshop or continuing-education course. Farmer, Monahan, and Hekeler (1984) give numerous techniques a person in a helping relationship might try in order to cope with the stresses and potential burnout of this position. Henderson and Bryan

(1984) caution those in helping relationships to keep the client's problems in perspective, to encourage self-help, and to use humor to help clients over rough spots. Their final comment may be the most important comment they make: "All helpers make mistakes when working with people with disabilities. They should learn from their mistakes and try not to repeat them" (p. 139).

Probe Questions for Speech-Language Pathologists

The questions in Table 6.3 can be used by speech-language pathologists to examine stress in their professional lives. This is not an exhaustive diagnostic tool, but may aid in establishing the presence of stress and therefore serving to initiate further self-evaluation or professional guidance.

TABLE 6.3
Probe Questions for Speech-Language Pathologists

Sources of Stress
1. What factors in my job do I find difficult?
2. How can I change these factors?
3. What kind and amount of personal and professional satisfaction do I receive from working with clients? families? other staff?
4. Are there opportunities for advancement?
5. What factors in my personal or family life are stressful?
6. Are my financial sources sufficient?
7. Is the institution I work in flexible and open to suggestions and change?

Effects of Stress
1. Does stress affect my physical well-being? How so? What are the symptoms?
2. Does stress affect my self-esteem and psychological well-being? How? What are the symptoms?
3. Does stress affect my everyday performance in therapy? diagnostics? family counseling? interactions with other staff? with my own family and friends?

Management of Stress
1. What do I do to cope with the causes and effects of stress?
2. Do I have a strong, meaningful support system? How do I use it?
3. Are there peers in my work environment with whom I can express my feelings?
4. Is professional help available to guide me through difficult stressful periods? Will I seek professional help and follow through with it?
5. Do I plan for time-out? vacations? personal time? recreation? physical exercise?

CASE STUDY

The following case study is offered to illustrate many of the concepts that have been developed in this chapter. It will serve as the concluding remarks for the chapter. Although the names of the principals have been changed, the story is true. The essence of this patient's story is that his speech problem extended far beyond the speech production difficulties he experienced. Both the patient and his family members were psychologically and emotionally affected by his situation, and the decision to institutionalize him was traumatic for all concerned. Working with this individual posed many complicated problems for the clinician.

Colonel Dick Canter was a 58-year-old retired army reserve officer who suffered a stroke with resultant mild aphasia and moderately dysarthric speech. Although his language skills improved quickly to nearly normal status, his speech remained dysarthric. Divorced 10 years prior to sustaining the stroke, Dick had lived alone in Washington, D.C. Two adult daughters resided in Dick's hometown—Buffalo, New York—and one son lived in California. Over the years, Dick had maintained little contact with his children, communicating with them only occasionally.

Following the stroke, Trisha, Dick's oldest daughter, assumed power of attorney for her father's affairs and became the primary decision maker in his life. She closed his apartment, sold most of his furnishings, and entered her father in a nursing home near where she lived. While in the nursing home Dick attended physical and speech therapy sessions, making excellent progress in physical therapy. His speech remained moderately dysarthric, however, and Trisha blamed that on the fact that her father had been a heavy drinker rather than on the fact that he had suffered a stroke.

Speech therapy sessions held twice weekly focused on improving Dick's speech intelligibility in sentences and conversation and emphasized self-monitoring of rate and articulatory clarity. During these sessions, Dick spoke of how unhappy he was in the nursing home. He perceived himself as a youthful, vigorous man in the company of a "bunch of old ladies." In reality, despite mild hypertension, he was physically fit and in good health. It was difficult for the speech clinician to focus therapy on improving the intelligibility of the patient's speech when Dick's primary concern (definition of the problem) was his need to live independently.

The social worker in the nursing home was sympathetic to Dick's problems but felt powerless to help him make changes in his living environment inasmuch as Dick's daughter was intent upon keeping her father in a controlled setting—the nursing home. Even though Trisha agreed that Dick might be motivated to improve his speech if he lived independently, she was afraid that if he left the nursing home he would begin drinking again. The speech clinician began to explore with Trisha the alternative living possibilities in the community, and it was during their discussions that Trisha revealed her long-held feelings about her father's drinking and his dominance over the family. At that time Trisha herself had several problems unrelated to her father's situation; her life was complicated by a pending divorce, a chronically ill preschooler, and her own need to return to work (multiple demands on caregiver). For Trisha, it was just easier to keep her father in the nursing home than to have him live elsewhere, regardless of his frustration and anger with that living arrangement.

Eventually Trisha agreed to move her father to a senior citizens health-related facility. Although this facility was less restrictive than the nursing home, Dick continued to perceive himself as "living with a bunch of old ladies." Moreover, during his stay in the nursing home he had established a personal relationship with a nurse there, and now he wanted a place where he could entertain her. During his weekly sessions with his speech clinician, he continued to focus on his need to live independently. His speech intelligibility improved somewhat, but he was preoccupied with changing his living environment, and that—not improvement of his speech—was his top priority. He told the clinician that in the setting in which he lived there was no one like him, no one with whom he could communicate, and therefore no real need for him to improve his speech communication (effects of institutionalization).

During the next year the speech clinician maintained close contact with Trisha, gently encouraging her to consider allowing her father to live alone in an apartment for a trial period. Dick was highly motivated to try this. Finally, when two years had passed since Dick sustained the stroke and he had had no alcohol during that time, Trisha agreed to look for a furnished apartment where her father could live for a 1-month trial period. She found such a place and this venture turned out to be successful. Eventually Dick moved to a small apartment close to shopping facilities and a bus line.

After he was settled in the apartment, Dick's motivation to improve his speech increased. At the present time, his speech, while not totally free of articulatory distortions, is very intelligible. He cares for all his needs except for his financial ones. Trisha continues to help in that area. Shortly after moving to his present home, Dick flew to California to visit his son whom he had not seen for several years. He reported that the visit was a successful one.

There is no doubt that Dick used his speech clinician as a primary communication partner during the therapy process. This was difficult for the clinician, since improving speech intelligibility seemed to be a secondary rather than a primary goal for Dick, and this was evident in every therapy session (clinician stress).

The clinician questioned her own role in the therapeutic situation—a role that extended far beyond that of a speech clinician. It was obvious that Dick and his daughter were using the clinician to work through their own personal difficulties. The clinician was faced with several alternatives: to terminate the case, to refer the family to a counselor, to focus therapy on speech production only, or to help the family work through its problems while continuing to work on the patient's speech production. Since both Dick and his daughter refused to seek counseling outside the speech therapy sessions, that was not a viable option. The clinician felt that the last alternative would be the most productive and, considering the positive outcome, it is apparent that the clinician chose the correct alternative. In fact, Trisha stated that she had not believed her father could live independently; it was the speech clinician's encouragement that convinced her to let him try.

Dick is no longer receiving formal speech therapy, but through follow-up telephone conversations the clinician has been able to determine that he is living successfully and is continuing to monitor his speech intelligibility. In this case, for the patient and his daughter, the definition of the problem did not include difficulty with speech production. Serious, long-term problems in their relationship, the effects of institutionalization, and personal demands on the daughter that were unrelated to her father's situation overshadowed the patient's speech problem. Until these other problems could be identified and solved, improving speech intelligibility was not a high priority for either the patient or his family. The speech clinician was willing to work with the client and his daughter within the framework of the problems that concerned them, and eventually that work resulted in the improvement of the patient's speech.

REFERENCES

Ainsworth, T. (1977). *Quality assurance in long-term care.* Germantown, MD: Aspen.

Baird, M., & Doherty, W. (1986). Family resources in coping with serious illness. In M. Karpel (Ed.), *Family resources: The hidden partner in family therapy* (pp. 359–383). New York: Guilford Press.

Bennett, R. (1963). The meaning of institutional life. *Gerontologist, 3,* 117–124.

Bernard, J., & Thompson, L. (1970). *Sociology of nurses and their patients in modern society.* St. Louis, MO: Mosby.

Bray, G. (1987). Family adaptation to chronic illness. In B. Caplan (Ed.), *Rehabilitation psychology desk reference* (pp. 171–184). Rockville, MD: Aspen.

Caplan, G., & Schecter, J. (1987). Denial and depression in disabling diseases. In B. Caplan (Ed.), *Rehabilitation psychology desk reference* (pp. 133–170). Rockville, MD: Aspen.

Committee on Aging. (1974). *Nursing home care in the U.S.: Failure in public policy.* Washington, DC: U.S. Government Printing Office.

Corey, G. (1982). *I never knew I had a chance.* Monterey, CA: Brooks, Cole.

Dunn, M. (1987). Social skills and rehabilitation. In B. Caplan (Ed.), *Rehabilitation psychology desk reference* (pp. 345–364). Rockville, MD: Aspen.

Farmer, R., Monahan, L., & Hekeler, R. (1984). *Stress management for human services.* Berkeley, CA: Sage.

Friedman, E. (1986). Resources for healing and survival of families. In M. Karpel (Ed.), *Family resources: The hidden partner in family therapy* (pp. 65–92). New York: Guilford Press.

Gerber, K., & Nekemkis, A. (1986). *Compliance: The dilemma of the chronically ill.* New York: Springer.

Goffman, E. (1961). *Asylums.* Garden City, NY: Anchor Books.

Goodstein, R. (1983). Cerebrovascular accident and the hospitalized elderly: A multidimensional clinical problem [Overview]. *American Journal of Psychiatry, 140,* 141–147.

Gottesman, L. (1973). Milieu treatment of the aged in institutions. *Gerontologist, 13,* 23–26.

Greenberg, S., & Valletutti, P. (1980). *Stress and the helping professions.* Baltimore, MD: Brooks Publisher.

Henderson, G., & Bryan, W. (1984). *Psychosocial aspects of disability.* Springfield, IL: Charles C. Thomas Publisher.

Hill, R. (1949). Generic features of families under stress. *Social Casework, 49,* 139–150.

Hudson, A. J. (1981). Amytrophic lateral sclerosis associated with dementia, Parkinsonism, and other neurological disorders: A review. *Brain, 104*(2), 217–247.

Imber-Black, E. (1986). Toward a resource model in systemic family therapy. In M. Karpel (Ed.), *Family resources: The hidden partner in family therapy* (pp. 148–174). New York: Guilford Press.

Jones, K. (1988). *The impact of C.V.A. on the family system.* Unpublished doctoral dissertation, State University of New York at Buffalo.

Jones, M. (1976). *Maturation of the therapeutic community.* New York: Human Sciences Press.

Kahana, E. (1973). The humane treatment of old people in institutions. *Gerontologist, 13,* 282–289.

Kastenbaum, R., & Candy, S. (1973). The four percent fallacy: A methodological and empirical critique of extended care facility statistics. *International Journal of Aging and Human Development, 4,* 15–21.

Kleemeier, R. (1961). *Aging and leisure.* New York: Oxford Press.

Koury, L. N., & Lubinski, R. (1991). Effective in-service training of a staff working with communication-impaired patients. In R. Lubinski (Ed.), *Dementia and communication* (pp. 279–291). Hamilton, Ontario: B. C. Decker Publishing.

Lemkau, J., Bryant, F., & Brickman, P. (1982). Client commitment to the helping relationship. In T. Wills (Ed.), *Basic processes in helping relationships.* New York: Academic Press.

Lieberman, M. (1969). Institutionalization of the aged. Effects on behavior. *Journal of Gerontology, 24,* 330–339.

Lubinski, R. (1981). Language and hearing programs in home health care and nursing homes. In D. Beasley & G. Davis (Eds.), *Aging: Communication processes and disorders* (pp. 339–356). New York: Grune and Stratton.

Lubinski, R. (1988). A model for intervention: Communication skills, effectiveness and opportunity. In B. Shadden (Ed.), *Communication behavior and aging* (pp. 294–308). Baltimore, MD: Williams and Wilkins.

Lubinski, R. (1991). Environmental considerations of elderly patients. In R. Lubinski (Ed.), *Dementia and communication* (pp. 257–278). Hamilton, Ontario: B. C. Decker Publishing.

Lubinski, R., Morrison, E., & Rigrodski, S. (1981). Perception of spoken communication by elderly and chronically ill patients in an institutional setting. *Journal of Speech and Hearing Disorders, 46,* 405–412.

Luterman, D. (1984). *Counseling the communicatively disordered and their families.* Austin, TX: PRO-ED.

Maslach, C. (1982). *Burnout: The cost of caring.* Englewood Cliffs, NJ: Prentice-Hall.

Maslach, C., & Jackson, S. (1982). Burnout in health professions: A social psychological analysis. In G. Sanders & J. Suls (Eds.), *Social psychology of health and illness* (pp. 227–254). Hillsdale, NJ: Erlbaum.

McCubbin, H., Boss, P., Wilson, L., & Lester, G. (1980). Developing family invulnerability to stress. In J. Trost (Ed.), *The family in change.* Vasters, Sweden: International Library.

McCubbin, H., & Patterson, J. (1983). Family stress process: A double ABC model of adjustment and adaptation. In H. McCubbin, J. Patterson, & M. Sussman. *Advancements and developments in family stress theory and research.* New York: Hayworth Press.

Miller, M., & Potter, R. (1982). Professional burnout among speech-language pathologists. *ASHA, 24,* 177–180.

Murgatroyd, S. (1985). *Counseling and helping.* London: British Psychological Society and Methuen.

Palmore, E. (1976). Total chance of institutionalization among the aged. *Gerontologist, 16,* 504–507.

Pines, A. (1982). Helpers and motivation and the burnout syndrome. In T. Wills (Ed.), *Basic processes in helping relationship.* New York: Academic Press.

Potter, R., & Rudensey, K. (1984). Coping with burnout. *ASHA, 26,* 35–38.

Power, P. (1985). Family coping behaviors in chronic illness: A rehabilitation perspective. *Rehabilitation Literature, 46,* 78–83.

Rauth, T. (1968). *Nursing homes.* Springfield, IL: Charles C. Thomas Publisher.

Rogers, C. (1951). *Client centered therapy.* Boston: Houghton.

Rosenstock, F., Goldman, M., & Rothenberg, R. (1969). Rehabilitation of the longterm patient: An action research program in milieu therapy. *Journal of Chronic Disabilities, 27,* 493–503.

Rossi, J., & Filstead, W. (Eds.). (1973). *The therapeutic community.* New York: Behavioral Publications.

Safilios-Rothchild, C. (1970). *The sociology and social psychology of disability and rehabilitation.* New York: Random House.

Satir, V. (1981). Family symptoms and approaches to family therapy. In G. Erickson & T. Hogan (Eds.), *Family therapy.* Monterey, CA: Brooks Cole.

Sussman, M. (1977). Dependent disabled and dependent poor: Similarity of conceptual issues and research needs. In J. Stubbins (Ed.), *Social and Psychological Aspects of Disability* (pp. 247–260). Baltimore, MD: University Park Press.

U.S. Department of Health and Human Services. (1983, August 11). *Advance data* (Public Health Services No. 91), pp. 1–4. Washington, DC: U.S. Government Printing Office.

PART III
Premotor Disorganization of Speech

CHAPTER 7

Apraxia of Speech Versus Phonemic Paraphasia: Theoretical, Diagnostic, and Treatment Considerations

Robert S. Pierce

> *Pierce discusses some current models of speech and language production. Breakdowns in different components of these models can lead to specific speech and language impairments in adults with aphasia and/or apraxia of speech. Special emphasis is placed on differentiating apraxia of speech from phonemic paraphasia with consideration given to diagnostic and treatment issues.*
>
> 1. *In the models discussed, where do breakdowns occur that lead to word retrieval problems and various types of paraphasias?*
> 2. *What patient behaviors are the most useful for differentiating apraxia of speech from phonemic paraphasias?*
> 3. *In reference to apraxia of speech, there is some thought that substitutions in the ear of the listener may actually be distortions in the mouth of the speaker. What do you think?*

The need to differentiate apraxia of speech from aphasia has echoed throughout the literature for more than a century. This distinction has gained fairly wide acceptance as professionals have recognized that the motor speech production errors of apraxia of speech are different from the word retrieval and grammatical formulation errors associated with aphasia. However, less clear are the behaviors encompassed by the term *apraxia of speech* and whether all errors that occur during speech production reflect disruption of the same underlying mechanism (Goodglass, 1975). It is the premise of this chapter that two distinct disorders exist, apraxia of speech and phonemic paraphasia, and that it is essential to differentiate between them, if for no other reason than because the treatment approaches for each disorder are different. This chapter begins with a discussion of models of speech and language production. Possible locations of errors within the production process are identified. The symptomatologies of apraxia of speech and paraphasias are compared and methods for their differential diagnosis are discussed. Finally, treatment considerations for each disorder are presented.

MODELS OF LANGUAGE PRODUCTION

In order to understand why different speech-language production errors occur, it is useful to review some recent theories of how words and sentences are produced. Toward this end, I will present a collage of ideas drawn primarily from the literature on the cognitive neuropsychology of language to further the understanding of where paraphasic and speech apraxic errors may originate. This discussion will focus on a psycholinguistic view of speech and language errors, emphasizing patient symptoms rather than syndromes. Figure 7.1 contains a visual image of this collage, based on models presented by several authors.

The overall framework, as indicated by the various levels, is based on the work of Garrett (1975, 1980). The process of constructing a sentence begins at the message level. The concepts and relationships aroused at this level activate a search through the mental lexicon for entries that represent those concepts (such as "girl," "boy," "hit") (Schwartz, 1987). The mental lexicon can be viewed as a store of contentive or open-class words. Each lexical entry contains three components, the syntactic, the semantic, and the phonological. The syntactic component contains information about the word's function, that is, whether it functions as a noun, verb, or adjective. The semantic component contains the word's meaning, including its categorical relationship, semantic features, and semantic relationships, along with associations for the word based on the speaker's personal experiences. The phonological component contains abstract representations of the phonemes

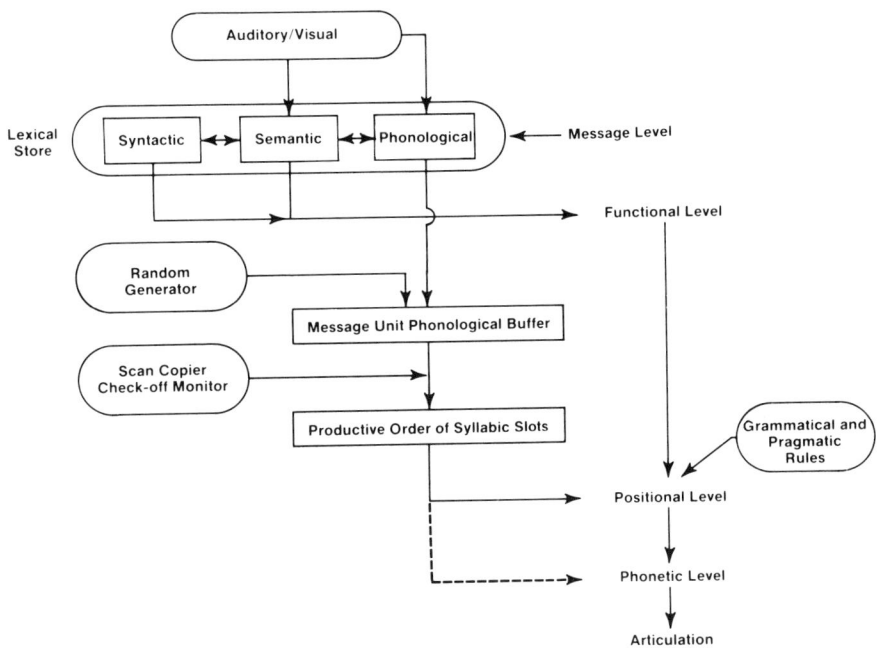

Figure 7.1 A model of language production.

that will comprise the eventual pronunciation of the word (Shattuck-Hufnagel, 1983). It is important to recognize that these components are independent of each other and that each component can be activated and acted upon independently of the others. It follows that these components can be differentially impaired resulting in disassociation of functions. This disassociation often is related to a specific site of neurologic lesion.

The entries activated by this search through the mental lexicon form the basis of the functional level where they are assigned roles in a predicate-argument structure (e.g., "girl hit boy") (Schwartz, 1987), and represent such relationships as agent, action, and object. Figure 7.2 delineates this stage. Two characteristics of the functional level are important. First, the predicate-argument structure is not specified as to its final grammatical form. For example, the relationship of "girl hit boy" can still be produced as an active or passive sentence. Second, the lexical entries are not specified as to their phonological form (Schwartz, 1987). Representation at the functional level is dependent on the syntactic and semantic components of the lexical entries only.

The phonological components of all lexical entries comprising the message unit (i.e., a phrase or clause) are activated and stored simul-

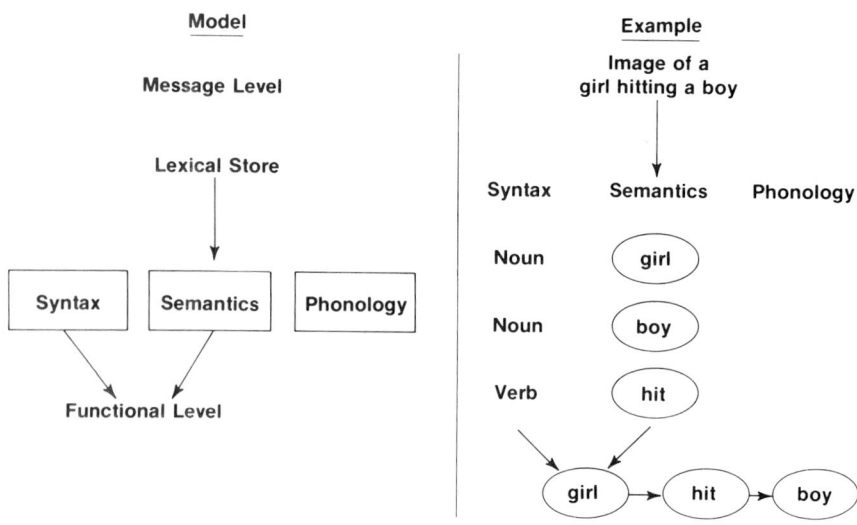

Figure 7.2 The evolution of the functional level from Figure 7.1.

taneously in a buffer (the message unit phonological buffer in Figure 7.1). The units that are stored here are phonemes (Shattuck-Hufnagel, 1983). As the positional level develops, two processes occur (see Figure 7.3). The phonemes contained in the buffer are selected and ordered into syllabic slots (Buckingham, 1987; Caplan, 1987), a process accomplished by a scan copier mechanism along with a checkoff monitor (Shattuck-Hufnagel, 1979, 1983). The scan copier scans the buffer, selects the appropriate phoneme, and copies or inserts it into its proper slot. Then the checkoff monitor either removes the phoneme from the buffer or identifies that it has been used. That the buffer contains phonological information from all of the contentive lexical entries of the message is important for two reasons. The first is that if the scan copier breaks down and selects phonemes in the wrong order, the errors can occur anywhere within the message unit (e.g., "the queer old dean" for "the dear old queen"). The second reason is that these slip-of-the-tongue errors occur primarily on content words (i.e., those activated at the functional level).

The second process at the positional level occurs when the lexical entries, with their ordered set of phonemes, are inserted into slots within a more fully outlined grammatical structure (Schwartz, 1987). It is at this level that grammatical rules are applied to form a specific phrase structure. As with lexical choice, the selection of appropriate grammat-

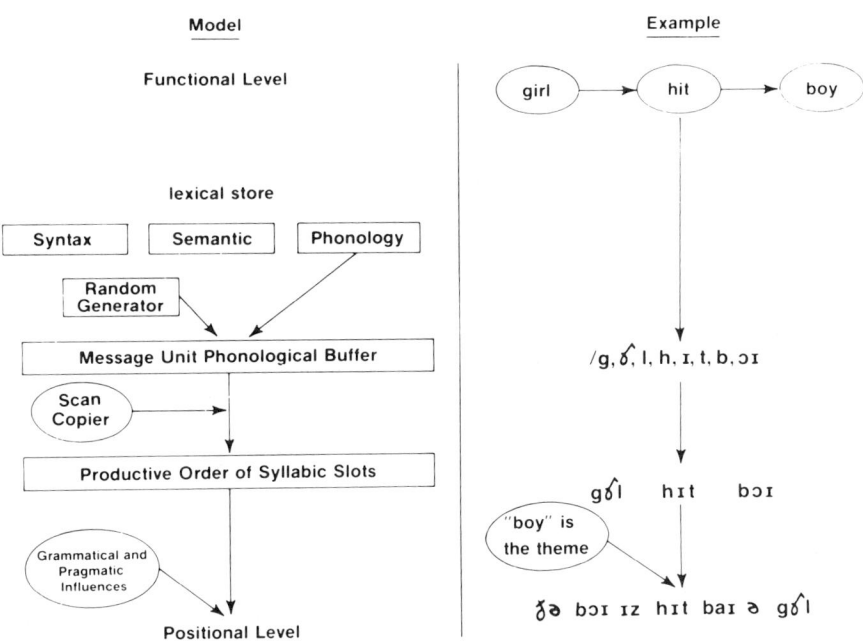

Figure 7.3 The evolution of the positional level from Figure 7.1.

ical form is directed by pragmatic and discourse considerations. For example, the predicate-argument structure "girl hit boy" can be expressed syntactically as either an active sentence ("The girl hit the boy") or a passive sentence ("The boy was hit by the girl") depending on the thematic requirements of the situation (i.e., who is being talked about). Other approaches to marking given-new relationships, such as the use of the definite versus indefinite article, also are applied at this level. Errors relating to the contentive lexical entries, such as reversals in word order or phoneme order, occur prior to morphosyntactic realization, since typically the final morphosyntactic form is appropriate for the incorrect output. For example, the correct article is used in "a money's aunt" even though the intended target was "an aunt's money" (Garrett, 1975).

While this discussion so far has related to sentence generation, the same procedures may be operative in single word productions and in oral reading, naming, and repetition. Single word productions remove the syntactic aspect of the event and can be extrapolated from Figure 7.1 as bypassing the positional level, with its grammatical influences, and going directly to the phonetic level designated by the dotted line.

Oral reading, naming, and repetition necessitate different inputs to the lexical store, bypassing the internal message level. The nature of these inputs is complex. In the normal course of events, the input (whether auditory as in repetition or visual as in reading and naming) activates both semantic and phonological components of the lexical entry. In fact, Caramazza, Berndt, and Brownell (1982) provide a model in which the semantic component plays an active role in the perceptual analysis of the input. Many other authors discuss similar top-down effects (see Pierce 1988 for a review of these contextual effects as they relate to comprehension processes in aphasia; see Vogel and Miller, Chapter 4 in this volume, for these effects as they relate to the treatment of dysarthric speech).

However, auditory or visual input can activate either the semantic or the phonological component alone. Activation of only the phonological component occurs in transcortical sensory aphasia where repetition is intact without comprehension (Goodglass & Kaplan, 1983) and in hyperlexia where oral reading occurs without comprehension (also seen occasionally in Wernicke's aphasia). Patients with dementia can read aloud and participate in confrontation-naming tasks without accessing the meaning component of the lexical store (Bayles & Kasniak, 1987). Activation of only the semantic component is seen clearly in word retrieval lapses where individuals demonstrate that they know the intended word but fail to retrieve the phonological form needed to produce it.

Communication Breakdown

Breakdown can occur at many points in the processes outlined in Figure 7.1 and will be discussed in the section that follows. Breakdown can occur in the retrieval of an appropriate semantic entry within the lexical store. When the word retrieved is semantically dissimilar to the target word but its phonological form is produced appropriately (e.g., "house" instead of "cat"), it is referred to as a verbal paraphasia. When the word retrieved is semantically similar to the target word and is produced in a phonologically correct form (e.g., "dog" instead of "cat"), it is referred to as a semantic paraphasia. Results of many studies have suggested that some individuals, particularly those with fluent aphasia, have a disrupted semantic representation that impairs the ability to retrieve accurate semantic components from the lexical store (Caramazza et al., 1982; Grober, Perecman, Kellar, & Brown, 1980; Whitehouse, Caramazza, & Zurif, 1978).

An individual may retrieve the semantic component of a word successfully but fail to retrieve the phonological form within the lexical store. This can happen to normal speakers, but they continue on by substituting a word, talking around the lapse (circumlocution), or in some way indicating that they cannot "think" of the precise word. This particularly frustrating event seems to occur often while working crossword puzzles or participating in games such as Scrabble or Trivial Pursuit. This "phonological" breakdown is more common in individuals with aphasia, regardless of syndrome, than it is in normal speakers. Some aphasic persons, especially those with Wernicke's aphasia, fill the empty space left by the lack of an appropriate phonological form with a randomly generated string of phonemes (Butterworth, 1979). This creates an unintelligible response referred to by Buckingham (1987) as an abstruse neologism. There is no known underlying phonological representation in an abstruse neologism. While the random generator proposed by Butterworth randomly selects phonemes for inclusion in the buffer, it is evident that the scan copier is sensitive to the phonotactic rules of the language, since phoneme sequences that are not permissible in English are seldom produced. The random generator also may become activated when the search for a semantic component fails completely and no phonological form is available. In Figure 7.1, the location of the random generator is between the phonological component of the lexical store and the phonological buffer associated with the message.

Breakdowns can occur in the functioning of the scan copier. It is at this level that phonemic paraphasias occur (Buckingham, 1987; Caplan, 1987). Phonological information is retrieved correctly from the lexical store and input into the message unit buffer. However, the scan copier fails to map a phoneme from the buffer accurately onto its appropriate production slot. Phonemes become juxtaposed, deleted, added, and sequentially misordered. While it is beyond the scope of this chapter to discuss the mechanics of the breakdown of the scan copier and the associated checkoff monitor, the interested reader is referred to Shattuck-Hufnagel (1979, 1987) for analyses of slips of the tongue and to Buckingham (1987; 1989) for analyses of phonemic paraphasias. What is important for our purposes is that the errors involve phonemes as abstract processing units and that they occur prior to stages of motor production. In addition, these errors should not be viewed as word retrieval errors, since the appropriate semantic and phonological information is retrieved from the lexical store. Because more than one lexical entry can exist in the message unit phonological buffer at one time, errors can occur across word boundaries. For example, one patient produced the sequence "his hat is on the ... shop ... /ʃe/ ... top ... shef ... shelf." The /ʃ/ phoneme from "shelf" was inaccurately mapped onto word initial position in "top." This is similar to what happens in slips of the tongue. Shattuck-Hufnagel (1987) states that word onset segments are more prone to interaction errors than are medial or final segments in slips of the tongue.

Breakdowns can occur in combinations. For example, the wrong word may be retrieved from the semantic component of the lexical store (e.g., "dog" for "cat"). It is then subjected to a phonemic paraphasia because of a faulty scan copier mechanism (e.g., dog → tog). The resulting utterance "tog" has little resemblance to the target word "cat." This is referred to as a target-related neologism because there is a known target word that has undergone several transformations (Buckingham, 1987). It reflects an underlying word retrieval deficit in addition to a disorder of the scan copier mechanism (Buckingham, 1981). Another example occurs on the audiotape *Motor speech disorders* (Darley, Aronson, & Brown, 1975). A female patient is asked to repeat a sentence containing the words "roast beef" and she responds, "road peach . . . peef . . . beef." A clear phonemic paraphasia is produced transforming "roast" to "road." Then she produces a semantic paraphasia substituting "peach" for "beef." In an attempt to correct this error, the patient retrieves the correct word, both semantic and phonological components, and inputs it into the message unit phonological buffer. However, apparently the phonological information from "peach" is still active and the two become combined by the scan copier. It is not clear whether the final position /f/ from "beef" combines with "peach" or whether the initial position /p/ of "peach" combines with "beef." In either case, the patient again recognizes the error and corrects it. One of the author's Wernicke's aphasic patients produced "tclebone" for "umbrella." Presumably the phonemic paraphasia (f → b) was overlaid on the verbal paraphasia (umbrella → telephone).

It is not always easy or even possible to identify the root causes of the errors produced by some patients. For example, a patient with Wernicke's aphasia produced "roll pickle" for "record player." This could reflect verbal paraphasias or severe phonemic paraphasias overlaid upon accurately retrieved semantic and phonological information from the lexical store. The same patient also told us of "pamples you can hold." The source of this error was not clear until she made us aware through gestures that she was discussing the parts of her glasses. No doubt the experienced clinician can recall many additional examples of similar errors.

The types of errors outlined above can be rank-ordered to reflect degrees of impairment. The abstruse neologism is the most severe because with this error complete failure occurs in retrieval of phonological information from the lexical store, and the resulting production provides the listener with no usable information for communication. Target-related neologisms caused by phonemic paraphasias overlaid upon incorrectly retrieved lexical items reflect somewhat less severe impairment; they show the retrieval of at least some lexical entry. Verbal and semantic paraphasias are less troublesome still. Although incorrect semantic forms are retrieved, the phonological components are correctly retrieved and produced. Semantic paraphasias are not as likely to impair communication as verbal paraphasias, since the semantic errors capture more of the meaning aspects of the target utterance and therefore convey more usable information to the listener. Phonemic paraphasias are the least detrimental to communication because they reflect a relatively intact lexical retrieval system with a breakdown in the scan copier mechanism. Frequently the error production is related closely enough to the target word so that the listener can use context to derive the intended meaning. As a patient begins to recover from aphasia, often the predominant error type evolves through these stages. Treatment is designed to facilitate this evolving process.

While neologisms and verbal and semantic paraphasias are characteristic of the speech of Wernicke's aphasics, and phonemic paraphasias are typically found in the speech of conduction aphasics, these two aphasic types are not mutually exclusive. Usually patients with either syndrome will produce most of these types of errors. However, for each syndrome certain error types predominate. One striking difference between Wernicke's aphasic patients and conduction aphasic patients is that patients with conduction aphasia are more successful at monitoring and correcting their errors (Joanette, Keller, & Lecours, 1980) and therefore may be more disturbed by their errors.

Referring again to Figure 7.1, for conduction aphasic patients the ability to self-correct may relate to the mechanism underlying phonemic paraphasias. These errors occur because of faulty functioning of the scan copier. The information in the message unit phonological buffer is intact and serves as a target. The patients realize that the phonemes they produced do not match the target, and so they try again. It has been this author's experience that often these patients are aware of their potential errors even before they attempt to produce the word. This suggests that they are able to compare the output of the scan copier (the productive order within the syllable slots) with the information in the message unit phonological buffer. In contrast, patients with Wernicke's aphasia frequently are not aware of their errors, and in cases where they are aware they have great difficulty correcting them. Usually these errors involve breakdowns in retrieval from the semantic and/or phonological components of the lexical store; therefore the information in the message unit phonological buffer is inaccurate and cannot serve as a reliable target. In fact, except for the phonemic paraphasias, the scan copier accurately passes all this information on to the next stage so the utterance actually matches the target as contained in the message unit phonological buffer.

The reader will note that patients with anomic aphasia have not been mentioned. In cases of anomic aphasia, while there is a breakdown in retrieval of semantic and/or phonological information from the lexical store, these patients do not demonstrate copious involuntary substitutions of incorrect words and sounds as do the patients who exhibit paraphasic errors.

From Planning to Production

Typically the production of speech utilizes three stages: planning, programming, and execution. A linguistic intent is developed based on the processes described in the previous sections of this chapter. The output of these processes is in the form of phonological goals that "represent the intent of the system to generate an acoustic output that is perceptually acceptable" (Abbs, 1986). Particular movements or actions of specific muscles are not dictated by these goals; rather, it is the role of the programming system to convert these goals into appropriate movement patterns. The programming system is represented by the phonetic level of representation in Figure 7.1.

The purpose of the programming system is to determine and coordinate movements across different muscle groups (e.g., larynx, tongue, lips, and palate) to achieve the perceptual goals (Abbs, 1986; Keller, 1987). For example, the programming system coordinates laryngeal activity with lip movement during bilabial productions or palatal activity with tongue movement during the production of nasals. This is the primary distinction between the programming system and the execution system (the articulation level in Figure 7.1), which acts on muscle groups relating to a single articulatory valve (e.g., the larynx or the tongue or the palate) (Keller, 1987). Electrical stimulation studies and work with primates support the concept that the primary motor cortex (Broadmann's area 4) activates individual muscle groups relating to a single articulatory value, while the premotor cortex activates multimovement gestures involving more than one articulator (Abbs, 1986; Keller, 1987).

The specific motor commands developed by the programming system do not have to be identical each time the same utterance is produced. There are many configurations of the vocal tract that can produce the same perceptually acceptable goals. This notion of motor equivalence related to the capacity of a motor system to obtain the same end-product despite considerable variation in the components that contribute to that output (Hughes & Abbs, 1976). Related to this notion is the finding that one muscle group will change its activity to compensate for changes in the activity of a different muscle group in order to maintain the integrity of the perceptual goal (Abbs, 1986; Folkins & Abbs, 1976). For example, limiting the movement of the jaw during bilabial closure will lead to greater movement of the lip to achieve the closure.

Based on the findings that coarticulation occurs across word boundaries (Daniloff & Moll, 1968), it is likely that the programming system coordinates multigesture movements across elements of the message unit exceeding a word. Whether or not the role of sensory feedback is a necessary component to the programming process is controversial. Although Borden (1979) states that speech production does not require feedback under typical, predictable circumstances, feedback is more important under unpredictable circumstances, for example, when the vocal tract is in an unusual position. Sensory feedback from the articulators is available to the motor programming system via the basal ganglia and cerebellum prior to the production of speech (Gracco & Abbs, 1987). A functioning programming system should be able to utilize this information to determine the best combination of motor commands depending on the specific vocal tract configuration.

Disruptions in the programming system result in apraxia of speech that is characterized by difficulty in determining and coordinating interarticulatory movements for the production of speech. Breakdowns in the execution of motor commands by one or more muscle groups cause dysarthria and usually are associated with some degree of weakness, slowness, incoordination, or alteration of muscle tone (Berry, 1983), symptoms that typically are absent in apraxia of speech.

CHARACTERISTICS OF APRAXIA OF SPEECH AND OF PARAPHASIAS

So far I have attempted to show that the characteristics of apraxia of speech can be very different from the characteristics of phonemic paraphasias. In general, paraphasias are incorrectly selected and sequenced phonemes that are subsequently articulated with normal amounts of effort and accuracy. Apraxia of speech reflects accurately selected phonemes that are articulated with a great amount of effort and inaccurate patterns of articulatory movement. Before proceeding, some cautionary comments are in order. Apraxia of speech and paraphasias are symptoms, not syndromes. They represent specific disruptions of components of the speech and language production system. For example, apraxia of speech is a symptom of the nonfluent aphasias such as Broca's aphasia, but is not symptomatic of the speech of all patients with Broca's aphasia.

Conversely, patients with Broca's aphasia have language deficits in addition to their motor programming difficulties (otherwise they would be apraxic but not aphasic). Accordingly, the errors these patients produce reflect those language difficulties in addition to their motor impairments. Thus it is not reasonable to automatically consider the speech errors of a Broca's aphasic patient to reflect apraxia.

Similarly, paraphasias typically are associated with the fluent aphasias, particularly the Wernicke's and conduction types. In fact, phonemic paraphasias are a prominent feature of conduction aphasia. It is known, however, that conduction aphasia may have at least two main varieties (Kempler et al., 1986). Consequently there may be a motor component of the speech errors produced by some patients with conduction aphasia. It should be realized, however, that in cases of conduction aphasia it is not reasonable to assign these motoric influences to paraphasias. It is important to remember that the two can coexist. Buckingham and Yule (1987) recently have suggested that motoric influences also may be evident in the speech of patients with Wernicke's aphasia. With these precautions in mind, the characteristics of the two symptoms will be discussed.

Effort

Probably the most prevalent distinction between apraxia of speech and phonemic paraphasia involves effort. While studies of effort per se are few, frequently effort is mentioned in the literature in connection with subject selection criteria. For example, Kent and Rosenbek (1983) stated their apraxic patients demonstrated "effortful trial and error groping, articulatory movements and attempts at self-correcting" and "obvious difficulty in initiating utterances" (p. 232). In a comparison of patients with apraxia of speech and patients with paraphasias, Hough (1978) found the primary distinction between the two was the presence of initiation difficulties manifested as audible groping by patients with apraxia of speech. Initiation difficulty with groping behavior as the patient searches for appropriate patterns of movements to articulate sounds correctly seems to be a natural result of a breakdown in motor programming skills.

While it is not unusual for patients with apraxia of speech to attempt to self-correct their speech errors, this behavior does not seem to differentiate them from paraphasic speakers. Joanette, Keller, and Lecours (1980) reported that patients with conduction aphasia were more successful at self-correcting consonant productions than were the Broca's or Wernicke's aphasic patients they studied. These authors observed that patients with conduction aphasia typically were more persistent in their correction attempts than were patients with Broca's aphasia. In addition, Kohn (1984) reported that patients with conduction aphasia produced a greater number and longer self-correction attempts than did patients with Broca's aphasia, but that the conduction aphasic patients were not more successful than the Broca's aphasic patients at producing the intended responses. These results demonstrated that for both types of aphasia—conduction and Broca's—the target word was intact and the internal feedback systems used remained operative to compare their utterances with the targets.

Another behavior that possibly may contribute to the perception of effort is syllable fragmentation. Kent and Rosenbek (1982, 1983) identified syllable segregation in the speech of apraxic patients. Syllables became separated by pauses and the intended word was not produced as a cohesive unit. This behavior can be observed in paraphasic speech also. Kohn (1984) reported that conduction aphasic patients produced word fragments in paraphasic speech. Although the tendency to break a word into syllables while speaking does not differentiate these two populations, presumably, the underlying reasons for this behavior are quite different. Because of their difficulty in generating coordinated movement patterns, apraxic speakers appear to use a syllable approach so that the programming demands are exerted over a smaller unit. They program the production of one syllable and pause before beginning to program the next syllable. They may do this because it is easier for them than programming at one point the movements for several syllables. In contrast, syllable segregation in patients with conduction aphasia may be a function of the patients' monitoring behaviors. That is, when patients become aware of producing a wrong phoneme, they stop at the next junction, possibly at the end of the syllable, to attempt to correct the error.

Other aspects of speech production such as coarticulation may differentiate apraxic and paraphasic speakers. Ziegler and von Cramon (1985, 1986) demonstrated a lack of coarticulation in a patient with apraxia of speech who showed a delay in the initiation of anticipatory vowel gestures. Similarly, apraxic speakers demonstrate prolonged articulations of both vowel steady states and transitions (Keller, 1984; Kent & Rosenbek, 1982, 1983) and tend to simplify their utterances so as to generate easier transitions between adjacent phonemes (Keller, 1984). They also show transitionalization errors during the production of consonant clusters, such as pauses between the consonants, intrusive vocalic sounds, and prolongations of the first consonant in the cluster (Canter, Trost, & Burns, 1985). These behaviors serve to separate the segments to be produced so that they can be programmed independently. These types of behaviors are not typically evident in the speech of paraphasic speakers. Therefore, while both groups of patients demonstrate breaks between syllables, apraxic speakers show disruptions within syllables.

Substitutions

When the listener applies a broad phonological transcription to both apraxic and paraphasic utterances, most errors are perceived as substitutions (Canter, Trost, & Burns, 1985; Monoi, Fukusako, Itoh, & Sasanuma, 1983; Nespoulous, Joanette, Ska, Caplan, & Lecours, 1987). However, there are important differences between the substitutions produced by the two groups of speakers. Usually the perceived substitutions of the apraxic speakers are only one distinctive feature from the target phonemes. Common error patterns observed include voiceless for voiced substitutions (Nespoulous et al., 1987; Trost & Canter, 1974) and changes in place of articulation for voiced consonants (Nespoulous et al., 1987). The most stable place of production is the alveolar ridge and the most stable production manners are stops and glides (Klich, Ireland, & Weidner, 1979). In contrast, the substitution errors produced by paraphasic speakers are frequently farther than one distinctive feature away from the target, that is, the errors can be two or three distinctive features away (Canter, Trost, & Burns, 1985; Monoi et al., 1983; Nespoulous et al., 1987). In addition, paraphasic errors are less stable or predictable (Nespoulous et al., 1987), that is, paraphasic speakers produce a greater variety of error phonemes for any specific target phoneme than do apraxic speakers. These results are consistent with the notion of a greater motor component for the apraxic errors than for the paraphasic errors.

Another aspect of apraxic errors is that the perceived substitutions may be just that—perceived rather than spoken. While apraxic speakers produce numerous errors of distortion, there is increasing agreement that apraxic speakers may distort their productions to such an extent that the acoustic features cross category boundaries and are perceived as representatives of a phonemic category different from the intended one. Thus the errors are not really substitutions of one phoneme for another but distortions of accurately selected phonemes. As stated previously, many of the errors demonstrated by apraxic speakers are perceived as voiceless for voiced substitutions. MacNeilage (1982) argues that it is considerably more difficult to produce voiced stops and fricatives than it is to produce their voiceless cognates. Accordingly, apraxic speech contains more voiceless than voiced sounds, and this rarely is observed in paraphasic speech. The acoustic feature of voicing is conveyed to a large extent by voice onset time, which requires precise coordination between laryngeal functioning and movements of the supralaryngeal articulators. Several studies of apraxic speakers have demonstrated that this coordination is impaired and leads to voice onset times that are inappropriate for the target sounds, sometimes occurring within the boundaries of the sound's cognate (Blumstein, Cooper, Goodglass, Statlender, & Gottlieb, 1980; Itoh et al., 1982; Kent & Rosenbek, 1983). Duffy and Gawle (1984) reported that apraxic speakers were impaired in their control of vowel duration preceding voiced or unvoiced consonants.

Vowel durations preceding voiced consonants were so aberrant that they were within the range expected for a subsequent voiceless consonant.

Similar difficulty in coordinating velar movement with other articulators was demonstrated by Itoh, Sasanuma, and Ushijima (1979) for an apraxic speaker but not for patients with Wernicke's aphasia (Itoh, Sasanuma, Hirose, Yoshioka, & Sawashima, 1983); Itoh, Sasanuma, Hirose, Yoshioka, and Ushijima (1980) reported the temporal disorganization of movements between the lips, tongue, and velum observed for an apraxic speaker. They concluded: "This finding seems to indicate that the motor programming for the temporal organization of different articulators becomes difficult in apraxia of speech under certain conditions resulting in inconsistent articulation errors" (p. 73). Also Fromm et al. (1982) reported a considerable degree of temporal disorganization between different muscle groups in apraxic speakers.

LESS COMMON TYPES OF ERRORS

Paraphasic speakers demonstrate some types of errors that are not common in apraxic speakers, for example, the sequencing of sounds in the wrong order in a word or transposition of sounds from one part of the utterance to an earlier or later part of the word (Canter et al., 1985; Monoi et al., 1983; Nespoulous et al., 1987). These errors can arise from the combination of a breakdown in the scan copier and a faulty check-off monitor (Buckingham, 1987). Several investigators have reported that apraxic errors occur more frequently on consonants while paraphasic errors occur relatively more frequently on vowels (Canter et al., 1985; Monoi et al., 1983). In contrast to the finding by Canter et al., McNeil, Hunter, Rosenbek, and Fennell (1987), using a narrow phonetic transcription, found that apraxic speakers demonstrate relatively equal numbers of errors on consonants and vowels. Paraphasic speakers may produce more errors at the end of the word than do apraxic speakers (Canter et al., 1985).

Repetition

It has been suggested that a hallmark of conduction aphasia is the inability to perform a repetition task accurately (Goodglass & Kaplan, 1983). Caplan (1987) found that for aphasic patients repetition, especially of nonsense words and multisyllabic words, was more impaired than oral reading. Similarly, Nespoulous et al. (1987) found a significantly poorer performance on repetition than on oral reading for patients with conduction aphasia, a finding that did not hold for patients with Broca's aphasia. In contrast, Canter et al. (1985) found no significant difference between repetition and naming of single syllable words, although they recognized that a difference was more likely to be found using multisyllabic words, phrases, and sentences.

The patient who demonstrates impairment in repetition may not be able to develop and maintain an internal phonological representation (Friedrich, Glenn, & Marin, 1984). Such a representation probably would be at the level of the message unit phonological buffer (see Figure 7.1). This phonological representation is unstable and fades rapidly; therefore the scan copier is deprived of information on which to work and errors result. This may explain why paraphasic errors occur with relative frequency toward the end of words. That is, the phonological information may decay before the copying occurs. If the initial stimulus remains constant and available, as in confrontation naming and oral reading tasks, the message unit phonological buffer can be reactivated continually. This would maintain appropriate target information to support the patient's tenacious attempts at self-correction. When the stimulus presented is momentary and fades rapidly, repetition is poor as is the ability to self-correct errors (Joanette, Keller, & Lecours, 1980).

To conclude this section, it is appropriate to reiterate the caution that apraxia of speech and paraphasias are symptoms only. A patient with Broca's aphasia probably will demonstrate linguistically based errors in addition to apraxia of speech. Similarly there may be a motor component in addition to the paraphasic substitutions of conduction aphasia. It becomes the speech-language clinician's responsibility to determine the symptom that is most detrimental to the patient's communication and to plan treatment accordingly.

DIAGNOSIS

In standard clinical practice, a complete evaluation is conducted in order to identify communication dysfunction. The interested reader is referred to Wertz, LaPointe, and Rosenbek (1984) for a description of a complete speech evaluation for patients with suspected motor speech disorders. This section will discuss those behaviors that can be used to differentiate between apraxia of speech and paraphasias.

No test exists presently that provides a tally of scores that differentiates apraxia from paraphasia. Currently the best approach for evaluation is to design verbal tasks that provide a sufficient number of examples on which to base the diagnosis. A number of these tasks are listed in the *Apraxia Battery for Adults* (Dabul, 1979) and in the *Motor Speech Evaluation* (Wertz et al., 1984). A sample of the tasks are the following:

1. A spontaneous speech sample including conversation and picture description
2. Oral reading of a standard paragraph
3. Vowel prolongation
4. Alternate motion rates (syllabic diadochokinesis)
5. Repetition of monosyllabic words with identical sounds in the initial and final position of a word, for example, "mom," "zoos"
6. One repetition of multisyllabic words
7. Repetition of several multisyllabic words several times each, for example, "artillery," "television"
8. Repetition of words of increasing length, for example, "flat," "flatter," "flattering"
9. Repetition of sentences containing multisyllabic words
10. Counting forward and backward

Performance on these tasks should reveal the presence of apraxia of speech; however, it will also reveal paraphasic difficulties. Therefore poor performance on these tasks does not guarantee the patient has apraxia of speech. Accordingly, it is necessary to observe carefully the behaviors exhibited.

To facilitate this process, it is useful for the clinician to examine certain behaviors in order to structure the observations during the evaluation. Table 7.1 contains the list of behaviors included in the *Apraxia Battery for Adults* (Dabul, 1979).

Dabul suggests that if five or more of the behaviors listed in Table 7.1 are present, apraxia of speech can be identified and that the more behaviors present, the greater the severity of the apraxia of speech. Based on the information discussed previously in this chapter, I believe that only three of these behaviors (difficulty in initiating speech, intrusion of a schwa, and abnormal prosodic features) are uniquely characteristic of apraxia, and so can be used to differentiate apraxia from paraphasia. Number 6, visible and audible searching, may be useful in differentiating the disorders depending on how the term *searching* is defined. Apraxic speakers search and grope for appropriate articulatory positions and movement patterns, while paraphasic speakers search for the correct phoneme to produce. The searching behavior by paraphasic speakers is both visible and audible but is not particularly groping in nature. The remaining 11 behaviors listed in Table 7.1 are characteristic of paraphasia as well as apraxic speech. Some (phonemic transpositions, vowel errors, off-target attempts at the word, and highly inconsistent errors) may be more characteristic of paraphasia than of apraxia. Accordingly, this particular inventory of speech characteristics does not effectively differentiate between apraxia and paraphasia.

TABLE 7.1
Inventory of Articulation of Characteristics of Apraxia

1. The subject exhibits phonemic anticipatory errors (*gl*een glass for *gr*een glass)
2. The subject exhibits phonemic perseverative errors (boo*b* for boo*t*)
3. The subject exhibits phonemic transposition errors (A*ri*fca for A*fri*ca)
4. The subject exhibits phonemic voicing errors (*b*en for *p*en)
5. The subject exhibits phonemic vowel errors (m*oa*n for m*a*n)
6. The subject exhibits visible and audible searching
7. The subject exhibits numerous and varied off-target attempts at the word
8. The subject's errors are highly inconsistent
9. The subject's errors increase as phonemic sequence increases
10. The subject exhibits fewer errors in automatic speech than in volitional speech
11. The subject exhibits marked difficulty initiating speech
12. The subject intrudes a schwa sound /ə/ between syllables or in consonant clusters
13. The subject exhibits abnormal prosodic features
14. The subject exhibits awareness of errors, and inability to correct them
15. The subject exhibits a receptive-expressive gap

Note. From *Apraxia Battery for Adults* by B. Dabul, 1979, Austin, TX: PRO-ED. Copyright 1979 by PRO-ED. Reprinted by permission.

Table 7.2 provides a list of questions that can be used to attempt to differentiate between apraxic and phonemic paraphasic errors. These are questions about behaviors typical of apraxic and paraphasic speech. In addition to these questions, other features can be considered. Typically apraxia of speech occurs in conjunction with the nonfluent aphasias and thus is associated with lesions of the left anterior cortex. Often there is a right hemiplegia. Paraphasias are associated with the fluent aphasias caused by lesions of the left posterior cortex. While a hemiparesis may be present, this occurs less frequently with a posterior than with an anterior lesion. Apraxia of speech is characterized by disturbed prosody (Kent & Rosenbek, 1982, 1983), while prosody is usually relatively intact in paraphasic speech. The disturbed prosody associated with apraxia may not represent a true impairment in the use of suprasegmental phonemes but may be a by-product of the reduction in the size of the message unit to single words or syllables for the purpose of facilitating motor programming demands. Finally, for globally impaired patients who produce no speech at all, determining whether or not apraxia is present is very difficult. As these patients begin to recover from their aphasia, however, apraxia may become evident. It is unlikely that paraphasia without apraxia would be observed.

TABLE 7.2
Questions to Differentiate Apraxia of Speech from Phonemic Paraphasia

Question	Apraxia	Paraphasia
1. Is there audible and visible groping for the initial articulatory positions of a word?	Yes	No
2. Does the patient produce errors within a syllable such as vowel and transition prolongations, reduced coarticulation, and pauses and/or vocalic sounds between consonant blends?	Yes	No
3. Are the perceived substitutions close to the targets and relatively consistent or predictable?	Yes	No
4. Are the perceived substitutions more off-target and unpredictable?	No	Yes
5. Does the patient produce many errors of phoneme sequencing and transpositions?	No	Yes
6. Is there the perception of a relatively high incidence of errors on vowels and in word final position?	No	Yes
7. Is repetition worse than nonrepetition, especially for multisyllabic words and sentences?	No	Yes

TREATMENT

Apraxia of Speech

The treatment of apraxic errors is dramatically different from the treatment of paraphasic errors. In general the treatment for apraxia of speech is based on imitation. Basing the treatment of paraphasic speech on imitation, however, would be like reading Wertz and Rosenbek without a degree in English literature, a dictionary, and a good sense of humor. There is no reason to expect that it could be done successfully.

Much has been written about treating apraxia of speech. Two particularly good sources are Wertz, LaPointe, and Rosenbek (1984) and Square-Storer (1989). In this section some traditional and some less than traditional approaches will be highlighted.

Apraxia of speech can be severe, moderate, or mild. When the apraxia is severe, the goal for treatment is the production of speech sounds in isolation, syllables, and words. If the patient is successful in producing sounds simply by imitating the clinician's verbal productions, then imitation can be considered the preferred technique. The eight-step continuum suggested by Rosenbek, Lemme, Ahern, Harris, and Wertz (1973) leads the patient from the production of speech by imitation to more spontaneous use of speech in role-playing situations. Deal and Florance (1978) suggest that the difficulty experienced by some patients, particularly with the middle steps in the eight-step continuum, can be alleviated by using an accumulative measure for reaching criteria at the lower steps before progressing to higher steps. Presumably, this accumulative measure may provide the patient with correct and stable responding in the early stages before moving on. Dabul and Bollier (1976) also outlined an imitative approach, although they emphasize nonmeaningful speech movements for improving the sequencing of speech movements. These authors suggest that individual consonants should be trained in isolation, and that the vowel /a/ should be added to the trained consonant to form syllables. Finally, the syllables are combined into sequences and words. Dabul and Bollier recommended nonmeaningful stimuli, reasoning that apraxic speakers need to learn movement patterns that can be applied to difficult words by using a sound-by-sound attack procedure.

When imitative approaches are not successful, other techniques can be tried. One technique is to substitute another stimulus for an auditory one or to combine an auditory stimulus with another type of stimulus. For example, some patients can produce words more accurately when reading (Collins, Cariski, Longstretch, & Rosenbek, 1980), and Simmons (1980) reported a case of a blind apraxic speaker whose verbal production improved when auditory and tactile (braille) stimuli were combined.

When treating severe apraxia, direct techniques may be needed. Wertz et al. (1984) suggest phonetic derivation, that is, observing the speech or nonspeech movements produced by the speaker and modifying the movements to form specific sounds. For example, humming can be used to generate voiced sounds, and placing the tongue behind the upper teeth and producing a clicking sound can lead to the production of /t/. A technique that is often coupled with derivation is phonetic placement, in which the clinician uses visual stimuli and describes and demonstrates how sounds are made in the mouth. In addition the clinician manually manipulates the patient's articulators to achieve appropriate positions and movements. Recently Square, Chumpelik, Morningstar, and Adams, (1986) reported success with a phonetic placement technique, the PROMPT system, used with adult apraxic patients. PROMPT stands for Prompts for Restructuring Oral Muscular Phonetic Targets and was developed by Chumpelik (1984) for use with developmentally apraxic children. It is a tactile-based program that employs a highly structured set of finger placements on the patient's face and neck to represent oral positions. These finger placements provide feedback to help the patient determine a target position toward which to move and, in addition, can cue aspects of production such as duration, continuance, and tongue tension. Chumpelik states that these placements can facilitate movements between phonemes in connected speech by chaining a series of prompts. The clinician can cue the position for each sound or for one sound that represents the primary target positions in a word. Square et al. (1986) reported that their adult apraxic patients improved production of sounds in multisyllabic words and short sentences with the use of PROMPT.

Stevens and Glaser (1983) described Multiple Input Phoneme Therapy for severely impaired patients who demonstrated an inability to imitate speech. In this program, the clinician uses whatever spontaneous output the patient provides (typically an involuntary utterance) and turns it into a voluntary utterance. The clinician "inputs" (verbally produces) the utterance and the patient is allowed to imitate the clinician's input only upon request. After the patient imitates the clinician, accurately, the clinician inputs additional words beginning with phonemes that were present in the original utterance. For example, if the patient involuntarily produces the word "one," the clinician would produce words such as "wash," "win," "wet," "walk," "white," "up," "us," "no," "new," "night," and "nose." Following successful completion of the Multiple Input Phoneme Therapy tasks, other tasks are used to strengthen the patient's volitional use of words and phrases. (See Wertz et al., 1984, for examples of these tasks.) Both PROMPT and Multiple Input Phoneme Therapy are discussed in Square-Storer (1989).

Melodic Intonation Therapy (MIT) is a procedure that has been recommended for use with patients who have good comprehension but very limited verbal output. It emphasizes the melodic pattern of a phrase or sentence; the patient is required to tap out the rhythm and intone or sing the words of the phrase or sentence. Subsequent steps in the program are used to shape these productions into natural speech. The procedure for MIT was outlined by Sparks and Holland (1976) and Sparks and Deck (1986). Several investigators have reported success with MIT after modifying the program (Dunham & Newhoff, 1979; Hyland & McNeil, 1987; Marshall & Holtzapple, 1976).

Unfortunately, functional speech is not an attainable goal for all patients, and for some it is necessary to consider nonverbal avenues of communication. These can range from gestural systems such as American Indian Sign (Amer-Ind) (Skelly, 1979) and finger spelling to language boards and electronic communication devices. Some nonverbal techniques have been used with success and some have not. It is important to recognize that the value of these nonverbal systems depends on whether a patient can use them successfully after leaving the treatment session. Of course the nature and extent of a patient's medical condition and the presence and severity of aphasia will have an impact on this process. The interested reader is referred to DiSimoni (1986), Rao (1986), and Beukelman, Yorkston, and Dowden (1985) for information concerning the use of nonverbal communication systems.

For treatment of moderate apraxia of speech, Wertz et al. (1984) discuss imitating contrasts. This involves imitating target consonants in a variety of vowel contexts (for example, contrasting /e/ → /ɛ/ in the word "pet" with the /a/ → /ɑ/ in the word "pot") and imitating target consonants in contrast to other consonants (for example, contrasting /s/ in the word "sigh" with the /t/ in the word "tie"). The degree of similarity between the contrasting phonemes can be manipulated to increase or decrease the difficulty of the task. Wertz et al. also discuss the use of contrastive stress drills. In these exercises the patient produces target sentences several times, varying the location of the primary stress in the sentence by either imitation or answering questions. For a complete description of this task and procedures for its use, see Chapter 9 in this volume.

Pairing speech with another activity such as gesturing (Rosenbek, Collins, & Wertz, 1976), tapping, using a pacing board (Helm, 1979), or finger counting (Simmons, 1978) has been reported to be successful for the patient with a moderate apraxia of speech. As patients begin to increase the accuracy of their verbal productions, the paired activity can be phased out. In addition, instructing moderately apraxic patients to prolong their speech and reduce their rate has led to improvement (Southwood, 1987). Dworkin, Abkarian, and Johns (1988) reported that an apraxic patient's speech improved when a hierarchy of nonspeech and articulatory tasks was paced using a metronome.

Wertz et al. (1984) provide several suggestions for treating the mildly apraxic patient. These include introducing a faster rate of speech, imposing increasingly longer delays, and providing a decreasing amount of assistance from the clinician. Tasks can be made more difficult by requiring the production of infrequently occurring words and by introducing unfamiliar topics. The responses required can range from answering simple questions and discussing familiar topics to participating in conversation and discussing unfamiliar topics. I have found that oral reading tasks are useful for treating the mildly apraxic patient. Finally, strengthening the patient's ability to self-monitor and correct errors is essential.

Case study. The following case study demonstrates how various procedures were used to treat a patient with apraxia of speech.

M. W. was a 65-year-old male who in May 1984 suffered a left hemisphere stroke that resulted in a mild right hemiparesis and aphasia. Due to recurring medical complications, M. W. received only 2 or 3 months of speech-language therapy during the first year postonset. In September 1985, approximately 16 months poststroke, he began speech and language therapy at the Kent State University Speech and Hearing Clinic.

Results of an initial evaluation with the *Boston Diagnostic Aphasia Examination* (BDAE) (Goodglass & Kaplan, 1983) revealed that M. W. was performing at the 80th percentile on the auditory and graphic subtests and at the 20th percentile on the verbal tasks. Oral apraxia was identified. His speech was limited to production of the syllable /ma/. M. W. also displayed a mild to moderate Broca's aphasia; he had difficulty in thought organization and a mild deficit in auditory and visual comprehension. His primary communication deficit was a severe apraxia of speech.

Oral motor tasks were introduced to increase agility of the oral musculature. Speech tasks included verbal imitation of vowels to initiate voicing and the use of integral (auditory plus visual) stimulation for consonant production in consonant-vowel combinations beginning with the phoneme with the easiest production manner (plosives) and the most visible placement (bilabials). Writing (of functional words and phrases) and gestures—specifically Amer-Ind—were incorporated into the therapeutic regimen as functional means of communication and as aids to increasing verbal output.

M. W.'s communicative ability was reevaluated in January 1986. *Communicative Abilities in Daily Living* (CADL) (Holland, 1980) was administered. Communication was primarily through writing, pointing, and production of one-word verbal responses. Humor, reading, writing, sequential relationships, and calculation all were within the normal range of performance.

Treatment tasks focused on increasing the accuracy and consistency of production of bilabials at the word and phrase level and on increasing nasal and fricative production in consonant-vowel (CV) and consonant-vowel-consonant (CVC) combinations using imitation with and without integral stimulation. Self-cuing strategies that were successful in initiating functional speech production included writing and preposturing of the articulators. M. W. was encouraged to use these cues to initiate spontaneous speech. He also was encouraged to transfer his written functional phrases to speech. The clinician asked M. W. questions or instructed the patient to request or provide information.

Reevaluation of the patient's communication skills with the *Minnesota Test for the Differential Diagnosis of Aphasia* (MTDDA) (Schuell, 1965) at 24 months postonset in May 1986 revealed that M. W. produced intelligible one- and two-word utterances. Treatment tasks at this time focused on continuing to increase articulatory accuracy of words and phrases through integral stimulation with particular emphasis on fricatives. A task aimed at prolonging vowels was implemented to improve sound and syllable transitions. Stress and intonation drills with accompanying visual cuing on words to be stressed were introduced to attempt to improve his verbal communication.

Administration of the BDAE in December 1986 at 31 months postonset revealed that M. W. produced three- and four-word utterances with labored, halting production and exaggerated articulatory postures. Blends, affricates, and some fricatives were consistently misarticulated (primarily distortions). An imitation task with visual cues was used to expand M. W.'s functional utterances. Placement cues, integral stimulation, and imitation alone were used to increase articulatory accuracy of affricates and fricatives in CV combinations and words. Oral motor activities were reintroduced to increase the speed and accuracy of labial and lingual articulatory movement.

Informal evaluation of M. W.'s apraxia in October 1987 (41 months postonset) yielded labored productions of five-word verbal utterances with frequent problems related to initiation and oral posturing. Therapy focused on increasing the accuracy of /ʃ/ and affricates in words and simple sentences through imitation. A task aimed at improving the rhythmic production of utterances was introduced to elicit a more automatic manner of production while speaking. This task used an "MIT-like" approach using hand tapping during the production of six- and seven-word utterances.

At present M. W. participates in a speech-language social group meeting once a week with other relatively high-level clients. M. W. attempts verbal communication, although he still has difficulty with speech initiation and accuracy of some sounds. Reduced speech naturalness is a problem and his speech generally has a halting quality.

Phonemic Paraphasias

In contrast to the wealth of information that exists for treating apraxia of speech, there is a virtual dearth of information concerning the treatment of paraphasic errors. This is understandable in that treatment for apraxia is direct and lends itself to the formulation of specific programs and procedures. Treating paraphasias is more indirect and there are few, if any, procedures that are specific to this disorder. Because of the lack of literature to draw on, I am taking the liberty of espousing some personal philosophies.

The information reviewed earlier in this chapter suggests that phonemic paraphasias come from a breakdown in the scan copier. The patient has difficulty selecting the correct phoneme to insert into the syllabic productive slots. Phoneme substitution and sequencing errors occur that subsequently are produced with minimal articulatory disruption. These occur most typically in patients with Wernicke's and conduction aphasias. These errors are readily recognized, especially by those patients with conduction aphasia, and attempts at self-correction are often zealous. If the task is not an imitative one, often attempts lead the patient closer to the target and eventual success is not uncommon.

Although imitation is often used successfully in treating apraxia of speech, this approach is not the best for treating paraphasic errors. Patients with conduction aphasia typically produce more errors on imitation than on spontaneous speech tasks. In fact, the repetition impairment often is viewed as a hallmark of this syndrome. Imitation also reduces patients' ability to self-correct errors. Since imitation plays such a small role in normal daily communication, it makes more sense during treatment sessions to emphasize patients' strengths (spontaneous speech) rather than weaknesses (imitation). This is not to say that patients should not repeat their response several times, especially if it contains an error. This type of repetition is beneficial for a patient although potentially frustrating as well. What should be minimized is asking patients to imitate something that has been presented only through the auditory channel. It is better for the response to be elicited in some other manner such as oral reading, answering questions, completing sentences, naming, describing pictures, and discussion. The severity of the aphasia will dictate the type and level of tasks that are appropriate. For example, Boyle (1989) reported a decrease in the number of phonemic paraphasias in a patient following a treatment program of structured oral reading tasks. Similar results were presented for a patient with conduction aphasia using sentence-level oral reading tasks with imposed delays (Sullivan, Fisher, & Marshall, 1986).

Since apraxia of speech is considered a speech motor control disorder that can occur along with various linguistic deficits, it is generally treated independently of the other deficits. In contrast, paraphasias are typically an integral part of a larger language disorder characterized by deficits in comprehension, word retrieval, thought formulation, and writing. Therefore treatment focuses on language impairment and the paraphasia problem is handled indirectly. Because it is difficult to predict whether a particular word will be subjected to phonemic paraphasia intrusions, treatment tasks should reflect variables that influence other aspects of the patient's performance. For example, variables that influence the accuracy of word retrieval, sentence formulation, or thought organization ability should guide the construction of the task. It is not uncommon for the visual input modality to be less impaired than the auditory input modality in patients with conduction aphasia. The clinician can capitalize on this difference by using visual along with auditory cues during auditory input tasks. As a paraphasia occurs, the patient can attempt to correct the error, then move on. A technique for reducing paraphasic intrusions involves instructing the patient to think of or write the first letter of a word or the entire word to be produced.

As other language skills improve, the number of paraphasias should decrease and the patient's ability to self-correct the paraphasic errors should increase.

It is important that successful communication be emphasized more and that phonemic accuracy be emphasized less. The patient should be encouraged to value the successful communication of a message even though it might contain a paraphasic error. Similarly, the listener should be counseled to appreciate the meaning of a patient's verbal message and to not demand phonemic accuracy. The listener can learn to utilize context to facilitate his or her comprehension of the speaker's message.

Case study. The following case study describes the treatment of a patient with paraphasic speech. F. R. was a 76-year-old male with a history of coronary bypass surgery and phlebitis who, in March 1987, sustained a left middle cerebral artery stroke with a resultant marked to moderate aphasia. No hemiparesis was present.

Results of the MTDDA revealed moderate auditory comprehension deficits, marked visual comprehension deficits, and significant writing impairment. Verbal output was characterized by word retrieval difficulties and a high prevalence of phonemic and verbal paraphasias that were noted in repetition tasks and spontaneous speech. His speech-language deficit was labeled conduction aphasia.

A variety of treatment tasks were employed. Several tasks were designed to improve auditory comprehension. The patient was required to answer yes or no questions, follow two- and three-step commands, and demonstrate an understanding of passages and paragraphs read by the clinician. The clinician used a variety of hand signals to indicate when the patient was to stop attempts at self-correction of verbal paraphasias. Tasks to improve word retrieval abilities were designed using sentence completion and questions and answers. Successful self-cuing strategies were identified in generative naming tasks in which the patient verbally listed items in a category and features of common objects.

The MTDDA was readministered in September 1987 at 6 months postonset. Results revealed mild auditory comprehension deficits and marked visual comprehension and writing impairments. There was a reduction in the word retrieval deficit, although phonemic paraphasias remained prevalent in the patient's speech. Attempts at self-corrections were reduced in number and they tended to lead to correct responses more often than was indicated at the previous assessment.

In therapy sessions conducted between September 1987 and January 1988, increased use of self-cuing strategies and improvement in auditory comprehension were emphasized. Results of the MTDDA administered in January 1988 revealed that phonemic paraphasias continued, and that mild auditory and moderate to marked visual comprehension deficits persisted.

Following the assessment in January, F. R. was discharged from therapy. He was moving to another state and planned to continue speech and language therapy after he relocated. We recommended that in the future F. R. concentrate on improving auditory comprehension of complex commands and on improving his understanding in conversations involving more than two conversation partners. Also we recommended therapy involve improving visual comprehension skills and self-cuing strategies.

CONCLUSION

Apraxia of speech and paraphasic speech are two distinct disorders. Apraxic errors result from difficulty in programming volitional articulatory movements, while paraphasic errors occur earlier in the production process and involve the faulty retrieval and sequencing of individual phonemes. Many of the behaviors displayed by apraxic and paraphasic speakers are similar, and therefore a differential diagnosis does not involve simply documenting failure on a test of apraxia of speech. Differential diagnosis is essential, however, because—as demonstrated in the two case studies—the approach to treatment is different for the two disorders. Future research must define treatment protocols more precisely with special emphasis on those tasks that facilitate carryover of the treated skills to functional communication.

REFERENCES

Abbs, J. (1986). Invariance and variability in speech production: A distinction between linguistic intent and its neuromotor implementation. In J. Perkell & D. Klatt (Eds.), *Invariance and variability in speech processes* (pp. 202–225). Hillsdale, NJ: Lawrence Erlbaum.

Bayles, K., & Kaszniak, A. (1987). *Communication and cognition in normal aging and dementia.* Austin, TX: PRO-ED.

Berry W. (Ed.). (1983). *Clinical dysarthria.* Austin, TX: PRO-ED.

Beukelman, D. R., Yorkston, K. M., & Dowden, P. A. (1985). *Communication augmentation: A casebook of clinical management.* Austin, TX: PRO-ED.

Blumstein, S., Cooper, W., Goodglass, H., Statlender, S., & Gottlieb, J. (1980). Production deficits in aphasia: A voice-onset time analysis. *Brain and Language, 9,* 153–170.

Borden, G. (1979). An interpretation of research on feedback interruption in speech. *Brain and Language, 7,* 307–319.

Boyle, M. (1989). Reducing phonemic paraphasias in the connected speech of a conduction aphasic subject. In T. Prescott (Ed.), *Clinical aphasiology: Vol. 18* (pp. 379–393). Austin, TX: PRO-ED.

Buckingham, H. (1981). Where do neologisms come from? In J. Brown (Ed.), *Jargonaphasia*. New York: Academic Press.

Buckingham, H. (1987). Phonemic paraphasias and psycholinguistic production models for neologistic jargon. *Aphasiology, 1*, 381–400.

Buckingham, H. (1989). Phonological paraphasia. In C. Code (Ed.), *The characteristics of aphasia*. New York: Taylor and Francis.

Buckingham, H., & Yule, G. (1987). Phonemic false evaluation: Theoretical and clinical aspects. *Clinical Linguistics and Phonetics, 1*, 113–126.

Butterworth, B. (1979). Hesitation and the production of verbal paraphasias and neologisms in jargon aphasia. *Brain and Language, 18*, 133–161.

Canter, G., Trost, J., & Burns, M. (1985). Contrasting speech patterns in apraxia of speech and phonemic paraphasias. *Brain and Language, 24*, 204–222.

Caplan, D. (1987). Phonological representation in word production. In E. Keller & M. Gopnik (Eds.), *Motor and sensory processes of language*. Hillsdale, NJ: Lawrence Erlbaum.

Caramazza, A., Berndt, R., & Brownell, H. (1982). The semantic deficit hypothesis: Perceptual parsing and object classification by aphasic patients. *Brain and Language, 15*, 161–189.

Chumpelik, D. (1984). The prompt system of therapy: Theoretical framework and applications for developmental apraxia of speech. *Seminars in Speech and Language, 5*, 139–156.

Collins, M., Cariski, D., Longstretch, D., & Rosenbek, J. (1980). Patterns of articulatory behavior in selected motor speech programming disorders. In R. Brookshire (Ed.), *Clinical aphasiology*. Minneapolis: BRK Publishers.

Dabul, B. (1979). *Apraxia battery for adults*. Austin, TX: PRO-ED.

Dabul, B., & Bollier, B. (1976). Therapeutic approaches to apraxia. *Journal of Speech and Hearing Disorders, 41*, 268–276.

Daniloff, R., & Moll, K. (1968). Coarticulation in lip rounding. *Journal of Speech and Hearing Research, 11*, 707–721.

Darley, F. L., Aronson, A. E., & Brown, J. R. (1975). *Audio seminars in speech pathology: Motor speech disorders*. Philadelphia: W. B. Saunders.

Deal, J., & Florance, C. (1978). Modification of the eight-step continuum for treatment of apraxia of speech in adults. *Journal of Speech and Hearing Disorders, 43*, 89–95.

DiSimoni, F. (1986). Alternative communication systems for the aphasic patient. In R. Chapey (Ed.), *Language intervention strategies in adult aphasia*. Baltimore: Williams and Wilkins.

Duffy, J., & Gawle, C. (1984). Apraxic speakers' vowel duration in consonant-vowel-consonant syllables. In R. Rosenbek, M. McNeil, & A. Aronson (Eds.), *Apraxia of speech: Physiology, acoustics, linguistics, management*. Austin, TX: PRO-ED.

Dunham, M., & Newhoff, M. (1979). Melodic intonation therapy: Rewriting the song. In R. Brookshire (Ed.), *Clinical aphasiology*. Minneapolis: BRK Publishers.

Dworkin, J., Abkarian, G., & Johns, D. (1988). Apraxia of speech: The effectiveness of a treatment regimen. *Journal of Speech and Hearing Disorders, 53*, 280–294.

Folkins, J., & Abbs, J. (1976). Additional observations on responses to resistive loading of the jaw. *Journal of Speech and Hearing Research, 19*, 820–831.

Friedrich, F., Glenn, C., & Marin, O. (1984). Interruption of phonological coding in conduction aphasia. *Brain and Language, 22*, 266–291.

Fromm, D., Abbs, J., McNeil, M., & Rosenbek, J. (1982). Simultaneous perceptual-physiological method for studying apraxia of speech. In R. Brookshire (Ed.), *Clinical aphasiology*. Minneapolis: BRK Publishers.

Garrett, M. (1975). The analysis of sentence production. In G. Bower (Ed.), *Psychology of learning and motivation* (Vol. 9). New York: Academic Press.

Garrett, M. (1980). Levels of processing in sentence production. In B. Butterworth (Ed.), *Language production* (Vol. 1). New York: Academic Press.

Goodglass, H. (1975). Phonological factors in aphasia. In R. Brookshire (Ed.), *Clinical aphasiology*. Minneapolis: BRK Publishers.

Goodglass, H., & Kaplan, E. (1983). *The assessment of aphasia and related disorders*, Philadelphia: Lea and Febiger.

Gracco, V., & Abbs, J. (1987). Programming and execution processes of speech movement control: Potential neural correlates. In E. Keller & M. Gopnik (Eds.), *Motor and sensory processes of language*. Hillsdale, NJ: Lawrence Erlbaum.

Grober, E., Perecman, E., Kellar, L., & Brown, J. (1980). Lexical knowledge in anterior and posterior aphasics. *Brain and Language, 10*, 318–330.

Helm, N. (1979). Management of palilalia with a pacing board. *Journal of Speech and Hearing Disorder, 44*, 350–353.

Holland, A. (1980). *Communicative abilities in daily living*. Austin, TX: PRO-ED.

Hough, M. (1978). *Frequency of specific types of phonological/motor errors produced by fluent and nonfluent aphasic adults*. Unpublished master's thesis, University of Florida, Gainesville, FL.

Hughes, O., & Abbs, J. (1976). Labial-mandibular coordination in the production of speech: Implications for the operation of motor equivalence *Phonetica, 44*, 199–221.

Hyland, J., & McNeil, M. (1987). The effects of an intoning therapy on the speech of a developmentally apraxic adult. In R. Brookshire (Ed.), *Clinical aphasiology*. Minneapolis: BRK Publishers.

Itoh, M., Sasanuma, S., Hirose, H., Yoshioka, H., & Sawashima, M. (1983). Velar movements during speech in two Wernicke aphasic patients. *Brain and Language, 19*, 283–292.

Itoh, M., Sasanuma, S., Hirose, H., Yoshioka, H., & Ushijima, T. (1980). Abnormal articulatory dynamics in a patient with apraxia of speech: X-ray microbeam observation. *Brain and Language, 11*, 66–75.

Itoh, M., Sasanuma, S., Tatsumi, I., Murakami, S., Fukusako, Y., & Suzuki, T. (1982). Voice onset time characteristics in apraxia of speech. *Brain and Language, 17*, 193–210.

Itoh, M., Sasanuma, S., & Ushijima, T. (1979). Velar movements during speech in a patient with apraxia of speech. *Brain and Language, 7*, 227–239.

Joanette, Y., Keller, E., & Lecours, A. (1980). Sequences of phonemic approximations in aphasia. *Brain and Language, 11*, 30–44.

Keller, E. (1984). Simplification and gesture reduction in phonological disorders of apraxia and aphasia. In J. Rosenbek, M. McNeil, & A. Aronson (Eds.), *Apraxia of speech: Physiology, acoustics, linguistics, management.* Austin, TX: PRO-ED.

Keller, E. (1987). The cortical representation of motor processes of speech. In E. Keller & M. Gopnik (Eds.), *Motor and sensory processes of language.* Hillsdale, NJ: Lawrence Erlbaum.

Kempler, D., Metter, E., Jackson, C., Hanson, W., Phelps, M., & Mazziotta, J. (1986). Conduction aphasia: Subgroups based on behavior, anatomy, and physiology. In R. Brookshire (Ed.), *Clinical aphasiology.* Minneapolis: BRK Publishers.

Kent, R., & Rosenbek, J. (1982). Prosodic disturbance and neurological lesion. *Brain and Language, 15,* 259–291.

Kent, R., & Rosenbek, J. (1983). Acoustic patterns of apraxia of speech. *Journal of Speech and Hearing Research, 26,* 231–248.

Klich, R., Ireland, J., & Weidner, W. (1979). Articulatory and phonological aspects of consonant substitutions in apraxia of speech. *Cortex, 15,* 451–470.

Kohn, S. (1984). The nature of the phonological disorder in conduction aphasia. *Brain and Language, 23,* 97–115.

MacNeilage, P. (1982). Speech production mechanisms in aphasia. In S. Grillner, B. Lindblom, J. Lubker, & A. Persson (Eds.), *Speech motor control.* Oxford, England: Pergamon Press.

Marshall, R., & Holtzapple, P. (1976). Melodic intonation therapy: Variations on a theme. In R. Brookshire (Ed.), *Clinical aphasiology.* Minneapolis: BRK Publishers.

McNeil, M., Hunter, L., Rosenbek, J., & Fennell, A. (1987, November). *Vowel errors and consonant distortions in apraxia of speech.* Paper presented at the annual convention of the American Speech-Language-Hearing Association, New Orleans, LA.

Monoi, H., Fukusako, Y., Itoh, M., & Sasanuma, S. (1983). Speech sound errors in patients with conduction and Broca's aphasia. *Brain and Language, 20,* 175–194.

Nespoulous, J., Joanette, Y., Ska, B., Caplan, D., & Lecours, A. (1987). Production deficits in Broca's and conduction aphasia: Repetition versus reading. In E. Keller & M. Gopnik (Eds.), *Motor and sensory processes of language.* Hillsdale, NJ: Lawrence Erlbaum.

Pierce, R. (1988). Language processing and the effects of context in aphasia. In M. Ball (Ed.), *Theoretical linguistics and disordered language.* London: Croom Helm.

Rao, P. (1986). The use of Amer-Ind code with aphasic adults. In R. Chapey (Ed.), *Language intervention strategies in adult aphasia.* Baltimore: Williams & Wilkins.

Rosenbek, J., Collins, M., & Wertz, R. (1976). Intersystemic reorganization in the treatment of apraxia of speech. In R. Brookshire (Ed.), *Clinical aphasiology.* Minneapolis: BRK Publishers.

Rosenbek, J., Lemme, M., Ahern, M., Harris, E., & Wertz, R. (1973). A treatment for apraxia of speech in adults. *Journal of Speech and Hearing Disorders, 38,* 462–472.

Schuell, M. (1965). *Minnesota Test for the Differential Diagnosis of Aphasia.* Minneapolis: Minnesota University Press.

Schwartz, M. (1987). Patterns of speech production deficit within and across aphasia syndromes: Application of a psycholinguistic model. In M. Coltheart, G. Sartori, & R. Job (Eds.), *The cognitive neuropsychology of language.* Hillsdale, NJ: Lawrence Erlbaum.

Shattuck-Hufnagel, S. (1979). Speech errors as evidence for a serial ordering mechanism in sentence production. In W. Cooper & C. Walker (Eds.), *Sentence processing.* Hillsdale, NJ: Lawrence Erlbaum.

Shattuck-Hufnagel, S. (1983). Sublexical units and suprasegmental structure in speech production planning. In P. MacNeilage (Ed.), *The production of speech.* New York: Springer-Verlag.

Shattuck-Hufnagel, S. (1987). The role of word-onset consonants in speech production planning: New evidence from speech error patterns. In E. Keller & M. Gopnik (Eds.), *Motor and sensory processes of language.* Hillsdale, NJ: Lawrence Erlbaum.

Simmons, N. (1978). Finger counting as an intersystemic reorganizer in apraxia of speech. In R. Brookshire (Ed.), *Clinical aphasiology.* Minneapolis: BRK Publishers.

Simmons, N. (1980). Choice of stimulus modes in treating apraxia of speech: A case study. In R. Brookshire (Ed.), *Clinical aphasiology.* Minneapolis: BRK Publishers.

Skelly, M. (1979). *Amer-Ind gestural code.* New York: Elsevier.

Southwood, H. (1987). The use of prolonged speech in the treatment of apraxia of speech. In R. Brookshire (Ed.), *Clinical aphasiology.* Minneapolis: BRK Publishers.

Sparks, R., & Deck, J. (1986). Melodic intonation therapy. In R. Chapey (Ed.), *Language intervention strategies in adult aphasia.* Baltimore: Williams and Wilkins.

Sparks, R., & Holland, A. (1976). Method: Melodic intonation therapy. *Journal of Speech and Hearing Disorders, 41,* 287–297.

Square, P., Chumpelik, D., Morningstar, D., & Adams, S. (1986). Efficacy of the PROMPT system of therapy for the treatment of acquired apraxia of speech: A follow-up investigation. In R. Brookshire (Ed.), *Clinical aphasiology.* Minneapolis: BRK Publishers.

Square-Storer, P. (Ed.). (1989). *Acquired apraxia of speech in aphasic adults.* New York: Taylor and Francis.

Stevens, E., & Glaser, L. (1983). Multiple input phoneme therapy: An approach to severe aphasia and expressive aphasia. In R. Brookshire (Ed.), *Clinical aphasiology.* Minneapolis: BRK Publishers.

Sullivan, M., Fisher, B., & Marshall, R. (1986). Treating the repetition deficit in conduction aphasia. In R. Brookshire (Ed.), *Clinical aphasiology.* Minneapolis: BRK Publishers.

Trost, J., & Canter, G. (1974). Apraxia of speech in patients with Broca's aphasia: A study of phonemic production accuracy and error patterns. *Brain and Language, 1,* 63–80.

Wertz, R., LaPointe, L., & Rosenbek, J. (1984). *Apraxia of speech in adults: The disorder and its management.* New York: Grune and Stratton.

Whitehouse, P., Caramazza, A., & Zurif, E. (1978). Naming in aphasia: Interacting effects of form and function. *Brain and Language, 6,* 63–74.

Ziegler, W., & von Cramon, D. (1985). Anticipatory coarticulation in a patient with apraxia of speech. *Brain and Language, 26,* 117–130.

Ziegler, W., & von Cramon, D. (1986). Disturbed coarticulation in apraxia of speech. *Brain and Language, 29,* 34–47.

ACKNOWLEDGMENT

The author gratefully acknowledges the assistance of Dr. Monica Hough on portions of this chapter.

CHAPTER 8
Acquired Neurogenic Dysfluency
Jon Deal and Michael P. Cannito

> *Deal and Cannito review existing literature, much of it case studies, on the problem of acquired neurogenic dysfluency. This disorder, while itself heterogeneous, is diagnostically differentiated from developmental stuttering, acquired psychogenic stuttering, and nonfluent aphasia. Potential sites of lesion are considered and a comprehensive framework for treatment is advanced.*

1. Describe diagnostic considerations for dysfluency in terms of differentiation from other superficially similar disorders and in terms of subcategories within this generic diagnostic label. Why is this differentiation significant for treatment?
2. What site(s) of lesion have been posited as underlying the phenomenon of acquired neurogenic dysfluency?
3. Outline treatment approaches for acquired neurogenic dysfluency. What kinds of considerations might figure in the selection of one approach as opposed to another?

In the context of this chapter, neurogenic dysfluency will refer to an onset of dysfluency in adult life that follows or is associated in some way with nervous system damage. There are three categories of acquired, adult onset dysfluency. First, the dysfluency may be a form of occult stuttering. Van Riper (1971) called this type of dysfluency interiorized stuttering, and implied that under conditions of great stress the dysfluency (stuttering) can no longer be hidden. The point is that adult onset of dysfluency may simply be the sudden appearance of stuttering that for years had been hidden or interiorized. This dysfluency is not a new problem, it is simply the sudden appearance of an old problem. If occult, or interiorized, stuttering can be ruled out, there are two other possible etiologies: the dysfluency may be of psychogenic or neurogenic origin.

When occult stuttering has been ruled out and there has been no demonstrable neurological insult and there are no neurological signs, then the dysfluency may be considered to be of psychogenic origin. Freund (1966) has described this type of dysfluency as a hysterical conversion neurosis. Psychogenic dysfluency has been discussed in the literature by a number of authors (Deal, 1982; Deal & Doro, 1987; Dempsey & Granich, 1978; Wallen, 1961; Weiner, 1981). These reports suggest that dysfluency which is neither developmentally nor neurologically based occurs in adulthood, is of sudden onset, and is temporally linked to some form of psychological trauma or cumulative psychological stress.

There is a third category, that of neurogenic dysfluency which also occurs in adulthood, may have a rapid onset, and is temporally linked to a demonstrable neurological insult or at least to demonstrable neurological signs. This chapter is concerned with the dysfluency of neurologic origin. The remainder of the chapter will attempt to define the characteristics of neurogenic dysfluency, to differentiate neurogenic from other types of dysfluency, to identify etiologies of neurogenic dysfluency, to differentiate different forms of neurogenic dysfluency, and to suggest treatment strategies.

TERMINOLOGY

It should be noted that the wording in the title of this chapter is "Neurogenic Dysfluency," not "Neurogenic Stuttering." *Dysfluency* is used instead of *stuttering* because there is some question as to the appropriateness of the term *stuttering* used in the context of neurogenic stuttering. Culatta and Leeper (1988) have made a rather eloquent case for not using the term *stuttering* in this context. Their basic premise is that all forms of dysfluency are not stuttering, and they urge that the term *stuttering* be reserved for "that well-defined and researched developmental dysfluency disorder, the causes of which remain unknown." Although much of the literature to be discussed uses the term *stuttering, dysfluency* will be substituted whenever possible. As Culatta and Leeper suggest, *dysfluency* may be the more appropriate term because there are differences between neurogenic dysfluency and developmental stuttering. *Dysfluency* may then be used as a descriptor without automatically, and perhaps subconsciously, drawing parallels to developmental stuttering.

By substituting *dysfluency* for *stuttering*, in an effort to avoid confusion with developmental stuttering, another confusion may arise. One of the etiologies associated with neurogenic dysfluency is stroke. Stroke may produce aphasia, and aphasia is often described along a fluent-nonfluent continuum. Thus a distinction must be made between dysfluency and nonfluency. Although dysfluency and nonfluency sometimes are regarded as synonymous, they are not. There are persons who demonstrate a nonfluent aphasia and who also demonstrate dysfluency. There are also those individuals who are dysfluent but are not nonfluent. Albert, Goodglass, Helm, Ruben, and Alexander (1981) describe nonfluency as follows: "Non-fluent speech is slow, laboriously produced, with abnormal speech rhythm and melody, poor articulation, shortened phrase length, and preferential use of substantive words (such as nouns and main verbs) rather than grammatical words (such as conjunctions and auxiliary verbs). Non-fluent speech, often called telegraphic or agrammatic, is frequently associated with anteriorly located lesions and is usually a feature of the anterior dysphasias" (pp. 4–5). Dysfluency implies stutteringlike behaviors such as sound and syllable repetitions, stutteringlike blocks, sound prolongations, and other stutteringlike phenomena. Dysfluency does not include articulation disorders, telegraphic speech, or agrammatic speech. Nonfluency implies a linguistic deficit; dysfluency implies a nonlinguistic motor control problem. Other aphasic symptomatology from which acquired neurogenic dysfluency should be differentiated includes the word-finding pauses and hesitations of anomia as well as reaproachment phenomena, wherein an aphasic patient repeatedly attempts pronunciation of a word, each time generating different phonological errors but progressively approximating the correct production. Although word-finding pauses and reaproachment behaviors are disruptive to the fluid ongoingness of speech, their underlying mechanisms are linguistic and they are part and parcel of the primary aphasia (see Chapter 7 of this volume for discussion).

THE CLINICAL REALITY OF NEUROGENIC DYSFLUENCY

There is no question that neurogenic dysfluency occurs. Rather, the question is: Is the dysfluency a clinically distinct and separate disorder, or is it a manifestation of other well-defined clinical syndromes? The literature does not provide an answer that is unambiguous.

Neurogenic dysfluency can occur following a variety of neurological insults, including stroke, head trauma, brain tumor, and certain disease processes. Considering the variety of etiologies, it is unlikely that neurogenic dysfluency is a unitary disorder. Yet there are enough descriptive reports and discussions in the literature to make the case that neurogenic dysfluency occurs as an isolated disorder, without concomitant aphasia, apraxia, or dysarthria. Reading the literature on neurogenic stuttering is like reading the literature on aphasia. Henry Head in 1926 described the literature on aphasia as "chaos." The same may be said of the more recent literature on neurogenic stuttering. Readers are confronted with concepts such as "stuttering in aphasia," "aphasic stuttering," "apraxic stuttering," "dysarthric stuttering," and "isolated stuttering." The conclusion to be drawn is that the dysfluency may be part of a larger clinical entity or it may be an entity unto itself. A rose by any other name may smell as sweet, but neurogenic stuttering may not be neurogenic stuttering, may not be neurogenic stuttering, etc.

NEUROGENIC DYSFLUENCY AND APHASIA

Luchsinger and Arnold (1965) and Schuell, Jenkins, and Jimenez-Pabon (1964) have pointed out that dysfluency may be present in the evolution of aphasia. This implies a transient phenomenon that is simply part of the natural history of aphasia and that there is nothing particularly unique or interesting about the dysfluency. Others have been more specific about dysfluency and its association with aphasia.

Arend and colleagues (1962), Helm and associates (1978, 1980), and Mazzuchi, Moretti, Carpeggiani, Parma, and Paini (1981) have provided more information about the relationship of dysfluency and aphasia. The following conclusions may be drawn from their reports:

1. Aphasia and dysfluency occur simultaneously and both persist.
2. Aphasia and dysfluency occur simultaneously and both are transient.
3. Dysfluency precedes aphasia, but both are transient.
4. Dysfluency precedes aphasia, but the dysfluency is transient and the aphasia persists.
5. Aphasia precedes the dysfluency, but the aphasia is transient and the dysfluency persists.
6. Dysfluency may be an isolated phenomenon, present without aphasia.

There are case reports supporting each of the situations listed.

This state of affairs would not present clinicians with any particular difficulty if we could predict when the dysfluency would persist; if we could predict when the dysfluency would be transient; if we could specify the time domain for "transient"; and if we could predict when the dysfluency would persist with or without aphasia. Unfortunately, at this point we are not able to predict the above with a comfortable level of certainty. An additional complication is the theory that the dysfluency is not neurogenic in origin at all. Rather, the dysfluency is the result of an emotional reaction to the communication difficulties resulting from the aphasia. Although they do not completely rule this out, Helm, Butler, and Benson (1978) do us the favor of presenting case reports that weaken the theory. They also suggest that dysfluency may persist when the dysfluent patient has difficulty drawing three-dimensional figures, copying block designs, and producing and sustaining sequential motor tasks. Neither of their patients who experienced transient dysfluency had these difficulties, but six of their eight patients with persistent dysfluency did.

DYSFLUENCY AS A COMPONENT OF MOTOR SPEECH DISORDERS

Dysfluency has been shown to be a component of aphasia. It may also be a component of certain motor speech disorders. As Rosenbek (1980) pointed out, Van Riper states that "the integrity of a spoken word demands great precision in the timing of its components. When, for any reason, that timing is awry or askew, a temporally distorted word is produced, and when this happens, the speaker has evinced a core of stuttering behavior" (Van Riper, 1971, p. 401). Certainly various motor speech disorders result in timing of speech production being "awry and askew." That being the case, it is no surprise that dysfluency has been a reported feature of motor speech disorders.

Apraxia of Speech

Various investigators note the marked prevalence of stutteringlike dysfluencies in association with articulatory programming problems of apraxia of speech (Johns & Darley, 1970; Trost, 1971; Yairi, Gintautas, & Avent, 1981) often accompanied by Broca's or motor aphasia. In their early observations on this subject, Johns and Darley (1970) noted that patients exhibiting apraxia of speech "as a group, do a creditable job of miming secondary stutterers, both acoustically and behaviorally" (p. 580), exhibiting circumlocution, word substitution, false starts, anticipatory struggle, blocks, and part word, word, and phrasal repetitions. No other disorder, motor or otherwise, produces such a strong temptation to theorize about stuttering (let alone dysfluency) as does apraxia of speech. The temptation stems from the similarities between apraxia of speech and stuttering. This temptation was too strong for Rosenbek to resist, and he wrote an article dealing with the relationship between the two disorders (Rosenbek, 1980).

The problem that arises is that it is tempting to regard stuttering as a form of apraxia of speech. Rosenbek was not able to support that thesis in 1980, and we will not attempt to support it now. We will simply refer clinicians to the literature of apraxia of speech, much of which can be found in the text by Wertz, Rosenbek, and LaPointe (1983).

Dysarthria

Certain forms of dysarthria are associated with dysfunction in neuromuscular substrates intimately involved with the timing of speech production. The hypokinetic dysarthria of Parkinson's disease or other extrapyramidal involvement (Darley, Aronson, & Brown, 1975) has been reported to produce dysfluency as a primary characteristic.

Canter (1971) included a patient with Parkinson's disease when he described characteristics of neurogenic stuttering, and Helm, Butler, and Canter (1980) also wrote of the dysfluencies associated with Parkinson's disease as neurogenic stuttering. Koller (1983) reported dysfluency associated with Parkinson's disease and other forms of extrapyramidal disease.

Palilalia

Palilalia is a form of motor speech perseveration. It has been described as multiple repetitions of a word, phrase, or sentence in a context of decreasing loudness and increasing rate (Critchley, 1927; LaPointe & Horner, 1981). In a recent acoustic study, however, Kent and LaPointe (1982) describe a palilalic patient whose reiterant utterances remained fairly uniform across a repetition train. These authors suggest that there may therefore be subtypes of palilalic disturbances. Palilalia has been reported in association with numerous neuropathologies including postencephalitic Parkinson's disease, pseudobulbar palsy, Alzheimer's disease, multiple infarct dementia, and idiopathic cerebral calcinosis (Helm, 1979). Rosenbek (1984) differentiates palilalia from "neurogenic stuttering" on the basis of infrequent syllable repetition in the former but pervasive syllable repetitions in the latter. Helm-Estabrooks (1986) points out that stuttering "involves repetitions, blocks, and prolongation of phonemes, whereas palilalia operates at the whole word/phrase level." Palilalia represents a distinctive subcategory of acquired neurogenic dysfluency (Horner & Massey, 1983).

Dysfluency as a Clinical Entity

The literature contains documentation that dysfluency is a component of aphasia, apraxia of speech, and dysarthria. Other neurogenic speech and language disorders have dysfluency as a component. The communication problems stemming from head injury and right hemisphere strokes also may have dysfluency as a characteristic (Andrews, Quinn, & Sorby, 1972; Horner & Massey, 1983; Lebrun & Leleux, 1985; Quinn & Andrews, 1977; Schiller, 1947). In the literature cited thus far and in the literature yet to be discussed, there are, we believe, sufficient case reports to support the concept of neurogenic dysfluency as a distinct clinical entity, albeit an uncommon one.

DIFFERENTIATING TYPES OF ACQUIRED NEUROGENIC DYSFLUENCY

When faced with a patient who presents with the putative diagnosis of acquired dysfluency, clinicians must be able to determine whether the dysfluency is a form of developmental stuttering, psychogenic dysfluency, or neurogenic dysfluency. Differentiating neurogenic dysfluency from developmental stuttering would seem to be a simple task. All we need to do is ask. If the patient denies stuttering as a child, we can assume that the present dysfluency is new and then determine whether it is neurogenic or psychogenic. Conversely, if the patient admits to stuttering as a child, we can assume that the dysfluency is the recurrence or exacerbation of a preexisting disorder. Unfortunately, as every clinician knows, it is not that simple.

This is not to imply that patients are not truthful. Stuttering has been difficult for professionals to define; it is too much to ask that our patients be as adept as we at defining it. We seem to know a great many people who say that they stuttered when they were children but outgrew it. Conversely, we know people (albeit a smaller number) who seem dysfluent but who would be offended to be called stutterers. Careful questioning of the patient, family, and others who know the patient may well resolve the issue.

The literature is not as helpful as we would hope, but some guidelines are available. Canter (1971) listed seven characteristics that he believed differentiated developmental stuttering and neurogenic dysfluency. Those seven characteristics were revised slightly and restated by Helm et al. (1980). The characteristics put forward as guidelines for differential diagnosis are the following:

1. The repetitions and prolongations are not restricted to initial syllables.
2. The phonemic foci of the dysfluencies may differ from those of developmental stuttering; specifically, the /r/, /l/, and /j/ sounds may be targets for dysfluency.
3. There is no particular relationship between dysfluency and the grammatical function of words, so that small functor words may be as troublesome as substantives.

4. Dysfluency is not necessarily in direct relationship to propositionality, so that self-formulated speech may be easier than more automatic speech tasks.
5. There is no observable adaptation effect.
6. The speaker may be annoyed but not necessarily anxious about his stuttering.
7. There may be no secondary symptomatology such as facial grimacing or fist clenching.

The literature does not support each of the seven guidelines equally. Rosenbek, Messert, Collins, and Wertz (1978) state that six of their subjects were not dysfluent on final consonants, and Lebrun, Leleux, Rousseau, and Devreau (1983) comment that this characteristic could also apply to developmental stuttering. Mazzuchi (1981) reported that a different group of phonemes produced more dysfluencies, and Caplan (1972) reported no phonemic specificity (Caplan did note that his five subjects were more dysfluent on initial consonants than on initial vowels). The first two guidelines seem to be the least supportable. The suggestion that the speaker may be annoyed but not anxious about speaking is directly contradicted by Rosenfield (1972) and Lebrun, Leleux, Rousseau, and Devreux (1983). In fact, exceptions can be found for each of the seven guidelines, including the lack of an adaptation effect (Koller, 1983; Mazzuchi et al., 1981; Quinn & Andrews, 1977; Rosenfield, 1972).

It is important to remember that even though exceptions exist, these seven guidelines were bold statements and should be considered by clinicians when attempting to differentiate developmental stuttering and neurogenic dysfluency.

Neurogenic Dysfluency Versus Psychogenic Dysfluency

Assuming that developmental stuttering has been ruled out, differentiating between neurogenic and psychogenic dysfluency also would seem to be a simple task. If there are neurological signs and symptoms or if there is a history of neurological dysfunction, the dysfluency would seem to be neurogenic in origin. If no neurological signs or symptoms are present, the dysfluency would seem to be psychogenic. The clinical reality is not so simple.

Nowack and Stone (1987) reported two cases of acquired dysfluency that suggested neurogenic and psychogenic dysfluency are not mutually exclusive. One patient had an episode of viral meningitis but had no speech symptoms for at least six years afterward. She began to experience neurological changes at the same time she was experiencing a series of psychological stresses. She also began to exhibit dysfluencies. When the neurological and the psychological problems resolved, so did the dysfluencies. The second patient suffered a left hemisphere stroke, apparently with aphasia but no stuttering. Several years later a right hemisphere stroke was followed by "persistent stuttering." When later she underwent a series of psychological stresses, the dysfluency was exacerbated.

Attanasio (1987) reported a case of what he considered to be a psychogenic dysfluency; however, his patient also had a history of epilepsy. Similarly, Deal and Doro (1987) described what they felt was a case of episodic, hysterical stuttering; however, their patient had sustained a head trauma more than 30 years prior to the onset of the dysfluency. It is not always easy to rule out a neurological component.

Guidelines for differentiating psychogenic and neurogenic dysfluency have, however, been provided (Deal, 1982). In psychogenic dysfluency the following guidelines apply:

1. The onset is sudden.
2. The onset is temporally linked to a significant episode(s) of psychological stress.
3. The pattern of dysfluency is primarily repetition of initial or stressed syllables.
4. Dysfluencies are not reduced by choral reading, masking noise, delayed auditory feedback (initially), singing, or different communicative situations.
5. There are no islands of fluency (initially).
6. The patient demonstrates no particular concern about the dysfluency.
7. There are usually no secondary symptoms.
8. The pattern of dysfluency is present during mimed speaking.

These guidelines suffer the same fate as those set forth for neurogenic dysfluency. They are not unequivocally supported in the literature. Rentschler, Driver, and Callaway (1984) described a dysfluent patient whose clinical features did not support the lack of masking effect, the lack of concern about the dysfluency, or the apparent dysfluency during mimed reading. Nevertheless, these are guidelines that clinicians may find helpful when attempting to determine whether dysfluency is of neurogenic or psychogenic origin.

FEATURES OF NEUROGENIC DYSFLUENCY

There is one statement about neurogenic dysfluency that may be difficult to contradict. That is, neurogenic dysfluency is not a unitary disorder. Descriptions of neurogenic dysfluency are not consistent. They vary in terms of the speech characteristics, the appearance with respect to the proposed neurological event(s) associated with the dysfluency, the persistence of the dysfluency, and the proposed neurological etiology. It is often difficult to find order in the literature.

Dysfluency and Vascular Lesions With and Without Aphasia

Lebrun, Leleux, Rousseau, and Devreau (1983) estimated that two-thirds of the reported cases of neurogenic dysfluency were subsequent to stroke. Aphasia is a frequent sequella of stroke and dysfluency is often associated with aphasia. Although often associated with left hemisphere lesions, dysfluency has been reported for patients with right hemisphere lesions and bilateral lesions as well.

Single Left Hemisphere Vascular Episodes

Caplan (1972) investigated the dysfluencies of five patients with anomia and apraxia. He felt that the dysfluencies were prominent enough to be called stuttering. Caplan provided a great deal of information about the dysfluencies, but little about the etiology or the course of the dysfluencies. Since he did not elaborate, we have assumed that the five patients had suffered single episode, unilateral left hemisphere stroke, inasmuch as these strokes usually are the culprits when aphasia is present. If our assumption is correct, then Caplan's report is of five patients who had neurogenic dysfluency and aphasia following a single, left hemisphere stroke. Donnan (1979) reported two cases of patients with acquired neurogenic dysfluency, one of whom had only a single left-sided vascular episode. The patient initially presented as having "complete expressive aphasia," but after 3 days she began to speak again—with stuttering. After 2 weeks, the stuttering had largely resolved and there was only slight word-finding difficulty.

Rosenfield (1972) described the sudden onset of stuttering in a 53-year-old female who suffered vascular headaches. Following one episode of headache, she began to stutter but without any aphasia, apraxia, or motor deficit. The stuttering gradually resolved over an 8-week period. Rosenfield's patient had no prior history of dysfluency. Rosenbek et al. (1978) reported seven cases of acquired dysfluency. Four of these patients apparently had single left hemisphere vascular episodes; one had a history of premorbid stuttering. Of the other cases reported, one had sustained a right hemisphere stroke, one had suffered multiple strokes, and one was reported to have possible generalized intellectual impairment. Fluency returned for only one of the four patients with a unilateral left hemisphere stroke. Mazzuchi et al. (1981) reported neurogenic dysfluency in 16 patients, 11 of whom had vascular events. Of these 11 patients, 3 had aphasia and dysfluency concurrently and both persisted, 2 had transient aphasia and persistence of the dysfluency, 3 had transient dysfluency and persistence of aphasia, and 3 had "isolated stuttering" without aphasia. Although in general the neurogenic dysfluency either disappeared or greatly decreased after weeks or months, several of the case descriptions indicate that the dysfluency persisted. Thus it would seem that (1) isolated neurogenic dysfluency does occur from single left hemisphere vascular episodes, and (2) neurogenic dysfluency and aphasia often occur together and either, both, or neither may persist.

Dysfluency and Bilateral or Multiple Vascular Episodes

Arend, Handzel, and Weiss (1962) described two patients with acquired neurogenic dysfluency, one of whom had two vascular events within a 2-year period. Both events seemed to involve the left hemisphere. Right hemiparesis that resolved in a few months was present following the first event, but no aphasia or dysfluency was observed. The second event produced "motor and amnestic aphasia with paraphasia and stuttering." After 4 months, the aphasia resolved but the dysfluency persisted. One of two cases reported by Donnan (1979) suffered several vascular episodes involving the left hemisphere. After the first, she had only right arm and hand parasthesia. The second episode, a few months later, produced right-sided parasthesia and weakness and sudden onset of severe stuttering. She eventually underwent left carotid endarterectomy and upon recovery was fluent. She was still fluent months later when a right carotid endarterectomy was performed, and at a follow-up examination 12 months later. One dysfluent patient discussed by Rosenbek et al. (1978) suffered multiple strokes. This person was reported to have a language disorder of an undetermined type (possibly aphasia), dysarthria, and stuttering. The dysfluency persisted at a 2-month follow-up session.

Helm et al. (1978) reported 10 patients with acquired neurogenic dysfluency, one of whom had sustained two left-sided vascular episodes. The patient with multiple episodes in the left hemisphere was aphasic following the first episode; the second episode produced aphasia and dysfluency. The aphasia persisted but the dysfluency was transient.

Bilateral Vascular Episodes

Five of the cases of dysfluency reported by Helm et al. (1978) were dysfluent following bilateral vascular episodes. For four of these patients, a right-sided vascular episode preceded the left-sided event. In three of these patients, dysfluency and aphasia were concurrent following the left (second) episode; dysfluency persisted in one patient. One patient suffered a left-sided episode first and was aphasic but not dysfluent. Following the subsequent right-sided episode, persistent stuttering was added to the aphasic component. Nowack and Stone (1987) report two cases of acquired dysfluency. One of the patients was a 55-year-old female who suffered a left hemisphere stroke and was apparently severely aphasic initially, but she recovered "good functional communicative ability." She suffered a second stroke involving the right hemisphere, with resultant persistent dysfluency. Carotid bypass surgery was attempted at that time but was unsuccessful. Several years later—14 years after the left hemisphere stroke and 6 years after the right hemisphere involvement—she experienced a series of psychological stresses that exacerbated the dysfluency. She was treated for the dysfluency problem. The authors report that after "several" sessions the dysfluency was decreased—but still present.

Dysfluency and Right-sided Vascular Episodes

Dysfluency also occurs following right hemisphere vascular episodes, although that has not been reported frequently. Of the seven cases of dysfluency reported by Rosenbek et al. (1978), one had sustained a right hemisphere stroke. Other than the dysfluency, speech and language were reported to be normal. The dysfluency appeared 96 hours after the stroke and was treated 24 hours later; after an additional 96 hours and six therapy sessions the dysfluency disappeared. Horner and Massey (1983) provide a detailed account of progressive dysfluency in a patient following a right hemisphere stroke. What makes this report especially interesting is that the dysfluency did not appear until 2 years after the occurrence of the stroke—for whatever the reason, the dysfluency did not manifest itself initially. When it finally did appear, the dysfluency had features of both stuttering and palilalia; however, palilalia seems the more appropriate descriptive label. In any event, the point is that the disorder persisted.

Fleet and Heilman (1977) described the onset of left hemiplegia and dysfluency in a 42-year-old female who sustained a right hemisphere stroke. The patient was bilingual and had a familial history of stuttering. Although her father and her brother stuttered, she had not. The dysfluency did not appear until several weeks following the stroke and the onset was described as gradual. Subsequently her left hemiplegia decreased. Her dysfluency decreased also but it did not resolve completely.

SUMMARY: DYSFLUENCY AND VASCULAR EPISODES

Based upon the literature cited, the following conclusions seem warranted:

1. Dysfluency occurs following vascular episodes.
2. Dysfluency often occurs with aphasia, but can occur in isolation. When dysfluency occurs in isolation, it tends to be a transient phenomenon.

3. Dysfluency can follow single left hemisphere lesions, bilateral lesions, multiple lesions within the same hemisphere, or right hemisphere lesions.
   a. Dysfluency associated with a single left hemisphere lesion tends to be transient.
   b. Dysfluency associated with bilateral lesions and with multiple unilateral lesions tends to persist.
   c. Dysfluency associated with right hemisphere lesions needs further study.

Not enough is known about this condition to draw conclusions regarding the persistence of the disorder.

Nonvascular Etiologies

Dysfluency has been reported as a sequella of head trauma (Quinn & Andrews, 1977; Helm et al., 1978; Helm et al., 1980; Baratz & Mesulam, 1981; Mazzuchi et al., 1981). Reviewing this literature, Helm-Estabrooks (1986) suggests features that differentiate head trauma from stroke-induced stuttering. She states that with head trauma there is less sudden onset, less likelihood of aphasia, greater likelihood of seizure disorder, greater likelihood of adaptation effect, and greater likelihood of secondary behaviors.

Progressive etiologies have also been reported. Parkinson's disease has been previously discussed. Other disorders associated with dysfluency include dialysis dementia (Rosenbek, McNeil, Lemme, Prescott, & Alfy, 1975), Alzheimer's disease (Quinn & Andrews, 1977), tumor (Helm et al., 1980), polysystemic central nervous system degeneration (Lebrun, Leleux, Rousseau, & Devreux, 1983) and upper motor neuron disease (Lebrun, Retif, & Kaiser, 1983). The latter case was peculiar in that stuttering was the original presenting symptom, followed only subsequently by other pyramidal motor signs. This course mitigates against an explanation of "psychogenic reactivity to neuropathology inasmuch as stuttering was the first salient symptom" (Lebrun, Retif, & Kaiser, 1983). Finally, dysfluency has been reported in association with drug usage (Quader, 1977; Elliot & Thomas, 1985; Nurnberg & Greenwald, 1981; McClean & McClean, 1988). Rentschler and colleagues (1984) report an interesting case of "stuttering" following lithium treatment for depression. This patient exhibited characteristics reminiscent of both acquired and developmental stuttering. Similarities to acquired stuttering included absence of adaptation effect, associated neuropsychological impairments (i.e., block design) and dysfluencies in all word positions and in function as well as content words. Similarities to developmental stuttering were speech anxiety, improvement with choral reading and masking noise, and secondary behaviors, including cheek puffing, head movement, and facial grimacing.

TREATMENT

Approaches to treatment of acquired neurogenic dysfluency have been many and varied. All can be generally subcategorized under two broad headings: managing the underlying pathology and direct symptom modification.

Managing the Underlying Pathology

Again, two generic divisions can be made for approaches that seek to manage the neuropathologies associated with dysfluent speech. First are such treatments as pharmacotherapy, surgery, or prosthetic devices which have attempted to enhance the physiological substrate of speech. Second are the speech-language therapies that address the primary communication deficit (i.e., aphasia, apraxia of speech, or dysarthria). Pharmacotherapy for acquired neurogenic dysfluency has not been widespread. Baratz and Mesulam (1981) used anticonvulsant medication to treat dysfluency in a 42-year-old female who exhibited stuttering and aphasia in association with multifocal brain damage and seizure disorder following closed head injury. Three hundred milligrams of phenytoin and 90 mg of phenobarbital daily were prescribed. Stuttering resolved and word-finding abilities improved within a week. Recurrence of seizurelike phenomena were associated with the return of stuttering. Stabilization of the seizures was eventually achieved using 200 mg of phenytoin and 800 mg of carbamazepine daily. In two cases described by Nowack and Stone (1987), in which acquired stuttering was associated with bilateral cerebral disease and seizure disorder, pharmacotherapy in combination with speech therapy (i.e., relaxation and airflow) was also effective.

Surgical intervention for acquired neurogenic dysfluency has been limited to one case reported by Donnan (1979). Severe stuttering was associated with repeated transient ischemic episodes. Word-finding difficulties were also noted. Carotid angiography revealed bilateral carotid artery stenosis, with greater stricture on the left side. Left carotid endarterectomy was performed successfully. When the patient regained consciousness, the stuttering had resolved and remained so at 2-month follow-up. Presumably restoration of cerebral blood flow restored speech-language function.

The use of a prosthetic or assistive device for neurogenic dysfluency was originally described by Helm (1979), who designed a pacing board for use with a palilalic patient with progressive Parkinson syndrome. This device was approximately 13 in. by 2 in. and consisted of eight colored sections separated by raised wooden dividers running the length of the board. Helm reported that the patient was able to speak syllable by syllable without dysfluency "while tapping his finger from left to right, from segment to segment" (p. 352). The technique was based upon Luria's suggestion that automatic movements can be replaced by intentional movements to increase motor control in Parkinson's disease. Because patients with palilalia appear to have a movement termination deficit, Helm felt that the pacing board imposed an external "stop-go control" that the patient could no longer generate internally. It is noteworthy that the patient continued to use the pacing board for real communicative interactions after being transferred to another facility. Since that time pacing boards and similar devices (e.g., a wood-mounted toggle switch) have also been found to be clinically useful with more stutteringlike forms of neurogenic dysfluency (Helm-Estabrooks, 1986).

Helm and Butler (1977) reported that use of external control stimuli can also be applied to dysfluent patients who require a more salient, ongoing stimulus. One patient exhibited persistent dysarthria accompanied by frequent blocks and occasional prolongation of initial and medial phonemes, following what appears to have been a series of transient cerebrovascular episodes. The patient was not aphasic, but some naming difficulty was noted. Use of a pacing board merely increased the speaking difficulty. In order to provide a more salient external stimulus, an electrolarynx was vibrated against the palm of her left hand during reading and conversation. Helm and Butler report that this technique reduced reading time by approximately 50%. The number of blocks dropped from 38 to 8. Similar effects were noted for the application of transcutaneous nerve stimulation to the bicipital groove of the left arm. When stimulation was removed, the dysfluencies returned. Attempts to use continuous auditory stimulation such as masking noise have not been as effective. Helm and Butler suggested that the effects of tactile stimulation on verbal output in acquired speech disorders warrant further investigation. Notable in this regard is a recent technological development that provides voice-actuated vibrotactile stimulation to the laryngeal area on the surface of the neck by means of a small portable stimulator unit. This Vocal Feedback Device was developed by Vocal Tech, Inc., for use with developmental stutterers (G. Shames, personal communication, 1988). It appears to provide a secondary cue that reminds the patient to use previously trained techniques such as slowed speech and laryngeal relaxation. While its utility for treating acquired neurogenic dysfluency has not been reported, by logical extension of Helm's findings its application to acquired neurogenic dysfluency may prove beneficial in some cases.

Another type of speech prosthesis that has proved useful in the management of some forms of neurogenic dysfluency is the portable delayed auditory feedback (DAF) unit. Such a unit is battery-powered and small enough to be carried in a shirt pocket. It employs a throat-mounted microphone that delivers binaural audiosignals via molded ear pieces (e.g., Aberdeen Speech Aid, manufactured by Malden Care). Variable gain and delay intervals are usually included. Clinical use of the portable DAF unit as a permanent speech aid was originally reported by Hanson and Metter (1980), who found it to provide long-term improvement in rate and loudness in a patient with hypokinetic dysarthria, secondary to progressive supranuclear palsy. This patient, however, was not described as being dysfluent. Subsequently, Downie, Low, and Lindsay (1981) experimented with DAF units with 11 Parkinsonian patients, 2 of which benefited significantly from the device. Both patients were dysfluent, exhibiting hesitations and blocks "akin to stammering." Speech improvement was said to come and go as "abruptly as the apparatus was switched on or off" (p. 852). A 50-msec delay time was found to be most optimal. One patient, the more severe, became habituated to the device after a year of continuous use. The other continued to find it a valuable aid to communication at 2-year follow-up. It should be recognized that the use of a portable DAF device as a permanent speech aid is quite different from the in-clinic use of DAF as an adjunct to a broader behavioral program of therapy (Hanson & Metter, 1980). It is possible that the use of delayed sidetone with such a short delay interval (in comparison with the 200–250 msec delay found most effective for developmental stutterers) might also constitute an external control stimulus akin to pacing. Thereby each echo would serve as a stop-go boundary for termination and initiation of the flow of speech.

Another set of therapeutic strategies that target the underlying disorder consists of the conventional speech-language therapies for the acquired neurogenic communicative disorders of aphasia, dysarthria, and apraxia of speech. The primary goal of traditional aphasia therapy is multimodality stimulation of the language system (Schuell et al., 1964). The primary goal of apraxia therapy is retraining of speech motor programming functions (Rosenbek, 1985), while the primary goal of dysarthria therapy is compensated intelligibility (Rosenbek & LaPointe, 1985). Implicit in these approaches is the assumption that dysfluency is a direct result of the primary communicative deficit and therefore dysfluency will resolve as the primary deficit resolves. Example cases illustrating such parallel variation in fluency and aphasia have been reported in the literature (Shtremel, 1963, cited in Rosenbek et al., 1978); however, so have counter examples of patients whose fluency did not improve (Andrews et al., 1972; Rosenbek et al., 1978). It does seem reasonable, at our present stage of knowledge, to initially target a primary deficit in cases for whom that deficit and acquired dysfluency appear to be closely linked. This is particularly true when the primary deficit is the overriding contributor to disruption of communication. In addition, prior remediation of the primary disorder may make direct symptom modification of dysfluency less complicated at a later stage of therapy.

Direct Modification of Dysfluent Symptoms

Approaches that target direct symptom modification of dysfluency as the treatment goal are borrowed in their entirety from the extensive developmental stuttering literature. These "stuttering therapies" can also be divided into two general classes: so-called fluency-shaping therapy and stuttering modification therapy (Guitar & Peters, 1980). Fluency-shaping involves establishing some form of fluency that is reinforced and modified to resemble normal speech, then generalized outside of the clinical setting to the patient's everyday environment. Fluency-shaping techniques have been applied to cases of acquired neurogenic dysfluency. Rosenbek et al. (1978) and Rosenbek (1984) describe a patient with intact language who stuttered following a right parietal lobe CVA. One day after onset he was placed on a program of "syllable timed speech." This involved rate reduction to approximately 50 wpm by increasing both articulation time (i.e., phoneme prolongation) and pause time. Treatment also included a significant counseling component. The patient was fluent after six sessions and remained so at follow-up one month later.

Delayed auditory feedback has also been used in the treatment of acquired neurogenic dysfluency. Marshall and Starch (1984) utilized DAF with a 32-year-old "acquired stutterer" to establish fluency at 4 years postonset of stuttering. To date, the most ambitious attempt at a treatment study involving DAF with neurogenic dysfluency was undertaken by Marshall and Neuburger (1987). These authors used single subject, multiple baseline designs with three severely dysfluent patients. Etiologies included closed head trauma, right parietal skull fracture with left temporal hematoma, and brainstem contusion. The patients were seen on an outpatient basis for 1 hour sessions, 2 to 3 times per week. Treatment followed conventional fluency therapy programs, in which an initial feedback delay of 250 msec is used to slow the speaking rate by requiring the patient to prolong each word to compensate for DAF; this delay interval is gradually reduced in 50-msec steps to zero. Frequency of stuttering events and reading rate were measured across baseline, treatment, and maintenance conditions for a variety of connected discourse tasks. The DAF treatment reduced dysfluencies in all three patients. Only one patient, however, sustained dysfluency reduction throughout the maintenance (i.e., treatment withdrawal) period. Generalization to nontreatment settings was not noted, but neither was any transfer training incorporated in the short-term experimental "therapy."

The authors conclude that "DAF has 'potential' as a treatment procedure in the management of acquired stuttering" (p. 363).

Stuttering modification therapy is based on interpretations of stuttering as learned avoidance and struggle behavior. Such therapies attempt to decrease avoidance behavior, improve negative attitudes toward speech, and reduce speech-related fear (Guitar & Peters, 1980). Stuttering modification therapy also has been applied to acquired neurogenic dysfluency. Nowack and Stone (1987) reported two cases of dysfluency associated with bilateral cerebral disease. As mentioned previously, neuropharmacological treatment was combined with a program of speech therapy which the authors regarded as broadly "anxiolytic." Both patients experienced marked speech anxiety. Treatment techniques included progressive relaxation and breathing exercises incorporating release of unphonated airflow in nonspeech tasks. The authors suggest that improvement in these cases followed alleviation of considerable psychological stress by speech therapy.

Electromyographic (EMG) biofeedback as an aid to relaxation during speech has been employed in the treatment of neurogenic stuttering (Helm-Estabrooks, 1986). Following a protocol originally developed for developmental stutterers, EMG treatment was used with a case of moderately severe "stuttering" secondary to a series of minor strokes. After a 4-month course of biweekly sessions, dysfluency was reduced to a mild level. Other forms of biofeedback therapy for more direct work on speaking variables also have been recommended (see Chapter 11 in this volume).

Finally, combined approaches drawing upon various treatment strategies also have been employed. Rosenbek (1984) indicates that therapy using syllable-timed speech, which was successful with one neurogenic dysfluent patient, also had a strong counseling component oriented toward reassurance that fluent speech was still possible. Nowack and Stone (1987) combined pharmacotherapy with relaxation-breathing techniques. Given the strikingly heterogeneous nature of the disorder, an eclectic approach toward treating acquired neurogenic dysfluency would seem advisable. The available literature provides a fertile basis for clinical experimentation with a variety of potential combinations and permutations.

CONCLUSION

In an effort to bring order to the diverse array of treatment approaches that have been employed with acquired neurogenic dysfluency patients, a classification scheme is provided in Figure 8.1. Selection of a particular treatment strategy is not simple, and may devolve into trial and error

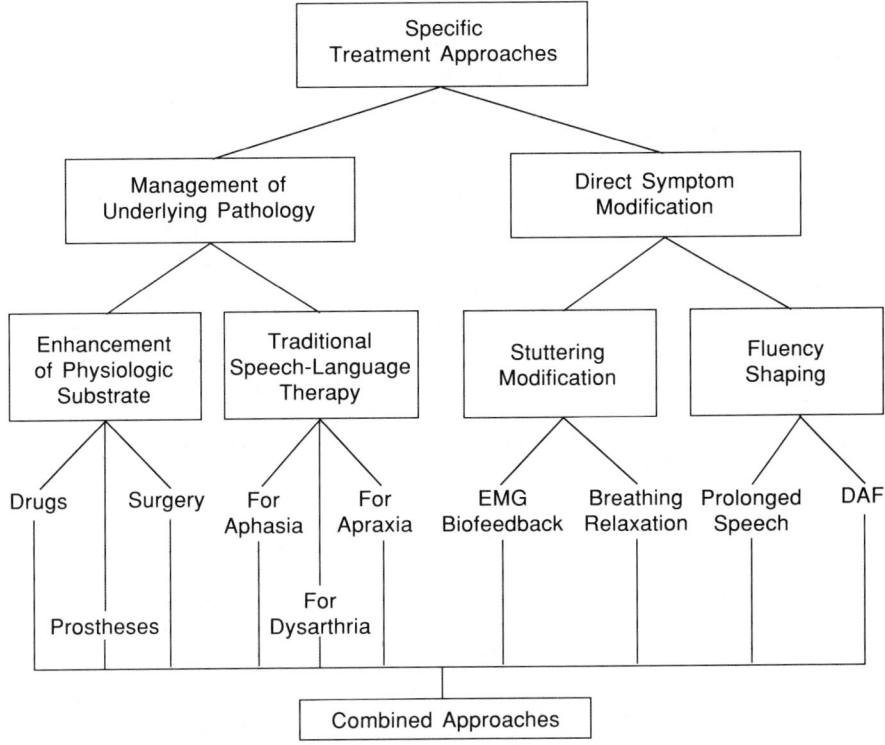

Figure 8.1 A framework for the treatment of acquired neurogenic dysfluency. The lowest labeled nodes represent treatments reported to have been successful in selected cases.

therapy in many cases. There remain no clear-cut guidelines. If medical management of the physiological substrate is indicated as part of an overall medical plan (e.g., for seizures or arterial circulation), one should attempt to monitor dysfluencies systematically before and after such intervention. There is at least some reason to be guardedly optimistic that physical intervention may decrease dysfluency. In most cases, however, it becomes the speech-language pathologist's responsibility to attempt to remediate the neurogenic patient's dysfluent speech.

The decision of whether to address the primary communicative deficit or to attempt direct symptom modification of dysfluency may be bolstered by a range of diagnostic information. Neurologic examination and brain-imaging studies may be useful in determining whether lesion loci are within the classic speech-language or motor control areas. Chronic neurogenic dysfluency, not associated with the classic neurogenic communication disorders, tends to stem from bilateral subcortical involvement (Helm-Estabrooks, 1986). Traditional aphasia and motor speech evaluations used in conjunction with the neurodiagnostic data will determine the presence of classical aphasias, dysarthrias, or apraxia of speech. Faced with dysfluency in the presence of these primary communicative deficits, addressing the primary deficit first may be the preferred procedure. If, however, dysfluency exists in isolation or is the most salient presenting problem, the clinician may elect to target direct modification of dysfluent symptoms. In such instances, an additional decision must be made as to whether to draw upon fluency-shaping or stuttering modification techniques or both. In cases in which there is little evidence of struggle behavior, avoidance, or speech anxiety, fluency-shaping may be indicated. Because these procedures are heavily operant in nature, they may also be preferable for patients with restricted cognitive capacity. In contrast, stuttering modification is intellectually demanding, rooted as it is in psychotherapeutic tradition. Contrary to popular belief (probably originating from Canter, 1971), many acquired neurogenic dysfluency patients do experience significant speech anxiety and exhibit nonspeech secondary behaviors such as grimacing or head nodding (Rosenbek et al., 1978; Nowack & Stone, 1987; Rentschler et al., 1984; Lebrun, Leleux, Rousseau, & Devreux, 1983). If cognitive capacity is adequate, stuttering modification therapies may be more appropriate for such patients. Assistive devices such as pacing boards and tactile stimulators may prove beneficial to some patients, and appear to be the treatment of choice for palilalia. As Helm-Estabrooks (1986) has stated, "Successful management of neurogenic stuttering requires differential treatment as well as differential diagnosis" (p. 211).

Yet we should not paint too rosy a picture. Many authors report cases of neurogenic dysfluency in which specific treatments either did not generalize (Marshall & Neuberger, 1987) or were generally ineffective (Rosenbek et al., 1978; Helm-Estabrooks, 1986). There are at present no proved prognostic indicators. As our knowledge of acquired neurogenic dysfluency increases, through controlled clinical experimentation, it seems likely that differential diagnostic profiling (incorporating data from neurology, psychology, and speech-language pathology) may come to guide selection of a therapeutic plan. In the meantime, it is encouraging to note that there is no shortage of field-tested approaches for remediation of acquired neurogenic dysfluency and that all of them have contributed successfully to the management of selected cases.

REFERENCES

Albert, M. L., Goodglass, H., Helm, N. A., Rubens, A. B., & Alexander, M. P. (1981). *Clinical aspects of dysphasia.* New York: Springer-Verlag.

Andrews, G., Quinn, P. T., & Sorby, W. A. (1972). Stuttering: An investigation into cerebral dominance for speech. *Journal of Neurology, Neurosurgery, and Psychiatry, 35,* 414–418.

Arend, R., Handzel, L., & Weiss, B. (1962). Dysphatic stuttering. *Folia Phoniatrica, 14,* 55–66.

Attanasio, J. S. (1987). A case of late-onset acquired stuttering in adult life. *Journal of Fluency Disorders, 12,* 287–290.

Baratz, R., & Mesulam, M. M. (1981). Adult-onset stuttering treated with anticonvulsants. *Archives of Neurology, 38,* 132.

Canter, G. J. (1971). Observations on neurogenic stuttering: A contribution to differential diagnosis. *British Journal of Disorders of Communication, 6,* 139–143.

Caplan, L. (1972). An investigation of some aspects of stuttering-like speech in adult dysphasic subjects. *Journal of South African Speech and Hearing Association, 19,* 52–66.

Critchley, M. (1927, July). On palilalia. *Journal of Neurology & Psychiatry,* 23–52.

Culatta, R., & Leeper, L. (1988). Dysfluency isn't always stuttering. *Journal of Speech and Hearing Disorders.*

Darley, F. L., Aronson, A. E., & Brown, J. R. (1975). *Motor speech disorders.* Philadelphia: W. B. Saunders.

Deal, J. L. (1982). Sudden onset of stuttering: A case report. *Journal of Speech and Hearing Disorders, 47,* 301–304.

Deal, J. L., & Doro, J. M. (1987). Episodic hysterical stuttering. *Journal of Speech and Hearing Disorders, 52,* 299–300.

Dempsey, G. L., & Granich, M. (1978). Hypno-behavioral therapy in the case of a traumatic stutterer: A case report. *International Journal of Clinical and Experimental Hypnosis, 16,* 125–133.

Donnan, G. A. (1979). Stuttering as a manifestation of stroke. *Medical Journal of Australia, 1,* 44–45.

Downie, A. W., Low, J. M., & Lindsay, D. D. (1981). Speech disorders in parkinsonism: Use of delayed auditory feedback in selected cases. *Journal of Neurology, Neurosurgery, and Psychiatry, 44,* 852–853.

Elliot, R. L., & Thomas, B. J. (1985). A case report of alprazolam-induced stuttering. *Journal of Clinical Psychopharmacology, 5,* 159–160.

Fleet, W. S., & Heilman, K. M. (1977). Acquired stuttering from a right hemisphere lesion in a right-hander. *Neurology, 35,* 1343–1346.

Freund, H. (1966). *Psychopathology and the problem of stuttering.* Springfield, IL: Charles C. Thomas.

Guitar, B., & Peters, T. J. (1980). *Stuttering: An integration of contemporary therapies.* Memphis, TN: Speech Foundation of America.

Hanson, W., & Metter, J. (1980). DAF as instrumental treatment for dysarthria in progressive supranuclear palsy. A case report. *Journal of Speech and Hearing Disorders, 45,* 268–276.

Head, H. (1926). *Aphasia and kindred disorders of speech.* London: Cambridge University Press.

Helm, N. A. (1979). Management of palilalia with a pacing board. *Journal of Speech and Hearing Disorders, 44,* 350–353.

Helm, N. A., & Butler, R. B. (1977). Transcutaneous nerve stimulation in acquired speech disorders. *Lancet, 8049,* 1177–1178.

Helm, N. A., Butler, R. B., & Benson, D. F. (1978). Acquired stuttering. *Neurology, 28,* 1159–1165.

Helm, N. A., Butler, R. B., & Canter, G. J. (1980). Neurogenic acquired stuttering. *Journal of Fluency Disorders, 5,* 269–279.

Helm-Estabrooks, N. (1986). Diagnosis and management of neurogenic stuttering in adults. In K. O. St. Louis (Ed.), *The atypical stutterer: Principles and practices of rehabilitation.* Orlando, FL: Academic Press.

Horner, J., & Massey, E. W. (1983). Progressive dysfluency associated with right hemisphere disease. *Brain and Language, 18,* 71–85.

Johns, D. F., & Darley, F. L. (1970). Phonemic variability in apraxia of speech. *Journal of Speech and Hearing Research, 13,* 553–583.

Kent, R. D., & LaPointe, L. L. (1982). Acoustic properties of pathologic reiterative utterances: A case study of palilalia. *Journal of Speech and Hearing Research, 25,* 95–99.

Koller, W. C. (1983). Dysfluency (stuttering) in extrapyramidal disease. *Archives of Neurology, 40,* 175–177.

LaPointe, L. L., & Horner, J. (1981). Palilalia: A descriptive study of pathological reiterative utterances. *Journal of Speech and Hearing Disorders, 46,* 34–38.

Lebrun, Y., & Leleux, C. (1985). Acquired stuttering following right-brain damage in dextrals. *Journal of Fluency Disorders, 10,* 137–141.

Lebrun, Y., Leleux, C., Rousseau, J. J., & Devreux, F. (1983). Acquired stuttering. *Journal of Fluency Disorders, 8,* 323–330.

Lebrun, Y., Retif, J., & Kaiser, G. (1983). Acquired stuttering as a forerunner of motor-neuron disease. *Journal of Fluency Disorders, 8,* 161–167.

Luchsinger, R., & Arnold, G. E. (1965). *Voice-speech-language.* Belmont, CA: Wadsworth.

Marshall, R. C., & Neuburger, S. I. (1987). Effects of delayed auditory feedback on acquired stuttering following head injury. *Journal of Fluency Disorders, 12,* 355–365.

Marshall, R. C., & Starch, S. A. (1984). Behavioral treatment of acquired stuttering. *Australian Journal of Human Communication Disorders, 12,* 87–91.

Mazzuchi, A., Moretti, G., Carpeggiani, P., Parma, M., Paini, P. (1981). Clinical observations on acquired stuttering. *British Journal of Disordered Communication, 16,* 19–30.

McClean, M. D., & McClean, A. J. (1988). Case report of stuttering acquired in association with phenytoin use for post-head injury seizures. *Journal of Fluency Disorders, 10,* 241–255.

Nowack, W. J., & Stone, R. E. (1987). Acquired stuttering and bilateral cerebral disease. *Journal of Fluency Disorders, 12,* 141–146.

Nurnberg, H. G., & Greenwald, B. (1981). Stuttering: An unusual side effect of phenothiazines. *American Journal of Psychiatry, 138,* 386–387.

Quader, S. E. (1977). Dysarthria: An unusual side effect of tricyclic antidepressants. *British Medical Journal, 9,* 97.

Quinn, P. T., & Andrews, B. (1977). Neurological stuttering: A clinical entity? *Journal of Neurology, Neurosurgery & Psychiatry, 40,* 699–701.

Rentschler, G. J., Driver, L. E., & Callaway, E. A. (1984). The onset of stuttering following drug overdose. *Journal of Fluency Disorders, 9,* 265–284.

Rosenbek, J. (1980). Apraxia of speech—Relationship to stuttering. *Journal of Fluency Disorders, 5,* 233–253.

Rosenbek, J. C. (1984). Stuttering secondary to brain damage. In R. F. Curlee & W. H. Perkins (Eds.), *Nature and treatment of stuttering: New directions.* Austin, TX: PRO-ED.

Rosenbek, J. C. (1985). Treating apraxia of speech. In D. F. Johns (Ed.), *Clinical management of neurogenic communicative disorders.* Austin, TX: PRO-ED.

Rosenbek, J., & LaPointe, L. L. (1985). The dysarthrias: Description, diagnosis and treatment. In D. Johns (Ed.), *Clinical management of neurogenic communicative disorders.* Austin, TX: PRO-ED.

Rosenbek, J., McNeil, M. R., Lemme, M. L., Prescott, T. E., & Alfrey, A. C. (1975). Speech and language findings in a chronic hemodyalysis patient: A case report. *Journal of Speech and Hearing Disorders, 40,* 245–252.

Rosenbek, J., Messert, B., Collins, M., & Wertz, R. T. (1978). Stuttering following brain damage. *Brain and Language, 6,* 82–96.

Rosenfield, D. B. (1972). Stuttering and cerebral ischemia. *New England Journal of Medicine, 287,* 991.

Rousey, C. G., Arjunan, K. N., & Rousey, C. L. (1986). Successful treatment of stuttering following closed head injury. *Journal of Fluency Disorders, 11,* 257–261.

Schiller, F., (1947). Aphasia studied in patients with missile wounds. *Journal of Neurology, Neurosurgery and Psychiatry, 10,* 183–197.

Schuell, H., Jenkins, J. J., & Jimenez-Pabon, E. (1964). *Aphasia in adults: Diagnosis, prognosis, and treatment.* New York: Harper & Row.

Shtremel, A. K. (1963). [Stuttering in left parietal lobe syndrome]. *Zhurnal Neuropatologii i Psikhiatrii imeni S. S. Korsakova, 63,* 828–832.

Trost, J. E. (1971, November). *Apraxic dysfluency in patients with Broca's aphasia.* Paper presented at the annual convention of the American Speech and Hearing Association, Chicago.

Van Riper, C. (1971). *The nature of stuttering.* Englewood Cliffs, NJ: Prentice-Hall.

Wallen, V. (1961). Primary stuttering in an 18-year-old adult. *Journal of Speech and Hearing Disorders, 16,* 394–395.

Weiner, A. E. (1981). A case of adult onset of stuttering. *Journal of Fluency Disorders, 6,* 181–186.

Wertz, R. T., Rosenbek, J. C., & LaPointe, L. L. (1983). *Apraxia of speech.* Philadelphia: Saunders.

Yairi, E., Gintautas, J., & Avent, J. R. (1981). Dysfluent speech associated with brain damage. *Brain and Language, 14,* 49–56.

CHAPTER 9
Neurogenic Disorders of Prosody

Donald A. Robin, Gayle V. Klouda, and Linda N. Hug

> *The authors discuss disorders of prosody in patients with focal cerebral lesions. After a review of the relevant literature, they detail the steps involved in diagnosis of prosodic disturbances. The discussion focuses on the importance of acoustic measures to complement perceptual judgments and on the need to examine both the production and the perception of prosody. A look at different treatment approaches and case descriptions follows the assessment section.*

1. Define the use of prosody as a communicative act and distinguish the different perceptual and acoustic components of prosody. What is gained by utilizing acoustic measures in diagnosing and treating prosodic disturbances?
2. How can acoustic measures be used to examine prosodic changes over time?
3. This chapter describes linguistic and emotive functions of prosody. How are these two functions similar and how do they differ? What stimuli should be used to assess and treat emotive and linguistic functions of prosody?

There has been a recent flurry of interest in the prosodic aspects of speech and language. However, statements about the role of prosody in disordered speech and language can be traced to Jackson (1874) and Pick (1919) (cited in Monrad-Krohn, 1947a, 1947b), who noted that language is more than words; it contains melodies through which humans convey meaning. Perhaps the first descriptions of neurologically impaired patients with prosodic disturbances can be found in the work of Monrad-Krohn (1947a, 1947b, 1963), who described different types of impaired speech prosody related to nervous system lesions. Yet given the historical significance of prosody in the literature, it remains a neglected area of clinical concern. Few clinicians routinely assess prosody and it is often treated as an afterthought.

It is important to stress that prosodic impairments may contribute to abnormal speech and language performance in patients with neurological disease. Prosody also serves important communicative functions that often override linguistic considerations. Myers (1984) and Robin, Jordan, and Rodnitzky (1986) have pointed out that patients and their families must be counseled as to the effect prosodic impairment has on communication successes and failures. In order to provide appropriate counseling, clinicians must have as detailed a picture as possible of a patient's prosodic profile.

This chapter examines prosodic disturbances related to neurological lesions. While the authors acknowledge impairments of prosody that accompany the various dysarthrias, the present chapter is aimed at "higher" level disturbances related to focal lesions of the cerebral hemispheres and the corpus callosum. Disorders of the production and perception of prosody will be described for various patient groups and related abilities will be discussed. Furthermore, the role of acoustic measures as clinical tools will be examined. It is our opinion that the clinician must make use of all possible knowledge that can be gained about a patient's speech and language and that acoustic studies of prosody are now mandatory in clinical practice.

The chapter is divided into an overview of normal prosody (including definitions, perceptual measures, and acoustic measures), a brief review of the history of prosody disorders from Monrad-Krohn to the present, suggestions for diagnosis of prosodic impairments, suggestions for treatment of prosodic disturbances, and case studies of patients with focal lesions of the nervous system and subsequent prosodic disabilities.

DEFINITION

Prosody has been called the melody of speech (Berry, 1969; Monrad-Krohn, 1947a, 1947b). It refers to changes at segmental and suprasegmental levels that convey meaning. Some functions of prosody operate above the linguistic level, while others serve specific linguistic functions. Netsell (1973) has defined three prosodic features: intonation, stress, and rhythm. These refer to variations in fundamental frequency and in the temporal structure of speech. Nation and Aram (1982) defined prosody as changes in the speech waveform that relate to intonation and stress patterns and changes that relate to timing and rhythm.

These perceptual contributions to communication through speech prosody are related to variations in three acoustic properties of the speech waveform: duration, amplitude, and fundamental frequency. Changes in these features give rise to variations in intonation or pitch patterns, stress patterns, and temporal (or rhythmic) patterns of speech that can alter the meaning of spoken language. While prosody is typically viewed as a suprasegmental feature (extending over the length of a word or utterance), segmental changes also can give rise to alterations in the melody or rhythm of speech and therefore can change intended meaning.

Communicative Functions of Prosody

A variety of communicative functions of prosody serve to signal meaningful differences between utterances. Prosody can be used to convey emotional states such as happiness, sadness, or anger (Cosmides, 1983; Monrad-Krohn, 1963; Nation & Aram, 1982; Scherer, 1986; Williams & Stevens, 1972). Prosodic changes also are used to convey linguistic distinctions. The difference between interrogative and neutral sentence forms may be conveyed by increasing fundamental frequency and duration over the final word of an utterance (Cooper, Eady, & Mueller, 1985; Eady & Cooper, 1986; Nation & Aram, 1982; Klouda, Robin, Graff-Radford, & Cooper, 1988). Perceptually this would be noted as a rising pitch at the end of a sentence during the asking of a question. The linguistic use of prosody also can be observed in the assignment of stress within an utterance (Selkirk, 1984; Cooper et al., 1985). In this case, a word might receive focus or stress, as in *"Don* shot the puck to Kent" versus "Don shot the puck to *Kent."* In the first sentence, "Don" is stressed and would be the appropriate answer to the question "Who shot the puck to Kent?"; in the second sentence, "Kent" receives stress and would be used to answer the question "Who did Don shoot the puck to?" Prosody also can be used to signal syntactic structure (Lea, 1973; Cooper & Sorensen, 1981). For example, the sentences "If Jerry kicked his mother, we'll be upset" and "If Jerry kicked, his mother will be upset" have different meanings depending on the position of the pause.

PROSODIC DISRUPTION DUE TO CEREBRAL INJURY

Monrad-Krohn (1947a, 1947b, 1963) discussed the role of prosody in speech and reported on patients with neurological insults who had impairments in speech melody. Monrad-Krohn described three types of prosodic breakdown. In the type of prosodic abnormality termed aprosody, a patient's melody of speech is flattened. The normal variation in prosody is generally reduced. When Monrad-Krohn described patients as hyperprosodic, he was referring to abnormally increased variations in the melody of speech. Recently, Shapiro and Danly (1985) have reported that patients with anterior right hemisphere lesions demonstrate reduced variations in fundamental frequency across sentences and are therefore aprosodic, while patients with lesions posterior in the right hemisphere are hyperprosodic, or have increased fundamental frequency variations. Monrad-Krohn's third disorder of speech melody is called dysprosody, in which patients have abnormal speech rhythm and seem to misuse prosodic cues. To support this observation, Monrad-Krohn (1947) described a subject with a "foreign accent syndrome" whose native accent (Norwegian) disappeared after a left hemisphere lesion. This subject reportedly sounded as if she had a German accent.

In the past 15 years, the study of prosodic disturbance related to neurological lesions has become more common. The modern study of prosody related to focal brain injury was initiated by the work of Ross (Ross & Mesulam, 1979; Ross, 1981), who described patients with right hemisphere lesions as aprosodic. The patients described in the Ross and Mesulam paper had a general flatness in their voices; they were unable to convey whether they were happy, sad, or angry, or whether they were asking a question or making a statement. Ross (1981) aptly points out that some patients may have difficulty in perceiving prosodic variations in speech in addition to their difficulty with production. Since the publication of Ross's two papers, a variety of studies have emerged examining the production and perception of speech prosody in patients with focal cerebral lesions. Most recently, acoustic studies have appeared in the literature that further our knowledge of the neural control of prosody and assist in our ability as clinicians to diagnose and treat such problems. In the remainder of this section, some studies in speech prosody will be reviewed and the role of prosody in the right hemisphere, the corpus callosum, and the left hemisphere will be discussed.

Prosodic Disturbances Due to Right Hemispheric Lesions

It is clear that unilateral damage to the right hemisphere can result in impairment in the production of prosody, the comprehension of prosody, or both (e.g., Heilman, Bowers, Speedie, & Coslett, 1984; Shapiro & Danly, 1985; Tompkins & Mateer, 1985). In regard to the production of prosody, Kent and Rosenbek (1982) reported that patients with right hemisphere lesions were aprosodic; spectral analyses of their speech revealed reduced fundamental frequency and intensity contours across utterances and limited variations in syllable durations. Shapiro and Danly (1985) found the typical fundamental frequency rise associated with yes-no questions was reduced in patients with right anterior lesions. Likewise, Cooper, Soares, Nicol, Michelow, and Goloskie (1984) found diminished use of clause and utterance lengths in patients with right hemisphere damage. In contrast to the aprosodia typically reported of right hemisphere patients, Shapiro and Danly reported that posterior right hemisphere lesions resulted in an exaggerated use of fundamental frequency cues. These patients were labeled hyperprosodic.

One critical point to remember is that the course of recovery from prosodic impairment in right hemisphere patients has not been addressed to any great degree. Colsher, Cooper, and Graff-Radford (1987) found that patients tested in the acute period following the insult were aprosodic and had reduced fundamental frequency contours, while patients tested at 6 months postonset appeared hypermelodic or normal. Further study of this issue is clearly warranted, as it is apparent that differences in the results of the studies on speech prosody following brain injury may be related to the time postonset that a particular patient is studied. In addition, the effects of treatment on recovery from prosody have never been examined. Another critical problem with the literature to date is that the neuroanatomical localization of the lesions have been poorly described. With better methods for analyzing lesion location and the use of magnetic resonance imaging and other scanning techniques, for example, results of future studies of prosodic disorders may be more consistent.

Patients who suffer focal right hemisphere lesions also may demonstrate impairments in the ability to perceive variations in speech prosody. Ross (1981) noted that patients with posterior right hemisphere lesions were impaired in their ability to perceive differences between happy, angry, and sad intonations, and whether a sentence was a question or a statement. Heilman and colleagues (Heilman, Scholes, & Watson, 1975; Tucker, Watson, & Heilman, 1977) found that patients with right hemisphere lesions were more impaired than left hemisphere patients in identification of sentences intoned as happy, sad, angry, or indifferent. Likewise, Tompkins and Flowers (1985) reported that males with right hemisphere lesions were impaired in the reception and recognition of emotionally intoned prosodic stimuli.

Disturbances of Prosody Due to Left Hemispheric Lesions

There have been relatively fewer studies of speech prosody in patients with left hemisphere lesions than of those with right hemisphere lesions.

Ryalls (1982) studied eight patients with Broca's aphasia and found that the fundamental frequency range was significantly more restricted for the patients than for normal controls. Danly and Shapiro (1982) reported that patients with Broca's aphasia had abnormally exaggerated fundamental frequency contours. It should be noted that the measures used in these two studies were different, which might account for the variation in the results (see Cooper & Klouda, 1987, for a discussion of this issue). Danly and Shapiro also found that patients with Broca's aphasia produce higher peak fundamental frequency on initial stressed words of long sentences than they did on short sentences. Cooper and Sorensen (1981) suggested that normal speakers increase fundamental frequency on the first stressed word of a long sentence compared to a short one to allow for a greater range of frequency declination across the utterance.

Kent and Rosenbek (1982), arguing that prosodic disturbance is a primary symptom of apraxia of speech, reported acoustic data on patients with left hemisphere lesions and apraxia. They found that apraxic speakers had a dissociated spectrographic pattern in which syllable durations were uniform and that the fundamental frequency pattern assumed a similar shape within syllables. The syllables tended to be separated by lengthy but consistent intervals.

Patients with posterior left hemisphere lesions and resultant Wernicke's aphasia have been studied by Danly, Cooper, and Shapiro (1983). In contrast to the clinical impression that prosody is normal in patients with Wernicke's aphasia, these researchers found that fundamental frequency contours across an utterance were normal, but that the use of fundamental frequency cues for specific syntactic structures was abnormal.

Disturbances of Prosody Due to Lesions of the Corpus Callosum

There is very little evidence to support a role for the corpus callosum in speech prosody. However, one might assume that any prosodic information processed in the right hemisphere must be transferred to the left hemisphere for the accurate production of speech and language. This transfer of prosodic information in all likelihood occurs across the corpus callosum (Ross, Harney, deLacoste-Utamsing, & Prudy, 1981; Speedie, Coslett, & Heilman, 1984). Watson and Heilman (1983) reported that a patient who had suffered callosal disconnection was unable to repeat affective tone. Speedie et al. (1984) studied prosody in two patients with left hemisphere lesions and mixed transcortical aphasia. Their patients were unable to repeat emotively intoned utterances. The authors argued that since lesions that result in transcortical aphasia spare the perisylvian speech regions, the impairment in emotive prosody had to be the result of a loss of communication between prosodic centers in the right hemisphere and speech centers in the left.

In a case that we will describe in detail in the case reports section, Klouda, Robin, Graff-Radford, and Cooper (1988) studied prosody of a patient who had suffered a pericallosal aneurysm that resulted in callosal disconnection. The patient was impaired in her ability to produce linguistic and affective prosodic variations. Acoustically, the most prominent changes were in fundamental frequency contour, while durational measures remained intact. Her fundamental frequency contours improved over the period of a year. This patient's inability to use fundamental frequency information for prosody initially suggested that the transfer of fundamental frequency contours from the right to the left hemisphere was disrupted.

Summary of Cortical Contributions to Prosody

This brief review of the literature on neurogenic disorders of prosody points out the need for special consideration of the ability of a patient to produce and comprehend prosodic variations in speech. Disorders of prosody have been documented in patients with right and left hemispheric lesions and in patients with lesions in the corpus callosum. The study of higher prosodic disturbances is still in its infancy, however, and numerous questions remain. For example, it is unclear if the prosodic disturbances found in right hemisphere patients are confined to emotional utterances or if they are present for linguistic distinctions as well. Some recent papers have addressed this issue (see Behrens, 1988; Ross, 1988; Ryalls, 1988; Tompkins & Flowers, 1985).

It is as yet unclear if the prosodic disorders we have described represent a high-level cognitive deficit in which patients are unable to meaningfully label the prosodic contour of an utterance, or if there exist some perceptual deficits that might account for the impairment. However, differential diagnosis might be possible in that the relative contribution of the right hemisphere to prosody may be related to the processing of fundamental frequency information and not to other prosodic features such as duration or intensity. Moreover, left hemispheric contributions to prosody may be related to durational aspects of prosody but not to the frequency aspects. Robin, Tranel, and Damasio (1990) reported that patients with right hemisphere lesions were impaired in their ability to perceive frequency information but were normal in their ability to perceive durational information. In direct contrast, patients with left hemisphere lesions were able to perceive frequency change but were abnormal in their performance of all tasks of temporal perception. It might be that this separation of processing capacities exists for prosodic stimuli as well. Moreover, the abnormal perceptual ability might be directly or indirectly related to the prosodic disturbances found in patients with focal cerebral lesions. Finally, Kent and Rosenbek (1982) found different spectrographic patterns depending on the site of the lesion in the nervous system, which suggests that differential diagnosis of the bases of acoustic parameters may be warranted.

What seems critical to the clinical endeavor is that carefully controlled evaluations of prosodic disturbances are performed. In order to do this successfully, clinicians need to consider using acoustic measures to define the specific parameters of prosody and develop stimuli that assess a range of emotive and linguistic conditions. Acoustic, coupled with perceptual, data may provide information needed for differential diagnosis and for the design of a specific therapeutic program.

ASSESSMENT OF PROSODIC PRODUCTION

The production of prosody can be measured perceptually, acoustically, and physiologically. We will focus on perceptual and acoustic measures for the reason that clinicians may find it easier to obtain the instrumentation for perceptual and acoustic measures than for physiologic measures. In addition to assessing prosody in speech production, clinicians should examine the patient's ability to perceive differences in prosody in the speech of others. This is an area of prosody that frequently has been overlooked.

Perceptual measures are those that rely on the ear of the clinician to determine prosodic accuracy and acceptability. It can be argued that if an impairment is not perceptually relevant, it does not constitute a disorder and should not be treated. However, it has been demonstrated that the human ear may be a poor judge of acoustic reality (Liberman, 1965; Breckenridge, 1977). That is to say, predictable prosodic changes are so ubiquitous in the language that we hear them even when they are absent from the acoustic signal, or we may not be able to judge which acoustic parameter is changing even when we accurately identify a prosodic change. The specific acoustic parameter that is disordered (duration, fundamental frequency, or intensity) cannot be determined without acoustic measures. Furthermore, although a patient may "sound" normal to the clinician during a treatment or diagnostic session, the clinician is operating in a restricted context. Often the patient or the family will complain that in other settings the patient seems to have lost the ability to convey humor or emotion through the voice. They may say that the patient's speech is "different" in that the tone of voice is no longer meaningful. The point is that both perceptual and acoustic measures of speech prosody should be used; they would complement one another and their combination would add an important dimension to the diagnostic effort.

In Table 9.1, the stimuli are listed that are used to examine the production of prosody in patients seen by our group at the University of Iowa (Cooper et al., 1985; Eady & Cooper, 1986; Eady, Cooper, Klouda, Mueller, & Lotts, 1986; Klouda et al., 1988; Robin et al., 1986; Robin, Klouda, Graff-Radford, Cooper, Damasio, & Hug, submitted). The battery is designed to assess emotive uses of prosody. The patient reads or repeats a sentence with happy, sad, or angry intonation. The linguistic distinction between question and statement also is assessed using these sentences. There are a total of four sentences and five intonation patterns for twenty items.

We further assess the linguistic use of prosody by examining a patient's ability to utilize prosody to convey emphatic stress placed on the initial or final words of a sentence. These stimuli also are shown

TABLE 9.1
Stimuli Used for Assessment of Prosody

I. Emotive intonation and question and neutral forms
   1. The bird flew away.
   2. Tomorrow I'm leaving for Chicago.
   3. My horse jumped over the fence.
   4. We sold our cottage last month.
II. Emphatic stress
   1. *Don* shot the *puck* to *Kent*.
   2. *Sheila* took the *money* from *Chip*.
   3. *Stan* paid the *check* for *Peg*.
   4. The *salesman* sold the *couch* to my *Father*.
   5. *Mary* typed the *paper* for *Kate*.
   6. *Chuck* ate *supper* with *George*.
III. Syntactic juncture sentence pairs
   1. If Harry went to the bank, Ann will be very angry.
      Uncle Harry went to the bank Ann went to yesterday.
   2. If Jerry kicked his mother, we'll be upset.
      If Jerry kicked, his mother will be upset.
   3. Roger went to the concert with Chuck, and Laura went with Rob.
      Roger went to the concert with Chuck and Laura and Rob.
   4. Ellen called Phillip, Bob called Jim, and Sally called Kate.
      Ellen called Phillip, Bob, and Jim, and Sally called Kate.
   5. If the teacher forgot, Jim would remind him.
      If the teacher forgot Jim, we'd remind him.
   6. I went skiing with Jack, and Mike met us there.
      I went skiing with Jack and Mike just last year.
   7. When John left Cindy, we were upset.
      When John left, Cindy was very upset.
   8. If Jimmy used the truck, Sharon will be angry.
      Cousin Jimmy used the truck Sharon used yesterday.

---

in Table 9.1. The patient is asked to read a sentence after being primed by a question. A set of three priming questions was composed for each of the sentences in Table 9.1. For example, for the sentence "Don shot the puck to Kent," we ask the patient: "Who shot the puck to Kent?" (to focus stress on the first word of the sentence); "Who did Don shoot the puck to?" (to focus stress on the final word of the sentence); and "What happened?" (to elicit a neutral version of the sentence).

A third prosodic production test was designed to assess a patient's ability to use syntactic juncture to convey meaning (Klouda, 1986). These stimuli also are listed in Table 9.1. Subjects are requested to read the sentences as they are written. They are told to read the sentences to themselves and to read them aloud only when they are sure of the responses. In summary, the use of these tests allows for examination of prosody across a variety of emotive and linguistic contexts in patients with neurological dysfunction.

The data obtained from patients on these production tests are analyzed utilizing two different measurement techniques: perceptual and acoustic. In order to assess the perceptual accuracy of the speech of the patient, we make an audio recording in which the patient's utterances are randomly interspersed with utterances from normal speakers who have performed the same task. A group of normal listeners judge the accuracy of each item. We digitize the sentences on a computer that randomly plays back the utterances. If such equipment is not available, clinicians can simply play back the tape of the patient's sentence production, leaving out identifying information such as the priming question. Listeners should be asked to listen to the tape and judge whether the intonation is happy, sad, or angry; whether a sentence is a question or a statement; where the linguistic stress in a sentence falls; and the meaning of the syntactic juncture sentences. It has been our experience that forced choice is the best way to obtain listener responses. Samples from our response forms for the perceptual analysis of the production tasks are shown in Table 9.2.

Acoustic measures also are made from the data obtained from the patients. Acoustic measures allow for an examination of fundamental frequency, durational, and relative intensity correlates of speech prosody. In our research protocols, we have been concerned with the measurement of fundamental frequency and durational elements of prosody. Clinically, however, we have begun recently to examine relative intensity changes related to prosodic variation. These acoustic measures necessitate the use of sound spectrographs or other commercially available equipment such as the Visipitch (Kay Instrumentation Company). A microcomputer to assist in data analysis is quite valuable, and clinicians should purchase instrumentation with this in mind. In our view these instrumental measures are critical to the clinical endeavor and provide a detailed sampling of the patient's speech.

TABLE 9.2
Listener Response Form Examples

I. Emotive intonation and question and neutral forms
Please circle the intonation pattern you think best describes a given sentence. Make sure to select one of the forms. If you are unsure, select your best guess and circle "Best Guess" along with your answer.

   Happy   Sad   Angry   Question   Neutral   Best Guess

   % Correct: _____   Total % correct: _____

II. Emphatic Stress
Please circle the word that is stressed or emphasized. If there is no stress, circle "Neutral." If you are unsure, select your best guess and circle "Best Guess" along with your answer.

   1. Don shot the puck to Kent.   Neutral   Best Guess

   % Correct initial stress: _____   % Correct final stress: _____

   % Correct neutral: _____

Table 9.3 lists the acoustic features we examine most often in the speech of our patients. To obtain fundamental frequency information we determine peak fundamental frequency over each word in the utterance by a time-domain pitch-detection algorithm described by Cooper and Sorensen (1981). Individual words of each sentence are located by viewing the waveform and simultaneously listening to the auditory signal. The peak fundamental frequency values for each word are then determined. We then plot the fundamental frequency contour and can visually inspect the plots for flattening or enhancement of the normal contours. This allows us to examine the specific contributions of frequency to the overall pattern as well. For example, an increase in fundamental frequency may be observed over stressed words in a sentence compared to the neutral condition in which words are not stressed. Eady et al. (1986) reported that fundamental frequency in normal speakers drops an average of 53 Hz following the first word stress in a sentence. These authors also found that when focus is placed on the final word of a sentence, the decrease in frequency between Word 1 and Word 2 is only 23 Hz, while there is an average increase of 12 Hz over the final word. Sentences with a happy intonation have higher mean fundamental frequencies than neutral utterances and a greater variability across the word than neutral utterances. Sad utterances are typically flat across the utterance and are lower in mean fundamental frequency than are neutral utterances. Question forms show a rise in fundamental frequency at the last word of the utterance to an average of 80 Hz; neutral

TABLE 9.3
Acoustic Measures

I. Fundamental frequency measures
   1. Peak fundamental frequency of each word
   2. Mean fundamental frequency of the sentence
II. Suprasegmental durational measures
   1. Sentence duration
   2. Word duration
   3. Pause duration
   4. Syllable duration
III. Segmental durational measures
   1. Voice onset time
   2. Vowel duration
   3. Formant frequency duration
   4. Closure duration
   5. Fricative duration
   6. Nasalization
   7. Spirantization

utterances, in contrast, have a drop in fundamental frequency over the terminal portion of the sentence (Eady & Cooper, 1986). Examples of fundamental frequency analyses of patient's speech are included in the case reports section of this chapter.

Both suprasegmental and segmental durational measurements of the utterances are made. At the suprasegmental level we examine total sentence, word, and pause duration. At this level normal speakers increase total utterance duration in emoting sad compared to neutral forms. Happy utterances typically are shorter in total sentence duration than are sad utterances. Also, the variability of duration within a sentence is greater for happy and angry utterances than for sad and neutral utterances. Colsher, Cooper, and Graff-Radford (1987) reported that the duration found in normal speakers for emotive conditions is 276 ms.

Questions typically are intoned with longer final word durations than are found in neutral utterances (Eady & Cooper, 1986). We have found an average increase of 45 ms for final words in questions produced by normal speakers. In regard to emphatic stress (sentence focus) in normal speakers, stressed words are longer than the same words in neutral utterances (Eady et al., 1986). Furthermore, most normal speakers deemphasize nonstressed final words following initial stressed words by decreasing final word durations in the initial stress condition compared to the neutral condition (Eady et al., 1986). Inserting pauses between words in an utterance and increasing word duration preceding the pause are tactics used by normal speakers to signal a clause boundary (Cooper & Sorensen, 1981).

Segmental analysis involves a variety of within word measurements. We obtain measures of voice onset time (VOT), which reflects the time between the initial onset of acoustic energy for a consonant and the onset of vocal fold vibration. It is well known that voiced sounds have VOTs in the 0= 3=ms range, while voiceless sounds have VOTs in the 40= 70=ms range. These numbers vary depending on context. Also, we measure vowel duration, formant frequency duration, closure duration (the time between the offset of acoustic energy associated with a vowel and the onset of energy for a following consonant), fricative duration, spirantization, and nasalization. These measures allow us to examine the integrity of detailed aspects of the speech waveform.

ASSESSMENT OF PROSODIC PERCEPTION

The complete assessment of prosody in patients includes the examination of perception of emotive and linguistic variations in speech. Currently, the neurologically impaired patients seen, both in our clinic and for our research protocols, are tested with these examinations. To this end, we have developed two tests to assess the comprehension of prosody. Stimuli used in these tests are similar to those used in the production tasks. For the first test, we assess the patient's ability to perceive differences in emotive utterances (happy, sad, angry) and the linguistic distinction between question and neutral. The second test is designed to examine the patient's ability to perceive differences in stress in a sentence. For this test, the patient listens to the utterances and reports which word in the utterance received relative stress. The patient's performance is compared to the performance of normal subjects who can identify the utterances with better than 95% accuracy.

Summary of Prosodic Evaluation

The results of these production and comprehension tests allow for systematic analysis of each patient's prosodic ability. A summary sheet of results is shown in Table 9.4. This sheet allows the clinician quick reference to the overall prosodic pattern demonstrated by a given individual.

TREATMENT OF PROSODIC DISORDERS

Myers (1984) pointed out the lack of literature regarding treatment of prosodic disturbances related to right hemisphere lesions. In fact, there are no reports of treatments for primary prosodic disturbances for focal cerebral lesions in general. However, suggestions for treatment of pro-

TABLE 9.4
Prosody Summary Sheet

I. Emotive stimuli
   Comprehension   % Correct
      Happy   _____
      Sad   _____
      Angry   _____
      Total   _____
   Production–perceptual   % Correct
      Happy   _____
      Sad   _____
      Angry   _____
      Total   _____
   Production–acoustic   Normal   Hypoprosody   Hyperprosody   Dysprosody
      Fundamental frequency   _____   _____   _____   _____
      Duration   _____   _____   _____   _____
      Intensity   _____   _____   _____   _____

II. Linguistic stimuli
   Comprehension   % Correct
      Question   _____
      Statement   _____
      Sentence focus   _____
   Production–perceptual   % Correct
      Question   _____
      Statement   _____
      Sentence focus   _____
   Production–acoustic   Normal   Hypoprosody   Hyperprosody   Dysprosody
      Fundamental frequency   _____   _____   _____   _____
      Duration   _____   _____   _____   _____
      Intensity   _____   _____   _____   _____

TABLE 9.4. Continued

	Normal	Decreased	Increased
III. Segmental duration measures			
VOT	——	——	——
Vowel duration	——	——	——
Formant frequency duration	——	——	——
Closure duration	——	——	——
Fricative duration	——	——	——

sodic disturbances of production in dysarthric and apraxic patients do exist in the literature and can serve to guide prosodic treatment with the types of neurogenically based prosodic disorders in this chapter. No approaches to treatment of prosodic perception deficits exist as far as we know. The following section focuses on counseling and treatment of disorders of prosodic comprehension and production.

Counseling

As noted in the introduction to this chapter, counseling of patients and their families about the effect of prosodic disturbances on communication success and failure is one goal of treatment. Myers (1984) and Robin, Jordan, and Rodnitzky (1986) have suggested that patients and their family members can benefit from counseling. Such counseling might inform the individuals that they can no longer rely on speech cues such as intonation to carry meaning. It has been our experience that many family members feel their relative no longer has a sense of humor or that they are no longer able to tell what the relative wants from the individual's tone of voice. We suggest to these family members that they need to specify the message clearly and that they cannot rely on prosodic cues. In this vein, patients and families are counseled to use the meaning of words, rather than tone of voice, to get their messages across.

Treating Disorders of Prosodic Perception

If a patient has difficulty understanding prosodically intoned utterances, this problem must be addressed before or concurrently with any attempts to remediate production deficits. The clinician should begin treatment by using very different prosodic contours (e.g., sad and happy) to facilitate the patient's discrimination of the patterns. Visual cues such as pictures of the various emotions can be used, then gradually faded. It is important to have the patient identify the prosodic contours of utterances spoken by a variety of different individuals and in different ways.

The use of a feedback device such as the Visi-Pitch can promote better understanding of differences in prosodically intoned utterances. For example, showing the fundamental frequency as it is spoken may facilitate better understanding of the pattern than relying on the auditory feedback alone. Contrasting the contours of two different sentence types (e.g., happy versus sad) also is useful in promoting increased understanding. Of course, eventually the visual cue should be faded.

Contrasting two different prosodic contours also can be useful for remediation of prosodic comprehension of linguistic stimuli. For example, the clinician can pair different types of linguistic stimuli (question versus statement or stress location differences) with visual cues to assess an understanding of these differences.

As research in the area proceeds, it may be that assessment of pitch and duration perception will be found to be essential in estimating the level of impairment (low-level perception versus high-level comprehension) and in planning a treatment program. If a patient has difficulty discriminating differences in pitch, the clinician may need to treat the pitch discrimination problem prior to treating the specific prosodic abnormality. Moreover, if the problem in understanding prosody is confined to one acoustic dimension, then the clinician can focus treatment on the one feature or on compensation for the loss of one feature by attending to another acoustic characteristic.

Treatment of Prosodic Production Deficits

As in the case of impaired comprehension of prosody, treatment of prosodic production disturbances should begin with two highly contrastive intonation types (e.g., happy versus sad). The clinician should begin by pairing visual and auditory stimuli. One stimulus might be a graphic representation of pitch contour associated with a particular utterance type. Using a device such as the Visi-Pitch that displays frequency, intensity, and timing information may be useful in facilitating prosodic change in patients. First, the clinician should model the prosodic contour, using a graphic cue as well as an auditory one. Next, the clinician and the patient should repeat the intonation type together. When an accepted level of accuracy is achieved, the clinician should instruct the patient to alter stress or prosodic patterns while answering different priming questions. Eventually the clinician should remove the visual cue and require the patient to alter prosodic patterns using self-monitoring skills.

In the absence of an available feedback device, the procedures outlined by Rosenbek and LaPointe (1985) may be useful in treating prosodic disturbances. These authors note that the stimuli should be selected to meet the needs of individual patients. Constraints to be considered include the complexity, length, and phonetic composition of the utterance. Initially the patient is instructed to imitate the clinician. Treatment then moves to the question and answer format described previously. Rosenbek and LaPointe suggest that once stress patterning is accurate in the contrastive stress drills, clinicians should move to a "preplanning activity," which is the first stage of carryover. In this stage, a conversation is instigated in which the questions and responses of the clinician elicit varying stress and prosodic patterns. Finally, real dialogues should be utilized in which the patient is asked to maintain stress patterns. It is important also to provide homework that is comprised of contrastive stress drills.

As part of the treatment process, clinicians must be able to monitor behavioral change objectively. Evaluation of prosody using acoustic measures may be useful in monitoring small changes over time. As part of our research protocol, we evaluate prosody in patients using the same stimuli we discussed previously. We evaluate during the acute phase (1–3 weeks postonset), at 3 months postonset, and at 1 year postonset. Of course the number of reevaluations in the clinic will depend on the needs of the individual patient. Thus subtle changes in frequency or durational cues that are not yet apparent to the ear may be detected by acoustic measures.

CASE STUDIES

In this section, we will present three case studies. These patients are presented in regard to their prosodic profiles.

Case 1: Right Hemisphere Lesion

Patient R. H. was a 63-year-old right-handed male who suffered a right middle cerebral artery stroke (Robin et al., submitted). The stroke compromised the anterior portions of the superior temporal gyrus, the insula, and the basal ganglia. Acute neurological symptoms included left hemiparesis, left homonomous hemianopsia, and left-sided neglect. All of these symptoms improved rapidly. A prominent symptom reported by the staff was that he was aprosodic. We evaluated R. H. three times (3 weeks, 3 months, and 1 year postonset). At all test periods, his ability to comprehend prosodic differences was relatively intact; initially, however, his production of prosody was quite flat. He was tested on the happy, sad, angry, question, and statement stimuli listed in Table 9.1. At the time his prosody was evaluated, we had not yet begun using additional tests for prosody.

Acoustic analyses of fundamental frequency and duration were performed on the measures. Figure 9.1 shows R. H.'s fundamental frequency contours for the emotive and neutral tone utterances for the three test periods. There is a clear flattening of the fundamental frequency contours at the time of the first test. It is interesting to note that there was very little variability with the happy utterance. Mean fundamental frequency for happy, sad, and neutral utterances are not different, and that is considered to be normal. Furthermore, inspection of the sad contour for the first time period suggests a pattern more similar to the question than to any other pattern. Perceptual indentification of these stimuli by normal listeners was markedly decreased. Changes in fundamental frequency were apparent over time. At Times 2 and 3, mean fundamental frequency was highest for happy utterances. Sad utterances did not increase at the end of the utterances as they did at Time 1. Mean values separated the utterance types and there remained little variability across some utterances.

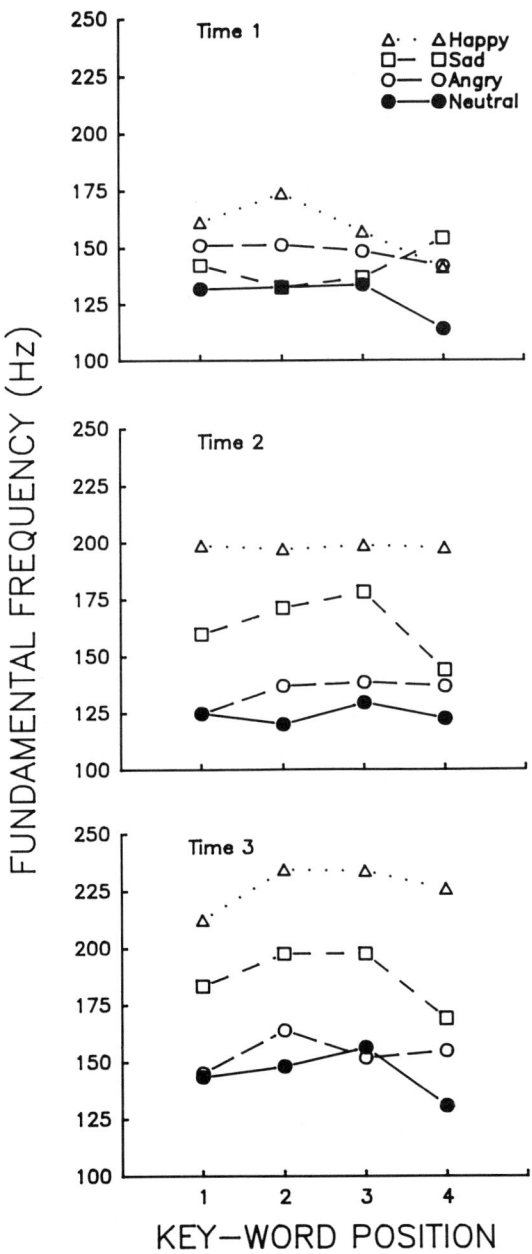

Figure 9.1 Average fundamental frequency peaks for emotionally intoned sentences at three different test times for R. H.

Analysis of suprasegmental durations for emotive utterance measures revealed that prosody for RH was essentially intact at all three test periods (Times 1, 2, and 3). When compared to neutral utterances, lengthening of total sentence duration for sad utterances was found. The duration of happy utterances was shorter than that of sad utterances. The difference between total sentence duration for sad utterances and neutral utterances increased at Times 2 and 3, suggesting some attenuation of this feature at Time 1. At Time 3, the distinction between happy and sad utterances was greater than at Times 1 and 2.

R. H.'s fundamental frequency contours for question and neutral utterances are shown in Figure 9.2. It can be seen in Figure 9.2 that at Time 1 the distinction between the two utterance types was minimal in that the normal terminal rise at the end of a question was diminished. This distinction, however, clearly improved to normal at Time 2 and was even greater at Time 3, suggesting a degree of hyperprosody at that time.

Durational cues for the question versus neutral utterances were essentially intact at all three test periods; lengthening for question utterances was apparent. The final word lengthening for question utterances was less at Times 1 and 3 than at Time 2. Lengthening at Time 3 was more apparent than at Time 1. This suggests that at Time 1 the use of this cue was somewhat diminished. Segmental durational analyses revealed intact measures at all three test periods.

In focusing treatment for R. H., several points were considered. Initially, increasing his ability to use fundamental frequency cues to alter tone was reasonable because his durational cues were essentially intact. There appeared to be changes in fundamental frequency over time that approached normal, and therefore we would not have attempted to teach the patient to compensate for the attenuation of fundamental frequency by using other prosodic cues. We might have begun treatment with question-statement utterances or some other linguistic distinction, as these abilities were less impaired than the emotive uses of prosody.

Case 2: Callosal Disconnection

Two of the authors of this chapter (Klouda and Robin) participated in the study of a patient with a callosal disconnection (Klouda et al., 1988). C. D. was a 39-year-old right-handed woman who suffered a subarachnoid hemorrhage from a left pericallosal aneurysm. The aneurysm was clipped. The lesion involved the anterior four-fifths of the corpus callosum but spared the splenium. Initially the patient was mute. By 4 weeks postonset she showed no focal neurological signs but spoke aprosodically. We tested her prosody at 4 weeks, 4 months, and 1 year postonset. Comprehension of prosody was intact at all test periods.

Neurogenic Disorders of Prosody   261

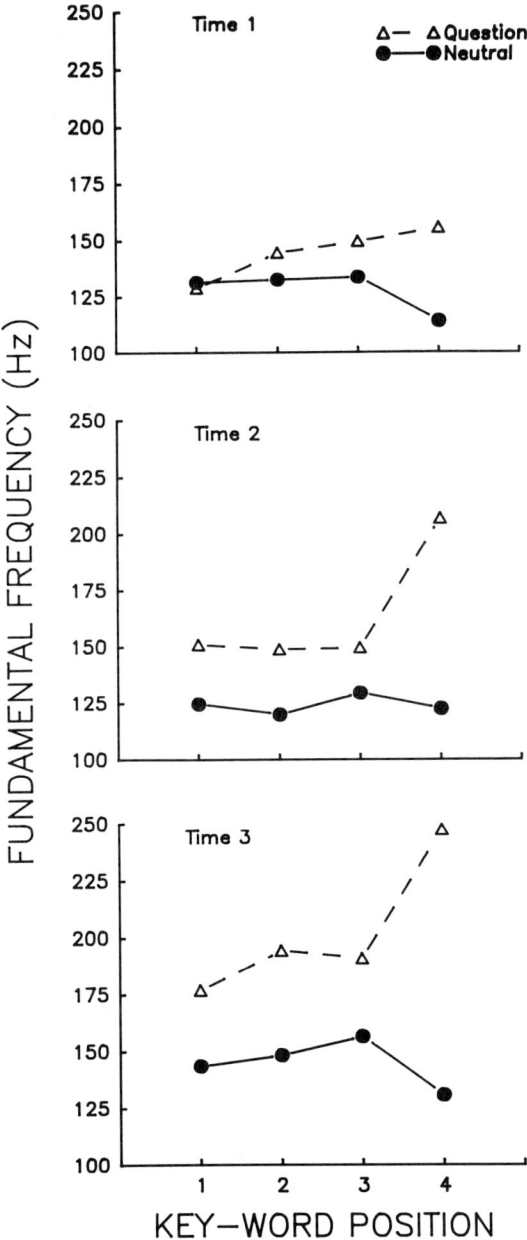

Figure 9.2 Average fundamental frequency peaks for questions and statement intonations at three different test times for R. H.

Figure 9.3 shows that, like R. H. at Time 1, C. D.'s fundamental frequency contours for emotive stimuli were relatively flat. However, at Times 2 and 3 her use of fundamental frequency had improved dramatically. It should be noted that this recovery did not reach normal levels: although normal listeners' perceptions of C. D.'s speech improved over time, at Time 3 listeners continued to make errors in their perception of C. D.'s speech (e.g., sad utterances were perceived with only 29% accuracy at Time 3). Suprasegmental durational measures for these items were intact at all three test periods.

Figure 9.4 shows fundamental frequency contours for the question and neutral forms. While C. D. made a distinction between them, it was clearly attenuated at Time 1, although improvement was noted at Times 2 and 3. Further, normal listeners' perceptions of question forms was less accurate (79%) at Time 1 than at Times 2 and 3. Durational cues for questions were intact.

Figure 9.5 shows C. D.'s fundamental frequency contours for the sentence focus tasks we described. At Time 1 the typical increase in fundamental frequency, when compared to neutral utterances associated with initial and final stress, is diminished. At Time 2, this improved somewhat but did not become normal. This distinction was more pronounced at Time 3 than at Time 2. The decrease in frequency following the initial stressed word was present, but was less than normal at Times 1 and 2 and nearly normal at Time 3. All durational cues were intact at all three test periods. Listeners were 100% accurate in judging stress in these stimuli, suggesting that durational cues were salient in producing sentence focus and might serve to compensate for the loss of frequency in these utterance types. Segmental durational elements were essentially intact.

This patient made such prominent changes in fundamental frequency control over time that if treatment had been initiated, one would have expected success with that feature of prosody. Whether treatment would have enhanced the normal recovery of this patient is not known. However, because at 1 year postonset listeners continued to have some difficulty perceiving her prosodic patterns, treatment might have been warranted for C. D.

Case 3: Left Hemisphere Lesion

Patient L. H. was a 58-year-old woman who suffered a left hemisphere stroke that involved the white matter of the frontal lobe and extended into the basal ganglia. We examined her at 4 weeks poststroke. At that time her ability to comprehend differences in prosody was impaired. She was 75% accurate in her comprehension of distinctions between happy, sad, angry, question, and neutral utterances but only 30% accurate in

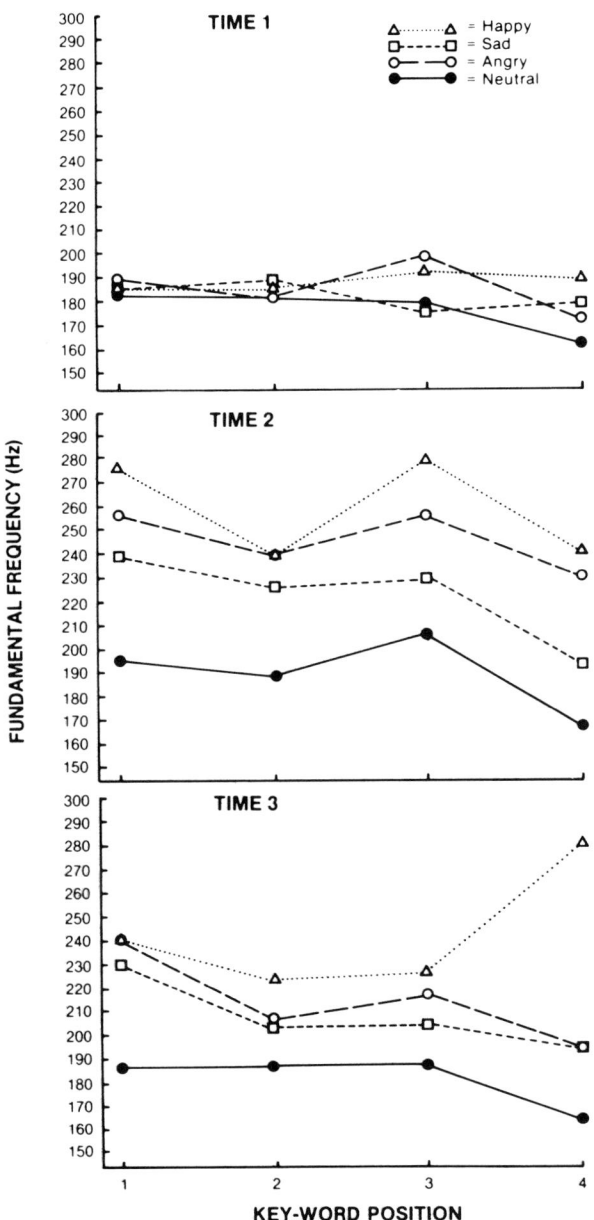

Figure 9.3 Average fundamental frequency peaks for emotionally intoned sentences at three different test times for C. D. From "The role of callosal connections in speech prosody" by G. V. Klouda, D. A. Robin, N. R. Graff-Radford, and W. E. Cooper, 1988, *Brain and Language, 35*(1), p. 160. Copyright 1988 by Academic Press. Reprinted by permission.

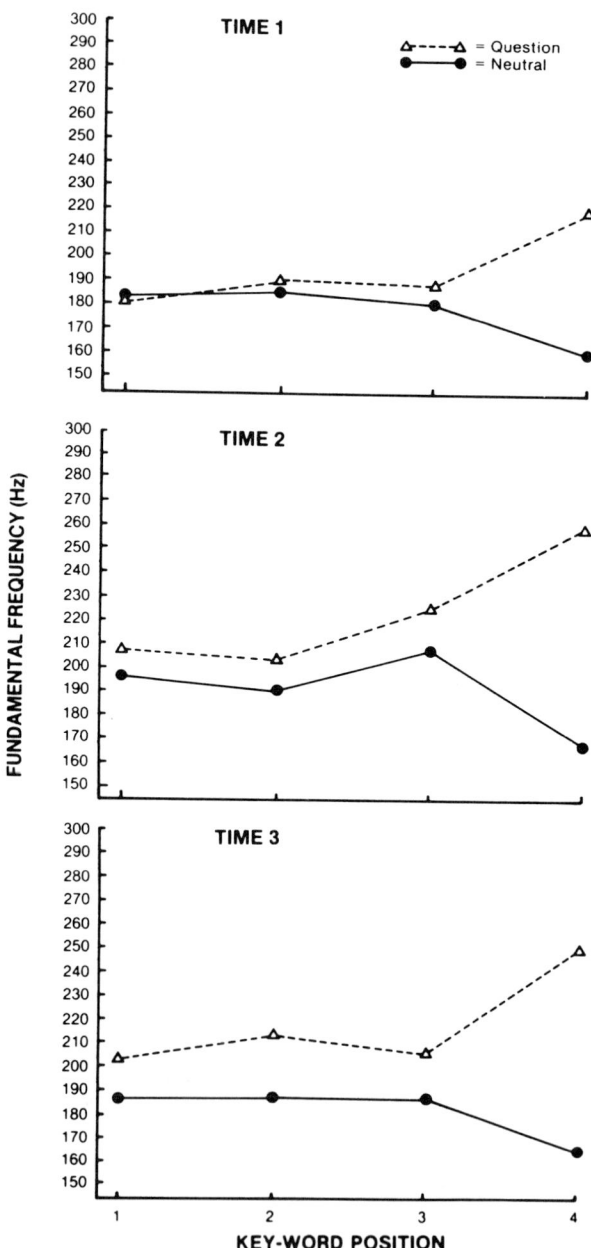

Figure 9.4 Average fundamental frequency peaks for question and statement intonations at three different test times for C. D. From "The role of callosal connections in speech prosody" by G. V. Klouda, D. A. Robin, N. R. Graff-Radford, and W. E. Cooper, 1988, *Brain and Language, 35*(1), p. 161. Copyright 1988 by Academic Press. Reprinted by permission.

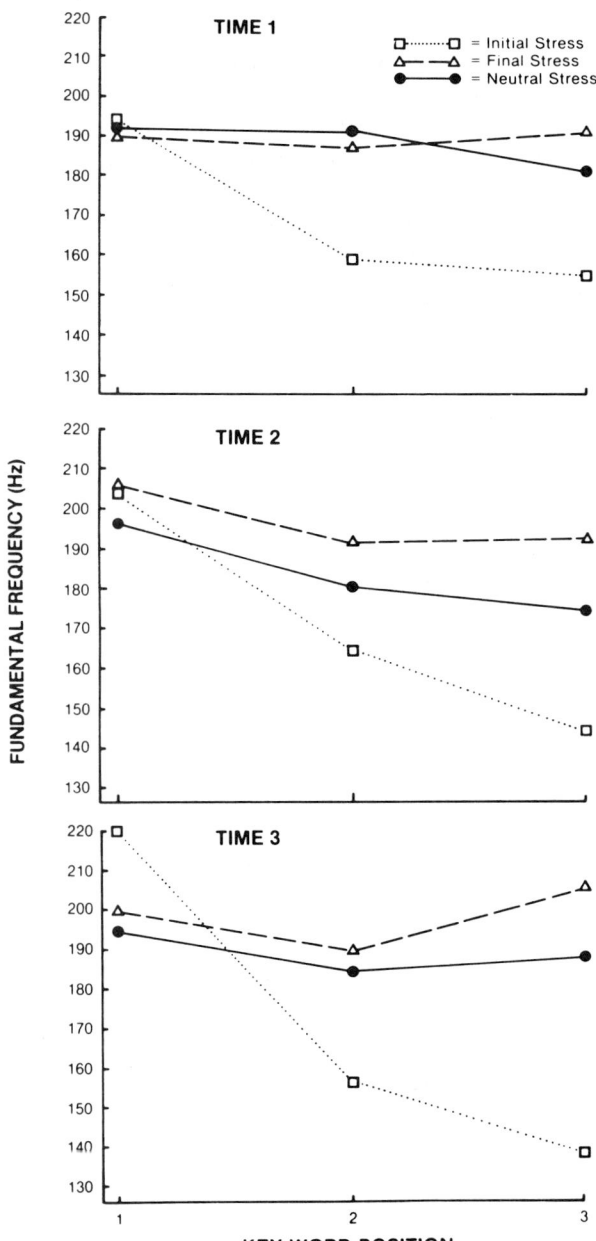

Figure 9.5 Average fundamental frequency peaks for sentences with different stress patterns at three different test times for C. D. From "The role of callosal connections in speech prosody" by G. V. Klouda, D. A. Robin, N. R. Graff-Radford, and W. E. Cooper, 1988, *Brain and Language, 35*(1), p. 163. Copyright 1988 by Academic Press. Reprinted by permission.

her identification of stress placement within sentences. Perceptually, her production was determined to be dysprosodic. She seemed to have a disorder of rhythmic organization of speech output.

Figure 9.6 represents L. H.'s fundamental frequency contours for happy, sad, angry, and neutral utterances. Generally her use of frequency to convey these distinctions was intact. The measure of happy intonation reveals greater variability than does the measure of sad intonation, and in general neutral utterances appear flat. Of interest is that for L. H. the neutral intonation did not exhibit the typical frequency decline across the sentence.

Figure 9.7 represents L. H.'s use of fundamental frequency to convey the distinction between question and neutral forms. Note that she accurately produced the question form as indicated by the rise in frequency at the last word. In summary, her use of frequency to convey prosodic information was generally intact.

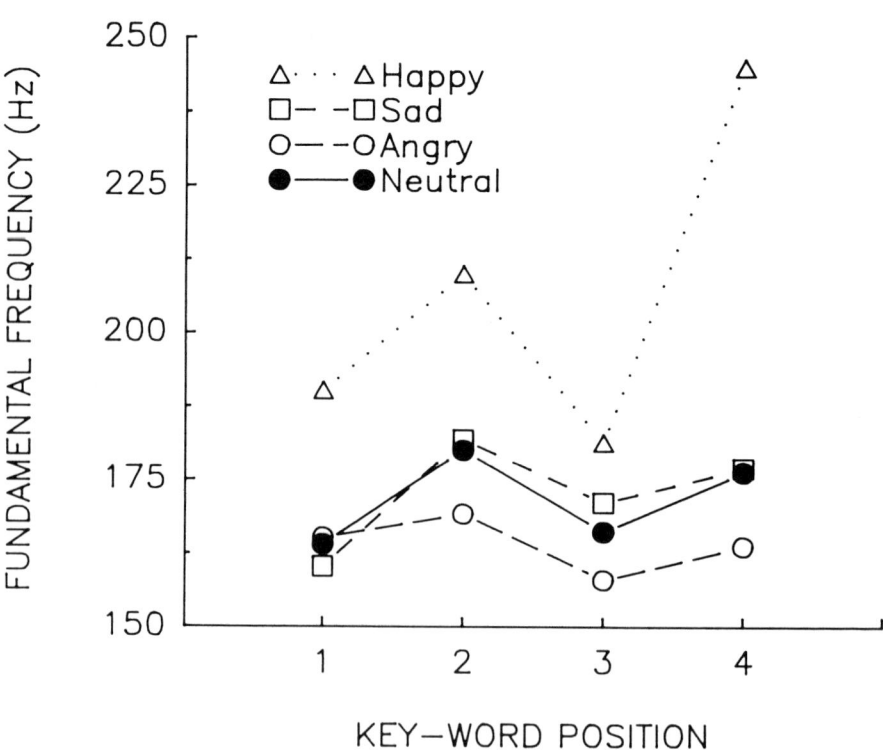

Figure 9.6 Average fundamental frequency peaks for emotionally intoned sentences at one test time for L. H.

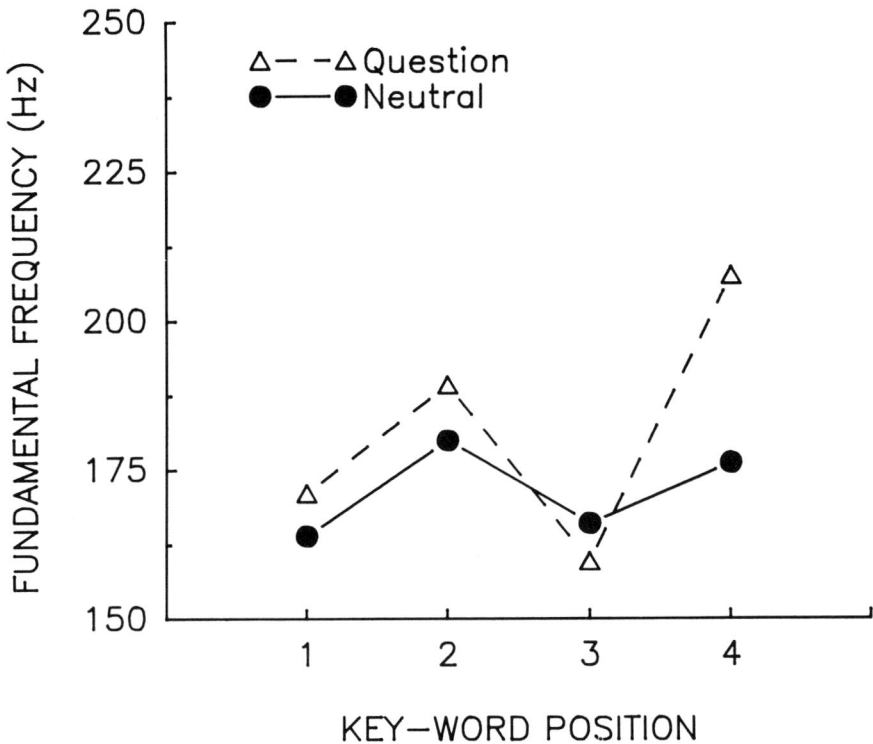

Figure 9.7 Average fundamental frequency peaks for question and statement intonations at one test time for L. H.

Measurements of durational cues revealed impairment of prosody. Measurement of total sentence duration indicated that L. H. tended to elongate sad utterances more than neutral utterances but to a lesser degree than most normal speakers. However, when final word duration of question forms was compared with final word duration of neutral utterances, on the average an increase in final word duration of question forms was found. Moreover, L. H.'s speech contained an increased number of pauses and increased pause lengths. Segmental analyses revealed prolongation of vowels and poor control of voice onset time.

Because this patient's prosodic problem was most evident in durational abnormalities related to the rhythm and timing of speech, treatment focused on those aspects of prosody. However, given her impairment of comprehension, we concentrated on the perception of sentence stress along with the treatment of production errors. In production, we would target some global features of prosody such as word and pause length. After her appreciation of stress placement improved, we would begin to add this type of stimulus to the session.

CONCLUSION

Patients with lesions of cortical areas often have disruptions of prosody. These problems may be in production or comprehension or both. Accurate assessment of these disorders is essential to realizing a complete picture of a given patient's communication profile and to the development of appropriate treatment strategies. Although the data are preliminary, it appears that right hemisphere lesions disrupt the control of fundamental frequency as used in prosody while left hemisphere lesions impair the use of durational information. However, this should be examined in each patient, as these laterality differences are variable in the population at large. It also appears that some patients with right hemisphere lesions do not recover from prosodic abnormalities and these cases may need specific treatment. Treatment of prosody should include counseling as well as therapies aimed at specific prosodic features.

REFERENCES

Behrens, S. J. (1988). The role of the right hemisphere in the production of linguistic stress. *Brain and Language, 33,* 104–127.

Berry, M. F. (1969). *Language disorders of children.* New York: Appleton-Century-Crofts.

Breckenridge, J. (1977). Declination as a phonological process. *Bell Laboratories Technological Memo.* Murry Hill, NJ: Bell Laboratories.

Colsher, P. L., Cooper, W. E., & Graff-Radford, N. R. (1987). *Intonational characteristics of right-hemisphere-damaged patients' speech and its perception by normal listeners.* Unpublished manuscript.

Cooper, W. E., Eady, S. J., & Mueller, P. R. (1985). Acoustical aspects of contrastive stress in question-answer contexts. *Journal of the Acoustical Society of America, 77,* 2142–2156.

Cooper, W. E., & Klouda, G. V. (1987). Intonation in aphasic and right-hemisphere-damaged patients. In J. H. Ryalls (Ed.), *Phonetic approaches to speech production in aphasia and related disorders* (pp. 59–80). Austin, TX: PRO-ED.

Cooper, W. E., Soares, C., Nicol, J., Michelow, D., & Goloskie, S. (1984). Clausal intonation after unilateral brain damage. *Language and Speech, 27,* 17–24.

Cooper, W. E., & Sorensen, J. M. (1981). *Fundamental frequency in sentence production.* New York: Springer-Verlag.

Cosmides, L. (1983). Invariances in the acoustic expression of emotion during speech. *Journal of Experimental Psychology: Human Perception and Performance, 9,* 864–881.

Danly, M., Cooper, W. E., & Shapiro, B. (1983). Fundamental frequency, language processing, and linguistic structure in Wernicke's aphasia. *Brain and Language, 19,* 1–24.

Danly, M., & Shapiro, B. (1982). Speech prosody in Broca's aphasia. *Brain and Language, 16,* 171–190.

Eady, S. J., & Cooper, W. E., (1986). Speech intonation and focus location in matched statements and questions. *Journal of the Acoustical Society of America, 80,* 402–415.

Eady, S. J., Cooper, W. E., Klouda, G. V., Mueller, P. R., & Lotts, D. W. (1986). Acoustical characteristics of sentential focus: Narrow versus board and single versus dual focus environments. *Language and Speech, 29,* 233–251.

Heilman, K. M., Bowers, D., Speedie, L., & Coslett, H. B. (1984). Comprehension of affective and nonaffective prosody. *Neurology, 34,* 917–921.

Heilman, K. M., Scholes, R., & Watson, R. T. (1975). Auditory affective agnosia: Disturbed comprehension of affective speech. *Journal of Neurology, Neurosurgery, and Psychiatry, 38,* 69–72.

Kent, R. D., & Rosenbek, J. C. (1982). Prosodic disturbance and neurologic lesion. *Brain and Language, 15*(2), 259–291.

Klouda, G. V. (1986). *Speech production in stutterers.* Unpublished doctoral thesis, University of Iowa, Iowa City, IA.

Klouda, G. V., Robin, D. A., Graff-Radford, N. R., & Cooper, W. E., (1988). The role of callosal connections in speech prosody. *Brain and Language, 35,* 154–171.

Lea, W. A. (1973). Segmental and suprasegmental influences on fundamental frequency contours. In L. M. Hyman (Ed.), *Consonant types and tone* (pp. 15–70). Los Angeles: University of Southern California Press.

Liberman, P. (1965). On the acoustic basis of the perception of intonation by linguists. *Word, 21,* 40–54.

Monrad-Krohn, G. H. (1947a). Dysprosody or altered "melody of language." *Brain, 70,* 405–415.

Monrad-Krohn, G. H. (1947b). Altered melody of language ("dysprosody") as an element of aphasia. *Acta Psychiatrica et Neurologica Scandinavica, 47*(Supp.), 204–212.

Monrad-Krohn, G. H. (1963). The third element of speech prosody and its disorders. In L. Halpern (Ed.), *Problems of dynamic neurology* (pp.101–117). Jerusalem: Hebrew University Press.

Myers, P. S. (1984). Right hemisphere impairment. In A. Holland (Ed.), *Language disorders in adults* (pp. 177–208). Austin, TX: PRO-ED.

Nation, J. E., & Aram, D. M. (1982). *Diagnosis of speech and language disorders* (2nd ed.). Austin, TX: PRO-ED.

Netsell, R. (1973). Evaluation of velopharyngeal function in dysarthria. *Journal of Speech and Hearing Disorders, 34,* 131.

Robin, D. A., Jordan, L. S., & Rodnitzky, R. L. (1986, February). *Prosodic impairment in Parkinson's disease.* Paper presented at the Third Biennial Clinical Dysarthria Conference, Tucson, AZ.

Robin, D. A., Klouda, G. V., Graff-Radford, N. R., Cooper, W. E., Damasio, H., & Hug, L. N. *Prosodic impairment following focal lesions of the right hemisphere.* Manuscript submitted for publication.

Robin, D. A., Tranel, D., & Damasio, H. (1990). Auditory perception of temporal events in patients with left and right cerebral damage. *Brain and Language, 39,* 539–555.

Rosenbek, J. C., & LaPointe, L. L. (1985). The dysarthrias: Description, diagnosis, and treatment. In D. F. Johns (Ed.), *Clinical management of neurogenic communicative disorders* (pp. 97–152). Austin, TX: PRO-ED.

Ross, E. D. (1981). The aprosodias: Functional-anatomic organization of the affective components of language in the right hemisphere. *Archives of Neurology, 38,* 561–569.

Ross, E. D. (1988). Right hemisphere's role in language, affective behavior and emotion. *Trends in Neuroscience.* Amsterdam: Elsevier Science Publications.

Ross, E. D., Harney, J. H., deLacoste-Utamsing, C., & Purdy, P. D. (1981). How the brain integrates affective and propositional language into a unified behavioral function. *Archives of Neurology, 38,* 745–748.

Ross, E. D., & Mesulam, M. M. (1979). Dominant language functions of the right hemisphere? *Archives of Neurology, 36,* 144–148.

Ryalls, J. H. (1982). Intonation in Broca's aphasia. *Neuropsychologia, 20,* 355–360.

Ryalls, J. H. (1988). Concerning right-hemisphere dominance for affective language. *Archives of Neurology, 45,* 337–339.

Scherer, K. R. (1986). Vocal affect expression: A review and model for future research. *Psychological Bulletin, 99,* 143–165.

Selkirk, E. O. (1984). *Phonology and syntax: The relation between sound and structure.* Cambridge, MA: MIT Press.

Shapiro, B., & Danly, M. (1985). The role of the right hemisphere in the control of speech prosody in propositional and affective contexts. *Brain and Language, 25,* 19–36.

Speedie, L. J., Coslett, B., & Heilman, K. M. (1984). Repetition of affective prosody in mixed transcortical aphasia. *Archives of Neurology, 41,* 268–270.

Tompkins, C. A., & Flowers, C. R. (1985). Perception of emotional intonation by brain-damaged adults: The influence of task processing levels. *Journal of Speech and Hearing Research, 28,* 527–538.

Tompkins, C. A., & Mateer, C. A. (1985). Right hemisphere appreciation of prosodic and linguistic indications of implicit attitude. *Brain and Language, 24,* 185–203.

Tucker, D. M., Watson, R. T., & Heilman, K. M. (1977). Discrimination and evocation of affectively intoned speech in patients with right parietal disease. *Neurology, 27,* 947–950.

Watson, R. T., & Heilman, K. M. (1983). Callosal apraxia. *Brain, 106,* 391–403.

Williams, C. E., & Stevens, K. N. (1972). Emotions and speech: Some acoustical correlates. *Journal of the Acoustical Society of America, 52,* 1238–1250.

ACKNOWLEDGMENTS

The preparation of this chapter and the research reported therein were supported in part by NINCDS Program Project NS19632. The authors acknowledge the support of Dr. Antonio Damasio. We thank Dr. Hanna Damasio for her interpretation of the neuroanatomical data discussed in this chapter. Drs. William C. Cooper and Neill R. Graff-Radford are acknowledged for their development of some of the stimuli. We also acknowledge the secretarial support of Ms. Colleen Thompson.

PART IV
Idiopathic Speech-Specific Disorders

CHAPTER 10
Neurobiological Interpretations of Spasmodic Dysphonia
Michael P. Cannito

> *In this chapter Cannito critically reviews the numerous potential sites of neurologic lesion that have been proposed as underlying the signs and symptoms of spasmodic dysphonia. Some are found to be more credible than others. When viewed in conjunction with other behavioral and neurophysiological research, a model of variable supranuclear pathology emerges as the most viable interpretation of this mysterious voice disorder. Clinical implications for both assessment and management, supported with an actual case study of spasmodic dysphonia, are presented.*

Questions
1. *Why are lower brain stem and peripheral nerve explanations of spasmodic dysphonia unjustifiable, given our present state of knowledge?*
2. *What aspects of spasmodic dysphonia symptoms are best explained by an appeal to limbic system function?*
3. *How might a supranuclear dysarthria model of spasmodic dysphonia influence treatment decisions in a manner that is differentiated from traditional hyperfunctional voice therapy? From psychotherapy?*

Spasmodic (spastic) dysphonia (SD) is an enigmatic disturbance of vocal motor control characterized by intermittent voice stoppage in a context of strained-strangled (laryngealized) and/or breathy (aspirate) phonatory perturbations (Cannito & Johnson, 1981). These disruptions are typically speech-specific, imparting a bizarre, labored, and dysfluent quality. Aronson (1978) catalogs a diverse assortment of perceptual-acoustic symptoms, characterizing SD voice productions as "staccato or stuttering-like, intermittent, jerky, grunting, squeezed, groaning and effortful" (p. 533). In contrast, the majority of SD patients exhibit a more normal voice quality for nonspeech vocal gestures such as singing, paralanguage, yawning, and laughing, and when phonating in the higher ranges of their fundamental pitch (Aronson, 1985; Freeman, Cannito, & Finitzo-Hieber, 1985a). Furthermore, the supralaryngeal articulatory aspects of speech production appear to be relatively unimpaired. It is both its apparent focality and function specificity that make SD one of the most puzzling and controversial disorders of human communication.

Because SD is an uncommon disorder, its precise incidence and prevalence remain unknown. It appears to affect men and women in approximately equal proportions. Onset has been reported as early as the teens and 20s, but the average age of SD patients falls nearer to 50 years (Aronson, 1985). Slow insidious onset is commonly reported, although some SD patients have experienced an abrupt initial deterioration of the voice. The disorder is notoriously resistant to speech therapy and other behavioral interventions (Boone, 1977); however, many patients report that they have acquired beneficial compensatory strategies as a result of the therapies they have explored (Freeman, Cannito, & Finitzo-Hieber, 1985b). For a few years it appeared that surgical treatment (recurrent laryngeal nerve resection) would solve the problem of SD; however, postoperative return of symptoms and other complications have been reported in a substantial subset of surgically treated SD patients (Aronson & DeSanto, 1983; Dedo & Izdebski, 1983).

Prior to 1973, voice clinicians tended to regard SD as a single clinical entity whose primary defining feature was "intermittent voice stoppage" (Aronson, Brown, Litin, & Pearson, 1968a) or periodic breaks in phonation (Fox, 1969), suggestive of involuntary muscular contraction at the level of the vocal folds.

More recently, attempts have been made to specify the perceptual acoustic characteristics of SD in greater detail. Aronson (1973) identified two forms of SD: the adductor and abductor types. He described the predominant characteristic of the adductor type as a strained-strangled hoarseness due to irregular hyperadduction of the vocal folds. The salient characteristics of the abductor type was described as intermittent breathy phonation or intermittent aphonia. To further objectify the acoustic characteristics of SD, a number of authors have conducted spectrographic case studies of these patient types (Wolfe & Bacon, 1976; Merson & Ginsberg, 1979; Zwitman, 1979; Cannito & Johnson, 1981). Review of these reports suggests a striking variability of vocal symptoms across patients (even within the same subcategory). Indeed, one is tempted to conclude that heterogeneity of vocal symptoms within SD is at least as great as that between SD and other voice pathologies from which it is differentiated. Such a conclusion, however, is probably unwarranted. Cannito and Johnson (1981) suggested that SD may be more parsimoniously considered a "continuum disorder" amenable to scaling along two continuous dimensions of harshness and breathiness, rather than to strict binary categorization. This hypothesis has been supported by subsequent research indicating that both variants of SD share many phonetic similarities as well as differences (Freeman, Cannito, & Finitzo-Hieber, 1985a; Freeman, Cannito, Finitzo, & Schaefer, 1985). In addition, Aronson (1985) suggests that the continuum hypothesis "is not only plausible, but one that would help to explain their similarities pertaining to nature of onset, factors influencing severity, and multiple etiologies" (p. 190). At present, however, the heterogeneity versus homogeneity issue continues to be controversial.

Other challenges to an explanatory model of SD include its dramatic intermittency and affect sensitivity, or waxing and waning of symptoms as a function of the emotional context. Because of the striking variability of SD symptoms, including (*a*) intermittency of dysphonia during connected speech, (*b*) vocal deterioration under psychological stress, and (*c*) marked improvement for nonspeech vocalizations, SD was long considered to be of psychogenic etiology (Traube, 1871; Murphy, 1964; Brodnitz, 1976; Aronson, 1978). It has often been suggested that SD patients are significantly depressed (Aronson et al., 1968a). Accumulating evidence, however, has linked SD with a variety of neuropathological symptoms (Aronson, Brown, Litin, & Pearson, 1968b; McCall, 1974; Feldman, Nixon, Finitzo-Hieber, & Freeman, 1984).

Acknowledging that, as with other motor speech disorders, a psychogenic "mimic" form of SD is at least possible (Darley, 1978), this chapter focuses upon explanations of a neurogenic etiology in SD. While the literature suggests that the neurogenic etiology is the more prevalent one, researchers disagree as to the specific type and localization of neuropathology underlying the symptom complex of SD. Hypothetical lesion loci have included peripheral nerve, medulla, midbrain, basal ganglia, cerebral cortex, and the limbic system. The levels of CNS involvement in SD that have been posited by various authors are summarized in Figure 10.1. Each of these levels will be discussed in detail in the remainder of this chapter. For a review of neuroanatomical structure and function, the reader is referred to Chapter 3 in this volume.

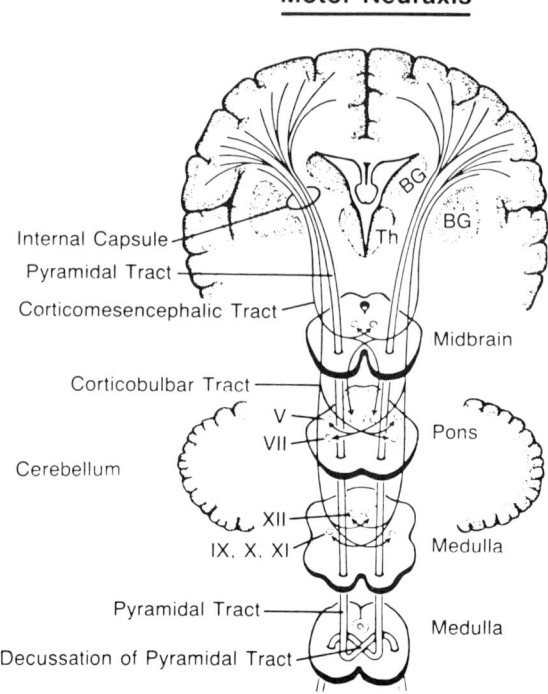

Figure 10.1 Possible sites of central nervous system lesions, proposed by various authors, to account for the pathology of spasmodic dysphonia. Drawing from "Neuropathologies of Speech and Language: An Introduction to Patient Management" by T. Wertz, in *Clinical Management of Neurogenic Communicative Disorders,* edited by D. F. Johns, 1985, Austin, TX: PRO-ED. Copyright 1985 by D. F. Johns. Adapted by permission.

It is clear, however, that an adequate neuropathological model of SD must account for its apparent focality, function specificity, heterogeneity, intermittency, and affect sensitivity. In the review that follows, it will be argued that infranuclear explanations implicating lower motor neurons or peripheral nerves are inadequate to account for vocal and other symptoms exhibited in SD. In contrast, supranuclear explanations, and particularly those involving the pyramidal/extrapyramidal voluntary motor system, do indeed provide a coherent basis for a model of this enigmatic disorder. Finally, implications of such a model for clinical management and an SD patient treated within a neuromotor framework are discussed.

PROPOSED LESION LOCI

Peripheral Nerve

In an effort to explain the positive response of SD patients to surgical sectioning of the recurrent laryngeal nerve, Dedo, Townsend, and Izdebski (1978) compared recurrent laryngeal nerves of SD patients with control recurrent laryngeal nerves taken at autopsy and at laryngectomy. Based on light microscopy and histological staining techniques, atypical fiber bundles were reported in the SD sample, but no active demyelinization or other abnormalities were found. Boccino and Tucker (1978) subsequently reported evidence of demyelinization in the recurrent laryngeal nerves of SD patients. These findings, however, were refuted by Ravits et al. (1979), who utilized more sensitive histometric and "teased fiber" morphology techniques in conjunction with electron microscopy. Results yielded "no significant difference between the disease and control groups in morphology, median fiber diameter, density or size distribution of fibers, or morphology of teased fibers" (p. 1380).

Explanations implicating peripheral neuropathy are inadequate on symptomatic grounds as well. It is well known that peripheral neuropathy can result in the slowing of conduction of neural impulses (in the case of demyelinization) or their complete disruption (Rowland, 1982). Disruption of the final common pathway to the intrinsic laryngeal musculature results in consistent adductor or abductor fixation of the vocal fold(s), rather than in an intermittent abnormality that is restricted to speech (Luchsinger & Arnold, 1965). It is generally felt at present that the neurologic locus of dysfunction underlying SD must be at least at the level of the brain stem within the central nervous system (Shipp et al., 1985).

Medulla

Evidence of abnormal reflex behavior mediated by brain stem (cranial) sensorimotor nuclei has been reported in SD for middle ear (stapedial) reflexes (McCall, 1974; Hall & Jerger, 1976; Hall, 1981), as well as parasympathetic efferent vagal stimulation of the stomach and the heart (Feldman et al., 1984). In addition, abnormal auditory brain stem responses (ABR) have been reported in SD patients (Sharbrough, Stockard, & Aronson, 1978; Hall, 1981; Finitzo-Hieber, Freeman, Gerling, Dodson, & Schaefer, 1981; Schaefer, Finitzo-Hieber, Gerling, & Freeman, 1983). These abnormalities potentially implicate cochlear, trigeminal, facial, and vagal dorsal motor nuclei of the pons and medulla, and the polysynaptic brain stem auditory pathway to the level of inferior colliculus in the midbrain.

These factors, combined with frequent somatic complaints by SD patients implicating a varity of cranially innervated structures, led Schaefer et al. (1983) to posit that SD may be a generalized brain stem syndrome involving multiple cranial nerve nuclei. Suggested mechanisms included either a "shared" lesion affecting adjacent structures or a "skip" lesion affecting more distal structures.

It is clear, however, that a lesion involving a significant portion of the cranial sensorimotor neuron pool would result in widespread, crippling consequences. A variety of such brain stem syndromes are well documented in the neurologic literature (Clark, 1975). A lateral medullary syndrome, for example, can be characterized by a loss of pain and thermal sense of the ipsilateral half of the face and contralateral half of the body, vertigo, nausea, disequilibrium, persistent hiccup, and vocal hoarseness (Carpenter, 1978). For the majority of SD patients these symptoms are simply not present. Because SD does not resemble the effects of a gross structural medullary lesion, a disease process implicated at this level must be both subtle and diffuse. For example, dysfunction of a number of specific neurotransmitter systems may be inferred (Schaefer, 1983). With respect to vocalization, however, medullary lesions are in general maximally disruptive of species-specific vocalization in monkeys (Kirzinger & Jurgens, 1985); therefore even a subtle and diffuse lesion at this level would seem inadequate to account for the selective disruption of speech that is apparently exhibited by patients with SD.

A second attempt at a brain stem localization hypothesis has been offered by Izdebski and Shipp (1985), who suggest dysfunction in an unspecified "comparator" mechanism localized to the brain stem. This comparator receives afferent somatosensory input from subglottal mechanoreceptors that are sensitive to air pressure and flow. The comparator then utilizes this information for regulation of efferent adductor laryngeal control. These authors hypothesize that in SD there is an enhancement of the threshold level for subglottal pressure necessary to trigger an adductory reflex response. Thus when the critical subglottal pressure value is exceeded during speech, the result is an immediate hyperadduction of the vocal folds. The positive response of many SD patients to recurrent laryngeal nerve resection, which reduces overpressure by fixation of one vocal fold, has been offered as evidence in support of this position.

There are, however, a number of problems associated with this hypothesis. It has been demonstrated in animals that the mechanoreceptors in question do indeed exist and that they project, along with other laryngeal somatosensory receptors, to secondary neurons housed primarily in the caudal portion of nucleus solitarius and secondarily in the main sensory and spinal nuclei of the trigeminal nerve (Dubner, Sessle, &

Storey, 1978). It is plausible that a disease process could affect these structures locally, resulting in an afferent hypersensitivity of the type proposed. Axelrod (1974), for example, has demonstrated hypersensitivity in postsynaptic pineal neurons, either by presynaptic denervation or long-term pharmacologic (reserpine) blockade, altering at a molecular level "the 'avidity' with which the receptor binds the neurotransmitters" (p. 9).

It seems unlikely, however, that a destructive process would be selective for only those cell bodies associated with subglottal pressure and flow detection. A destructive lesion should logically implicate other functions mediated by the brain stem nuclei in question. Nucleus solitarius mediates taste, visceral pain, and general laryngopharyngeal proprioception; the trigeminal nuclei mediate general somasthesia for the head and neck (Dubner et al., 1978). Abnormalities of these functions (i.e., taste, vocal tract somasthesia, and visceral pain) have not been reported typically in the SD literature (cf. Schaefer et al., 1983). Cannito (1986) found no difference in oral stereognosis, oral 2-point discriminations, or facial tactile number recognition between 18 SD females and matched normal controls.

On the aerodynamic side, the afferent hypersensitivity hypothesis would predict an increased frequency of vocal perturbations in SD specific to phonetic environments in which subglottal pressure is particularly increased. Two obvious instances of this include the early portions of sustained vowels and the vocalic nuclei of strongly stressed syllables. No published studies have reported such distributions. Further, some SD patients exhibit quite the opposite effect. Thus the afferent hypersensitivity hypothesis is dissatisfying on both anatomic and aerodynamic grounds.

A third theory implicating the brain stem focuses on the medullary reticular formation. The reticular formation is a phylogenetically primitive structure that traverses the length of the brain stem and forms its inner core. In addition to its role in the reticular activating system, which subserves arousal, the reticular formation functions as an interneuronal pool analogous to the intermediate gray area of the spinal cord (House, Pansky, & Seigal, 1979). Maximal overlap of afferent fibers from different sources occurs in the medullary reticular formation and subserves associative sensory functions. For example, parvicellular reticular nucleus receives fibers from secondary cranial nerve nuclei including the cochlear, trigeminal, solitary, and vestibular. At this level, reticular interneurons participate in control of autonomic cardiovascular and respiratory responses (House et al., 1979). Because of its important role as a lower center for cranial sensorimotor convergence, some authors have logically inferred that a lesion in the medullary reticular formation could explain the diversity of symptoms associated with SD. As early as 1965, Kiml speculated on a possible role of brain stem reticular formation in SD due to its enormous cytoarchitectural possibilities for interaction. Among more recent neural models considered for SD, Schaefer (1983) also hypothesizes a lesion of reticular formation neurons of the brain stem predicated on the role of reticular formation in mediating respiration and interneuronal convergence.

Despite its logical appeal, a gross lesion in medullary reticular formation is probably unsupportable as an underlying etiology of SD. Experimentally induced lesions of the lateral medullary reticular formation surrounding nucleus ambiguous (as well as lesions in nucleus ambiguous itself) have been shown to abolish all elicited species-specific vocalizations in squirrel monkeys (Jurgens & Pratt, 1979a, 1979b). These primitive mammalian vocalizations are more comparable to human vocal gestures such as laughing and crying than to speech (Jurgens & Ploog, 1981). Therefore a lateral reticular lesion would most likely predict either a total loss of phonatory function or a loss of nonspeech vocal function. In addition, clinical neuropathology of lateral brain stem reticular formation frequently results in loss of consciousness, accompanied by respiratory and cardiovascular disturbances that often become fatal (House et al., 1979). Thus, while the medullary reticular formation remains of interest to an understanding of SD, abnormalities at this level may reflect abnormal neuronal processing interactions that occur under the modulating influence of impaired supranuclear structures.

Midbrain

Another locus that potentially has some explanatory power in relation to SD is the reticular formation of the midbrain tegmentum. This region houses a number of critical nuclear masses that might be implicated in the symptom complex of SD. These include (*a*) auditory nuclei and pathways of the lower midbrian thought to be major contributors to wave five of the auditory brain stem response (Stillman, 1980); (*b*) the periaqueductal gray, a midline reticular nucleus that is a coordinating center for mammalian species-specific vocalization (Kelley, Beaton, & Magoun, 1946; Jurgens & Pratt, 1979a; Jurgens & Ploog, 1981); (*c*) midbrain reticular substance, wherein experimental lesions in primates have been associated with postural tremors, spasmodic torticollus, and intermittent losses of postural muscle tone (Foltz, Knopp, & Ward, 1959; Bril, Sharpe, & Ashby, 1979; Pechadre, Larochelle, & Poirier, 1976); (*d*) the substantia nigra, associated with movement control and motor deterioration in Parkinson's disease (Carpenter, 1978); and (*e*) mesencephalic nucleus of the trigeminal nerve, thought to be associated with jaw proprioception (House et al., 1979). While the reputed functions of all these structures may appear related to SD symptoms, lesions in even a subset of them would produce more striking clinical abnormalities than are typical of the SD patient. For example, a midbrain lesion should result in severe abnormalities of more rostral components of the auditory brain stem response, while a periaqueductal lesion would abolish all species-specific vocalizations (Jurgens & Pratt, 1979a, 1979b; von Cramon, 1981). The auditory brain stem response of the SD patient is not markedly abnormal, but rather exhibits merely a prolongation of wave five latency at higher repetition rates of acoustic stimulation; and vocal perturbations are intermittent and specific to purposeful speech. Although it is possible that a very subtle and diffuse lesion in these areas may not have such gross consequences as have been portrayed, even a minimal lesion at the midbrain level would seem unable to explain the functional specificity and focality that is characteristically attributed to SD.

Because of the synaptic possibilities it offers for diverse interneuronal processing interactions among multiple midbrain and other rostro-caudal structures, midbrain reticular formation seems to be a reasonable candidate for localization of dysfunction, if not a structural lesion, in SD. Actual lesions of midbrain reticular formation frequently produce coma and are associated with large-amplitude slow waves in the cortical EEG (House et al., 1979). Thus it again appears that if there are abnormalities at this level they are probably restricted to deviant interneuronal processing, again perhaps under the modulating influence of impaired higher-level structures. One such structure, the globus pallidus of the basal ganglia, projects a major outflow (via the ansa lenticularis) to the pedunculopontine nucleus of the midbrain reticular formation. This is the only directly descending output of the basal ganglia, and may mediate basal gangliar modulation of motor function (House et al., 1979). Along similar lines, Jankovic (1983) has reported two cases of blepharospasm in humans secondary to focal midbrain lesions, resulting in denervation hypersensitivity of the facial nucleus. While spasmodic blinking is obviously not a speech-specific disorder, the parallel with a midbrain interpretation of SD is intriguing. Clinical cases of aphonia and dysphonia secondary to midbrain lesions have also been reported (Botez & Barbeau, 1971; Vogel & von Cramon, 1982). In any case, a midbrain locus would indicate a supranuclear disorder with respect to laryngo-pharyngeal motor neurons subserving vocal function.

Basal Ganglia and Related Structures

Although the term *extrapyramidal* is unfortunately ambiguous, in routine clinical parlance it has come to be associated with the basal ganglia (caudate, putamen, and globus pallidus) and other intimately related subcortical motor centers of the diencephalon and midbrain including the subthalamic nucleus and substantia nigra. Disorders of the extrapyramidal motor system result in a variety of dyskinesias wherein the smoothly modulated control of voluntary movement is impeded by fast or slow spontaneous alternations of muscular tone. For definitions of the extrapyramidal movement disorders and a discussion of their pathophysiology, the reader is referred to Chapter 5 in this volume. A variety of hyperkinesias affecting oral-facial-cervical structures have been described in the neurology literature (Marsden, 1976; Jankovic, 1981). These include blepharospasm, oral-mandibular dystonia, spasmodic torticollus, and essential tremor. Cooper (1976) has suggested a model for the dystonias that involves a variety of lesions disrupting complex motor feedback circuits that subserve communication among subcortical motor programming structures. These structures include the globus pallidus, red nucleus, midbrain reticular formation, brachium conjunctivum (cerebellar-cortical pathway) and dentate nucleus. What these lesions have in common is that they all affect the pathways of convergence upon the ventrolateral nucleus of the thalamus.

Interestingly, there is a high incidence of SD among such movement-disordered subgroups (Jankovic & Ford, 1982). When spontaneous onset of oral-facial-cervical dystonia occurs, the disorder is termed Meige's syndrome (also known as Breugel's syndrome). According to Jankovic and Ford, "Spasmodic dysphonia, usually described separately, is now considered a focal dystonia occasionally associated with other features of Meige's syndrome . . . [which] may begin as blepharospasm, oromandibular dystonia, tongue protrusion, or spasmodic dysphonia and over a period of months or years may progress to a more generalized dystonia" (p. 410). In a study of 12 SD patients referred for routine neurologic examination, Dedo et al. (1978) reported that 50% exhibited dyskinetic movement disorders including postural tremor, blepharospasm, idiopathic torsion dystonia, and buccolingual dyskinesia. Similarly, Rosenfield (1988) reported that of 41 patients referred for SD, 59% exhibited essential tremors external to the larynx or Meige's syndrome or both. The view that SD represents a focal dystonia resulting from extrapyramidal motor pathology has been aired by many (Critchley, 1939; Aronson et al., 1968b; McCall, 1974; Marsden & Sheehy, 1982; Freeman et al., 1985a). In addition, SD has been noted as an early symptom of adult onset torsion dystonia (Jankovic & Ford, 1982) and a late symptom in Gilles de la Tourette syndrome (Lang & Marsden, 1983). SD has also been likened to dystonic writer's cramp, with the implication that as a dystonia it must be a basal ganglia disorder (Blitzer, Lovelace, Brin, Fahn, & Fink, 1985). It must also be acknowledged, however, that the

CNS pathophysiology underlying dystonic writer's cramp and similar function-specific dystonias remains essentially unknown.

In a series of studies of extrapyramidal motor involvement in SD, McCall (1974) utilized a combination of fluoroscopic, acoustic-phonetic, and electromyographic measures. Fluoroscopic assessments indicated that SD "can occur as a manifestation of apparent isolated, phonatory-related laryngospasms or may appear in association with a more general problem that affects the behavior of the larynx, hypopharynx, tongue and soft palate" (p. 127). Electromyography was performed on eight SD patients with non-tremor-related dysphonia. Recordings were obtained from bipolar hooked wire electrodes inserted in the cricothyroid, sternothyroid, and thyrohyoid muscles. Results indicated that intermittent voice stoppage in the acoustic records was associated with sharp, burstlike increases in electromyographic activity in the cricothyroid muscle and occasionally the sternothyroid and thyrohyoid muscles. McCall interpreted these findings as suggestive of laryngeal dystonia "consistent with the hypothesis of involvement of the extrapyramidal motor system" (p. 136). Abnormal fluctuations in laryngeal EMG activity in the interarytenoid, thyroarytenoid, and cricothyroid have also been demonstrated in one SD patient by Shipp et al. (1985).

Considerable similarity of symptoms has been noted in SD and essential tremor (Aronson et al., 1968b). Aronson and Hartman (1981) demonstrated that SD patients with rhythmic voice arrests during vowel prolongations share many commonalities with essential voice tremor patients including virtually identical voice tremor frequencies of 5 to 6 Hz, high incidence of extralaryngeal tremor, and a high percentage of other associated neurological soft signs. The resemblance is so striking that they suggest that this subgroup be differentiated diagnostically as "spastic dysphonia of essential tremor" (p. 57).

Although the precise underlying mechanisms of essential tremor remain unknown, converging physiologic evidence suggests a more central rather than peripheral site of origin (Jankovic & Fahn, 1980). A high incidence of postural tremor reminiscent of benign essential tremor has been noted throughout the spectrum of dystonic disorders (Marsden, 1976). Thus laryngeal tremors have been viewed as consistent with a diagnosis of focal dystonia in many patients with SD. A focal dystonia model of SD is appealing in that it establishes the notion that disruption at various locations within an integrated system of feedback loops can have similar consequences for the output of the system. A focal dystonia model does not explain, however, the speech specificity of SD or some of the associated sensory findings, nor the fact that a subset of SD patients does not appear to have associated dystonias, vocal tremors, or extralaryngeal tremors.

Cerebral Cortex and Its Projections

The classical pyramidal motor system has its cell bodies in the fifth and sixth layers of the perirolandic (frontoparietal) sensorimotor cortex, and descending axons project via the internal capsule and cerebral penduncles to brain stem and spinal lower motor neuron pools. Lesions in this system result in supranuclear palsy, spastic paralysis, and associated spastic dysarthria when the crianial musculature subserving speech is involved (Darley, Aronson, & Brown, 1975). It is quite possible to obtain a truly "spastic" dysphonia as an early symptom of a gradual onset dysarthria (Aronson, 1978) or as a chronic residual of dysarthria that has otherwise resolved.

A significant number of neurologic signs suggestive of pyramidal motor dysfunction have been reported in SD. Aronson et al. (1968a) reported hyperreflexia, dysdiadochokinesis of tongue and extremities, increased jaw and sucking reflexes, and asymmetry of face and palate as symptoms in their SD group. However, pyramidal soft signs were less common than extrapyramidal soft signs and were more typical of older patients. A similarly high incidence of pyramidal soft signs, in excess of five per patient, were reported by Robe, Brumlik, and Moore (1960), in contrast to a comparatively low incidence of other potentially localizing signs (i.e., cerebellar or brain stem symptoms).

In an effort to explore the possibility of cortical involvement in SD, a number of researchers have utilized electroencephalographic (EEG) techniques. The results of these studies are equivocal. In the early study of Robe et al. (1960), 9 of the 10 EEGs obtained were interpreted to be abnormal. The types of deviations noted were quite heterogeneous; however, 50% of the patients exhibited "burst-like" discharges in the absence of clinical history of seizures. Electrical deviations tended to arise from the posterior temporoparietal electrode placement, but results were not particularly informative with respect to lateralization. These results are problematic due to the fact that the EEG technique employed is obsolete (pre-International 10–20 standardization) and therefore not directly comparable to more contemporary research. (This does not imply, a priori, that in the hands of an experienced clinican the technique was necessarily invalid). More recent reports of EEG activity in SD patients have been less impressive. Kiml (1965) reported EEG abnormalities of various types in 4 of 10 SD patients. Aronson et al. (1968a) reported EEG abnormalities in 5 of 22 SD patients. Four of these exhibited "mild nonspecific dysrhythmia" while one was clearly abnormal (i.e., bilateral, independent spike foci during sleep). Dedo et al. (1978) reported normal EEG recordings in all 12 SD patients studied. Taken in combination, these later studies suggest approximately 20% incidence of EEG abnormalities in SD. The absence of control group data obfuscates interpretation of the findings.

In an important but neglected study, Maroun, Jacob, and Gowing (1970) reported dysphonic symptoms reminiscent of SD in patients undergoing surgery for neoplasms involving left frontoparietal and supplemental motor cortices. Based largely on the work of Penfield and Roberts (1976), these authors posited that a disruption of corticothalamic feedback loops involved in motor programming might provide the mechanism underlying vocal perturbation in SD. They write: "The dysphonia in these patients was clearly not due to edema or other local lesions in the larynx or pharynx, nor was there evidence of pseudobulbar palsy or dysfunction of lower cranial nerves. Therefore, the disturbance in phonation was considered to be 'cerebral' dysphonia" (p. 673). Subjective impressions of the patients' tape-recorded speech suggested a "strained hoarseness" at times associated with "explosive speech" and "facial flushing" during vocal efforts.

Other cortical areas that have been shown to be related to vocalization in subhuman primates include the prefrontal motor cortex, the anterior temporal cortex, and the anterior cingulate gyrus. Franzen and Myers (1973) observed a dramatic reduction in socially directed vocalizations in free-ranging macaques secondary to bilateral ablations of either the prefrontal or anterior temporal cortices that spared subcortical structures (e.g., amygdala and uncinate fassiculus). Anterior cingulate lesions did not have this effect. Combined bilateral lesions of the frontal and anterior temporal regions almost completely abolished naturalistic vocal responses. Because of the massive interconnections of the frontotemporal regions via the uncinate fassiculus, these authors speculate on a functional system subserving vocalization for social interaction. A striking disassociation is seen in the work of Sutton, Larsen, and Lindeman (1974), who demonstrated that anterior cingulate lesions abolish voluntary initiation of a conditioned vocalization in response to a "go signal," whereas lesions in the homologues of the human anterior and posterior speech areas had little effect. These findings have been replicated and extended by Kirzinger and Jurgens (1982).

Pathological involvement of vocalization cortex may be implicated in some patients with SD. It is potentially interesting that the anterior cingulate gyrus is intimately related, developmentally and anatomically, to the supplemental motor cortex that was discussed in relation to SD by Maroun et al. (1970). Supplemental motor cortex has been hypothesized by some authors to mediate the connection between the limbic "drive to speak" and the motor speech programmer in Broca's area (Freedman, Alexander, & Naeser, 1984; Rubens & Kertesz, 1983). It is also known, however, that large acute structural lesions in the supplemental motor area typically result in transcortical motor aphasia while prefrontal lesions result in Broca's aphasia (Benson, 1979) rather than SD. Yet it is among the "higher cortical" disorders (e.g., alexia without agraphia) that one expects the degree of functional specificity for language behavior that seems characteristic of SD, due to the increased spatial separation of functional centers on the convoluted surface of the hemispheres.

Evidence for a cortical motor component in SD can also be gleaned by analogy from electrical stimulation experiments performed in monkeys. Hast and Milojevic (1967) stimulated the laryngeal motor cortex of the inferolateral frontal operculum and recorded laryngeal muscle responses via strain gauge on a graphic-level recorder. Characteristic of their era, they delivered exaggerated voltage levels to the stimulating electrodes, effecting grossly aberrant movement patterns within the larynx. These consisted of sustained, synchronous oscillatory adduction-abduction of the vocal fold ending in complete adduction and a transient respiratory arrest. A subsequent study using microelectrode stimulation at low-current levels (Hast, Fischer, Wetzel, & Thompson, 1974) yielded no such aberrant oscillatory movements but did elicit differentiated contractions of the thyroarytenoid and cricothyroid muscles from discrete electrode placements in the laryngeal motor cortex. Curiously, however, cardiac slowing was also simultaneously obtained from those electrode placements effective in contracting the cricothyroid. These experiments suggest that in primates both visceral motor responses and laryngeal tremor phenomena can be linked to a single cortical locus of abnormal electrical discharge. One is reminded that abnormal cardiac slowing and abnormal cricothyroid EMG activity have been demonstrated in patients with SD (Feldman et al., 1984; McCall, 1974). A cortical locus of motor dysfunction might account for some apparent visceral and "extrapyramidal" findings reported among SD patients. Upper motor neuron pathology may also account for pyramidal symptoms (e.g., hypertonus, hyperreflexia) sometimes reported in association with SD, due to disinhibition of lower motor neuron pools deprived of regulatory supranuclear input.

Limbic System

Current concepts in neurophysiology stress the significance of multiple parallel sensorimotor pathways subserving related but unique processing activities within a given functional modality (Kelso & Tuller, 1981). Such afferent systems have been described with respect to audition, vision, and somesthesia (Diamond, 1979; Merzenich & Kaas, 1980). Multiple parallel systems have also been elucidated for extremity movement (Kuypers, 1982).

A growing body of converging evidence demonstrates the existence of multiple parallel pathways, apart from the classical pyramidal motor system, for mammalian species-specific vocalization (Kelley et al., 1946; Jurgens & Ploog, 1970; Sutton et al., 1974; Jurgens, 1976; Jurgens &

Pratt, 1979a, 1979b). According to Jurgens and Ploog (1981), in primates the cortex of the anterior cingulate gyrus is considered the highest level of the system because it is required for learned vocalization. Reticular formation surrounding nucleus ambiguous is regarded as the lowest level of the system, since stimulation at this level yields phonation, while direct stimulation of the motor neurons yields only vocal fold movement. Intermediate levels of this system include subcortical limbic structures (i.e., dorsomedial and lateral hypothalamus, basal amygdaloid nucleus, and midline thalamus) that are necessary structures for involuntary vocal emotional reaction, as well as the periaqueductal gray of the caudal midbrain. This latter structure serves as a synaptic processing station that integrates diverse internal and external stimuli which result in the generation of a vocal call.

Clinical reports of dysphonia associated with midbrain lesions in humans reinforce the distinction of volitional motor versus limbic vocalizations. Botez and Barbeau (1971) report three patients with lesions of the periaqueductal gray region of the mesencephalic-pontine tegmentum resulting in total mutism and reduced faciovocal activity. A recent series of eight patients with dysphonia secondary to midbrain trauma has also been reported (von Cramon, 1981; Vogel & von Cramon, 1982). These patients were initially mute and unable to perform voluntary adduction of the vocal folds, whereas they did phonate reflexively during coughing and choking. Subsequently these patients recovered relatively normal affective vocalizations, but remained completely speechless, or anarthric. Later in recovery these patients presented a profile of pseudobulbar dysarthria with speech-specific vocal characteristics that the authors considered to be reminiscent of SD. Symptoms included frequent laryngealization, monopitch, and hard glottal attacks. These defects were attributed to "a transitory lesion of the periaqueductal gray" causing "temporary inhibition within the brainstem vocalization system" (von Cramon, 1981, p. 804).

Alluding to this limbic vocalization literature, Schaefer (1983) has posited a "direct model" for spasmodic dysphonia involving "a lesion along any of these pathways or in the region of the periaqueductal gray or reticular formation" (p. 1199). Such an interpretation is contraindicated by the fact that lesions of the periaqueductal gray and its descending pathway abolish all species-specific vocalizations in primates (Jurgens & Ploog, 1970; Jurgens & Pratt, 1979a), whereas pyramidal system lesions are specifically disruptive to human speech. Regarding this phenomenon, Jurgens and Ploog (1981) write: "Speech must be learned, whereas monkey vocalizations are essentially innate—that is, genetically programmed motor patterns. If this explanation is correct, then genetically preprogrammed vocal patterns in man, such as laughing and crying, should be preserved, even after bilateral lesions in cortical face area" (p. 137).

In summary, the parallel limbic vocalization pathway offers an explanation for the normal or nearly normal nonspeech vocalizations exhibited in SD, rather than the converse. This concept has been invoked in the recent neurologic literature to explain the positive affect-sensitivity and preservation of nonspeech vocalizations seen in other speech disorders including pseudobulbar palsy (Meyers, 1976; Jurgens & Ploog, 1981), traumatic midbrain dysphonia (Vogel & von Cramon, 1982), and stuttering (Rosenfield, 1982, 1984) in addition to SD. This interpretation lends support to the view that speech-specific vocal perturbation in SD results from impairment of the volitional motor system rather than limbic or lower brain stem centers for vocal motor control.

COMPARISON OF SD WITH THE DYSARTHRIAS

It is plausible that disruption of neural structures subserving laryngeal motor control at various levels in the central nervous system could result in perceptually similar dysphonic symptoms. Dedo et al. (1978) have suggested that SD symptoms could result from various pathologies of the peripheral or central nervous system that were sufficient to cause "selective disturbances in conduction and control of neural impulses to the larynx" (p. 879). In addition, the possibility of multiple sporadic brain stem lesions, analogous to multiple sclerosis, has been suggested as a potential explanation of SD (Schaefer, 1983). According to these views, SD may be considered a selective dysarthria representing "several etiologically different disorders having similar voice signs" (Aronson, 1985, p. 168).

It has long been acknowledged that SD shares many vocal symptoms with dysarthrias that have more specific lesion localizations (Aronson et al., 1968b). According to Aronson et al. (1968a), the distinguishing feature differentiating SD from dysarthria in general is the lack of clinically significant involvement of the supraglottal articulators. Despite this now clinically accepted dogma, articulatory abnormalities have been reported in SD. Aronson et al. (1968a) state that "rate and fluency of articulation were profoundly influenced by the occurrence of spasm" (p. 210). Other abnormalities that the authors perceived included phoneme repetition and prolongation. Spectrographic verification of prolonged phoneme duration in SD has been reported (Merson & Ginsberg, 1979; Cannito & Johnson, 1981). Spectrographic evidence of variable consonantal errors in SD, including substitutions, omissions, and distortions, has also been presented by Freeman et al. (1985a). All of these authors have attributed the articulation difficulties to a loss of coordination among laryngeal and supralaryngeal structures associated with the dysphonic episodes. It should be acknowledged that this explanation represents a logical inference and not a quantitatively supported result. In contrast to this view, Cannito (1989) has demonstrated an abnormal degree of vocal tract unsteadiness in SD subjects who were sustaining vowels with an artificial voice source.

The failure of earlier Mayo Clinic studies (Aronson et al., 1968b) to provide a clear-cut indication of the relationship of SD symptoms to those exhibited by patients with dysarthrias is felt to stem from the dichotomous method of comparison that was employed. The occurrence of a particular symptom in SD and in other neurogenic voice disorders was simply indicated using a plus or minus scoring system. This type of approach obscures potentially valuable information regarding a symptom's relative prevalence and severity within any given disorder.

In order to clarify the relationship between SD and the dysarthrias, a reanalysis of the Mayo Clinic dysarthria data (Darley et al., 1975) was undertaken by this author, using the published mean perceptual ratings of subgroups of dysarthrics as the dependent measures. To accomplish this, 10 vocal symptoms characteristic of SD were selected from among the 38 dysarthric symptoms originally studied. These are listed in order of importance vertically in Table 10.1 (dyarthric subgroups are listed horizontally). Selection of SD vocal symptoms was based upon careful literature review coupled with clinical experience. A cross-check of this selection against the vocal symptoms of SD described by Aronson et al. (1968a) revealed good agreement with the symptoms reported in that study (see particularly the summary on page 209). The first five symptoms may be characterized as cardinal, or differentiating, symptoms of SD. The last five may be viewed as frequently associated symptoms. For each of these symptoms, the mean perceptual ratings of the dyarthric groups (reported in the original study) were ranked and tabulated.

Inspection of Table 10.1 reveals that all dysarthrias except cerebellar ataxia and bulbar palsy occurred among the highest ranked for various SD-related symptoms. Some groups, however, appear to exhibit relatively more frequent distribution of the higher ranks than others. To quantify these relationships, the extension of the median test, a nonparametric equivalent of one-way ANOVA for independent samples (Siegel, 1956), was computed. If the rankings were randomly distributed among dysarthric subgroups, the frequency of occurrence of the higher rankings would not differ significantly across the subgroups. A chi-square statistic was derived from the frequency of occurrence of the observed rankings in excess of the overall median among dysarthric groups. Cardinal and associated symptoms were tested alone and in combination. Resultant chi-square statistics were significant in all cases, $p < .005$. Paired comparisons (Mann-Whitney U) were computed for both

TABLE 10.1
Rank Ordering of the Mean Severity Ratings of Dysarthric Groups
Across 10 Vocal Symptoms of Spasmodic Dysphonia

Spasmodic Dysphonia Symptoms	Pseudo-Bulbar Palsy	Dystonia	Huntington's Chorea	Amyotrophic Lateral Sclerosis	Parkinson's Disease	Cerebellar Ataxia	Bulbar Palsy
Cardinal symptoms							
Vocal stoppages	6	7	5	2.5	2.5	2.5	2.5
Strain-strangle	7	6	4	5	1.5	3	1.5
Voice tremor	6	7	5	3	1.5	4	1.5
Transient breathiness	7	5	6	2	4	2	2
Monopitch	6	3	4	5	7	1	2
Associated symptoms							
Reduced rate	6	4	2	7	3	5	1
Forced respiration	3.5	3.5	7	3.5	3.5	3.5	3.5
Harsh voice	7	5	4	6	2	3	1
Low pitch level	7	3	2	6	5	1	4
Reduced loudness	5	6	1	4	7	2	3

Note. Based on a reanalysis of the Mayo Clinic dysarthria data in *Motor Speech Disorders* (Appendix C) by F. Darley, A. Aronson, and J. Brown, 1975, Philadelphia: W. B. Saunders. Copyright 1975 by W. B. Saunders. Adapted by permission.

the combined SD symptoms and for cardinal symptoms only. For combined symptoms, the results indicated that pseudobulbar palsy and dystonia were significantly different from cerebellar ataxia and bulbar palsy, $p<.05$. Amyotrophic lateral sclerosis was significantly different from cerebellar ataxia. Figure 10.2 illustrates the total number of SD symptoms falling above the combined dysarthric median for each group.

Inspection of Figure 10.2 reveals a high degree of association between the vocal symptoms of SD and pseudobulbar palsy and dystonia, reflecting upper motor neuron and basal gangliar (pallidal) pathology, respectively. A moderate degree of association with the symptoms of SD is exhibited by chorea, also a basal gangliar (striatal) pathology. Relatively low association with SD was exhibited by amyotrophic lateral sclerosis, a variable disorder with both upper and lower motor neuron components, and parkinsonism, a midbrain (nigral) disorder. Virtually no association with SD was exhibited by cerebellar ataxia or bulbar palsy. The conclusion that emerges from this analysis is that the higher one ascends

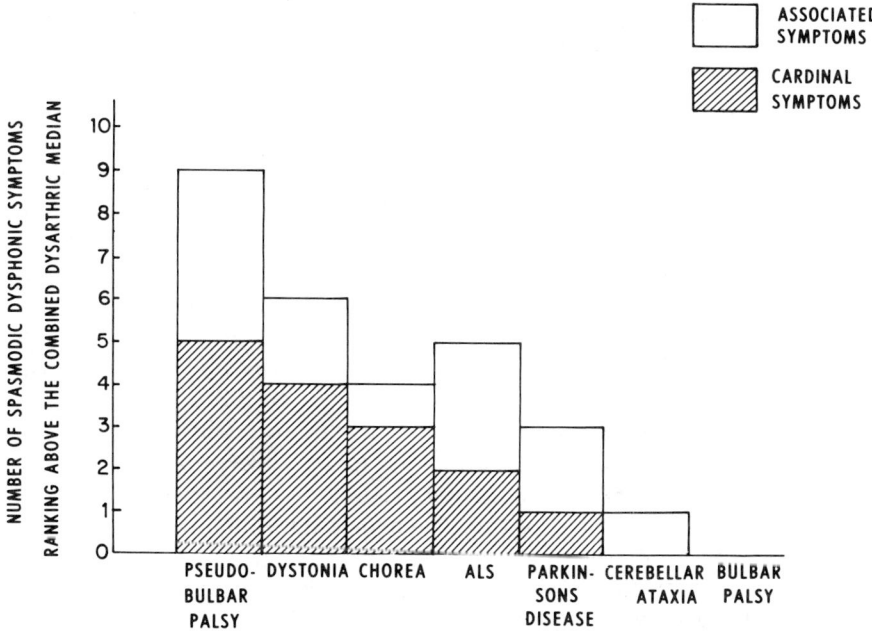

Figure 10.2 Comparison of dysarthrias on the basis of vocal symptoms of spasmodic dysphonia. Based on a reanalysis of the Mayo Clinic dysarthria data in *Motor Speech Disorders* (Appendix C) by F. Darley, A. Aronson, and J. Brown, 1975, Philadelphia: W. B. Saunders. Copyright 1975 by W. B. Saunders. Adapted by permission.

within the central nervous system, with respect to anatomical lesion locus, the more similar are the vocal symptoms to SD. This outcome argues not for multifocal pathogenesis of SD, but for a variable supranuclear lesion locus involving the pyramidal/extrapyramidal motor cortex and underlying basal ganglia structures deep within the cerebral hemispheres.

EXTRALARYNGEAL MOTOR FUNCTIONS IN SD

A variable supranuclear lesion model of SD, involving extrapyramidal motor cortex and basal ganglia or their interconnections, would appear to account for many of the speech and nonspeech motor symptoms associated with SD. Although numerous investigations have reported a high incidence of abnormal pyramidal and extrapyramidal motor signs and symptoms in SD patients, such findings are usually based on the subjective evaluation of one examiner, typically a neurologist. The major studies of this type are summarized in Table 10.2. In an attempt to more objectively quantify such clinical observations, Cannito (1986) compared upper extremity and vocal tract motor performance in 18 female SD subjects with that of a group of 18 closely matched normal controls. Subjects were equated for sex, age, and handedness. Care was taken to rule out subjects with significant neurological or psychiatric histories (other than SD). Performance on 19 motor variables was measured using a computer-automated-assessment battery approach. See Table 10.3. It was hypothesized that the SD subjects would perform more poorly than controls on complex voluntary serial motor activities and sustained positional steadiness (as predicted by a higher-level motor-processing model of SD), but would not differ from controls for simple isolated ballistic movements. All measures were found to be sufficiently reliable, with test-retest reliability coefficients (estimated from the intertrial correlations using the Spearman-Brown procedure) ranging from .85 to .98.

Multivariate analyses using Hotelling's T^2 statistic indicated a significant between-groups effect in the anticipated direction for those measures for which differences had been predicted ($T^2 = 36.51$; $df = 2, 27$; $p = .045$), but no difference for those measures for which similar performance had been predicted ($T^2 = 12.34$; $df = 8, 27$; $p = .441$). A stepwise discriminant function analysis revealed that a linear combination of four of the nonspeech motor measures was able to differentiate the subject groups with 86% accuracy ($F = 7.22$; $df = 8, 27$; $p < .001$). The measures included in the discriminant equation were finger-lift reaction time (dominant hand), finger-tapping speed (dominant hand), Purdue pegboard test (nondominant hand), and visual pursuit ramp tracking (mandibular). The resultant classification matrix is presented in Table 10.4.

TABLE 10.2
Summary of the Primary Studies Yielding a High Incidence of
Pyramidal-Extrapyramidal Neuromotor Signs in Spasmodic Dysphonia

Study	N	Incidence (%)
Critchley, 1939	3	100
Robe, Brumlik, and Moore, 1960	10	100
Aronson, Brown, Litin, and Pearson, 1968	27	74
Aminoff, Dedo, and Izdebski, 1978	12	50
Rosenfield, 1988	41	59
Total	93	68[a]

[a]Total percentage is weighted for variations in number of spasmodic dysphonia subjects across samples.

It is important to note that the SD group was characterized by a differential performance pattern with relatively poor performance on speed of finger tapping and peg placement, but relatively good performance on finger reaction time and slow ramp tracking. Although the results were striking, the a priori predictions were not entirely supported. Repeated-measures ANOVA ($p < .05$) indicated that significant differences were limited to rapid sequential movements of the upper extremities and vocal tract and vocal tract steadiness (Cannito, 1989; Cannito & Kondraske, 1990). Slow ramp visual pursuit tracking and sustained upper extremity steadiness remained unimpaired, as did the isolated ballistic movement tasks. In addition, the findings could not be accounted for on the basis of impaired affect (e.g., psychomotor retardation) inasmuch as the differentiating motor variables were uncorrelated with standardized psychometric tests of anxiety and depression (Spielberger, Gorusch, Lushene, Vagg, & Jacobs, 1983; Zung, 1967) that had also been administered. While the findings are compatible with earlier observations of extralaryngeal motor abnormalities in SD, a selective impairment in speech motor behaviors and rapid sequential manual skills seems to imply a defect of very high levels of motor information processing within the CNS (Cannito & Kondraske, 1990).

With respect to extralaryngeal motor functions in SD, it is of considerable interest that quantitative measures of laryngeal motor performance have yielded analogous results. Reich and Till (1983) found that SD subjects' phonatory reaction times were abnormally prolonged for productions of a two-syllable word but not for an isolated vowel. Ludlow and Connor (1987) also demonstrated significant delays for phonation onset in their SD subjects; however, laryngeal movement initiation time was normal. It was complex coordination for voicing rather than

TABLE 10.3
Extralaryngeal Motor Variables and Hypotheses

Hypothesis Number	Variable Number	Experimental Task	Impaired Function Predicted in Spasmodic Dysphonia
H1:		*Simple Versus Complex Movement*	
	1	Finger reaction time (dominant hand)	No
	2	Finger reaction time (nondominant hand)	No
	3	Finger-tapping speed (dominant hand)	Yes
	4	Finger-tapping speed (nondominant hand)	Yes
H2:		*Complex Movement Sequences*	
	5	Pegboard speed (dominant hand)	Yes
	6	Pegboard speed (nondominant hand)	Yes
	7	Whispered trisyllable speed	Yes
H3:		*Slow Visual Pursuit Tracking*	
	8	Slow ramp tracking (dominant hand)	Yes
	9	Slow ramp tracking (nondominant hand)	Yes
	10	Slow ramp tracking (jaw)	Yes
H4:		*Maintenance of Sustained Position*	
	11	Upper extremity steadiness (dominant hand)	Yes
	12	Upper extremity steadiness (nondominant hand)	Yes
	13	Second formant frequency steadiness	Yes

TABLE 10.3. Continued

Hypothesis Number	Variable Number	Experimental Task	Impaired Function Predicted in Spasmodic Dysphonia
H5:		*Ballistic Visual Pursuit Tracking*	
	14	Step track initiation time (dominant hand)	No
	15	Step track initiation time (nondominant hand)	No
	16	Step track initiation time (jaw)	No
	17	Step track movement time (dominant hand)	No
	18	Step track movement time (nondominant hand)	No
	19	Step track movement time (jaw)	No

Note. From *Extralaryngeal Functions in Spasmodic Dysphonia: Vocal Tract and Manual Control* (unpublished doctoral dissertation, University of Texas at Dallas, 1986) by M. P. Cannito. Printed by permission.

TABLE 10.4
Classification of Subjects as Spasmodic Dysphonic or Control on the Basis of the Stepwise Discriminant Function for Four Motor Variables

Actual Group	N of Cases	N Predicted	
		Group I (control)	Group II (spasmodic dysphonic)
Group I: Control	18	16 (89%)	2 (11%)*
Group II: Spasmodic dysphonic	18	3 (17%)**	15 (83%)
		$X^2 = 18.84$	$p < .001$

Note. A total of 86% of cases were correctly classified.
* Probability of misclassification is .111.
** Probability of misclassification is .167.

vocal fold movement per se that was impaired. These authors also suggest a supranuclear abnormality to explain the pattern of findings that was observed. Taken together, studies of laryngeal and extralaryngeal motor performance suggest that many SD subjects exhibit difficulty with coordination of rapid voluntary movements when task demands become sufficiently complex.

NEURAL IMAGING IN SPASMODIC DYSPHONIA

Preliminary support for the variable pyramidal/extrapyramidal lesion explanation of SD has also been provided by a series of neural imaging studies completed during the last several years by Freeman, Finitzo, and their associates (including the author) at the University of Texas at Dallas and Southwestern Medical Center. Among various techniques employed were nuclear magnetic resonance imaging (MRI) and brain electrical activity mapping (BEAM). This research is summarized in Finitzo and Freeman (1989). See Chapter 3 in this volume for technical descriptions of these techniques.

MRI is a signal-processing technology that records perturbations induced in an electromagnetic field around the head and reconstructs images of brain slices analogous to those obtained from computerized tomography (CT) scans. Preliminary findings in SD subjects have been reported by Schaefer et al. (1985). Both abductor and adductor patients were represented in their SD sample. Subsequently Cannito et al. (1986) described a 25-patient series resulting in 16 normal and 9 (36%) abnormal MRI scans. Sites of lesion in the abnormal studies included one right thalamocortical gliosis (post-thalamotomy onset of SD), one enlarged pineal body (probably tumor), one cerebellar malformation (Arnold-Chiari malformation, type I), and deep supratentorial white matter lesions in six patients. The deep white matter lesions were typically multiple and of small volume. Example MRI scans of one such patient are presented in Figure 10.3. A breakdown of the distribution of these lesions by subject is provided in Table 10.5. A total of 30 deep white matter lesions were identified. Working closely with the neuroradiologist, the author has plotted the distribution of the 30 deep white matter lesions on conventional CT templates (patterned after those of Naeser and Hayward, 1978). The composite brain slices showing the distribution of these lesions are depicted in Figure 10.4. Primary involvement was noted in the frontal white matter, with secondary involvements in the basal ganglia/internal capsule and parietal-occipital juncture areas. It may be significant that the greatest lesion density underlies the frontal lobes. This finding corresponds well to the localization hypothesized on the basis of a comparison of SD with the dysarthrias.

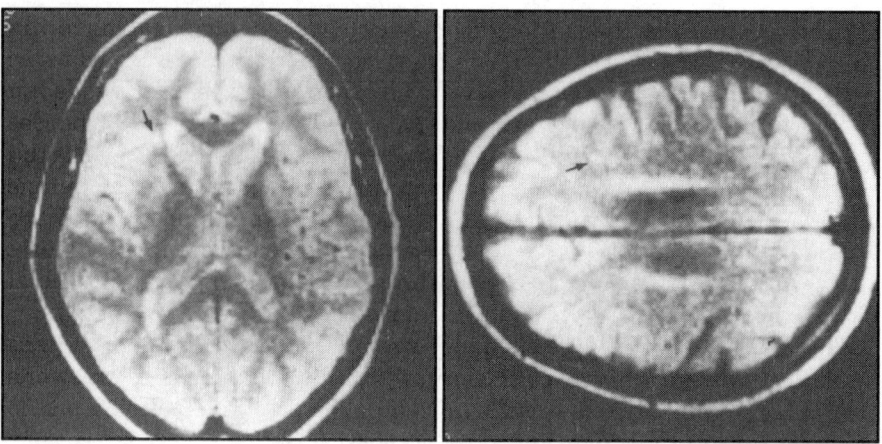

Figure 10.3 MRI of horizontal brain sections of an SD subject illustrating deep frontal white matter lesions. Left, callosal projection (forceps minor) level; right, corona radiata level. From *Extralaryngeal Functions in Spasmodic Dysphonia: Vocal Tract and Manual Control* (unpublished doctoral dissertation, University of Texas at Dallas, 1986) by M. P. Cannito. Printed by permission.

Lesions in the white matter adjacent to the left frontal horn may disrupt the motor outflow from the face area (Ross, 1980) and have been implicated in articulation problems associated with aphasia (Freedman et al., 1984). Lesions in the posterior corpus callosum cause disruption of bilateral sensorimotor integration or dyspraxia (Volpe, Sidtis, Holzman, Wilson, & Gazzaniga, 1982). It is possible that either or both of these mechanisms might result in loss of volitional laryngeal control. Despite careful scrutiny of lower regions, with the exception of a single cerebellar malformation, no brain stem lesions were observed. Radiological interpretation of probable etiologies included demyelinating, traumatic, vascular, neoplastic, and developmental causes. These results suggest that some SD patients exhibit gross lesions in supranuclear subcortical structures.

Cannito, Finitzo, Freeman, and Pool (1985) examined patterns of electrical brain activity thought to represent cerebral processing functions in 10 normal-hearing adductor SD patients using the recent BEAM technique. The equivocal nature of earlier EEG studies of SD may have reflected shortcomings of the traditional subjective method of visual inspection of the EEG recording. In contrast, the fully automated and probabilistic measurement strategy offered by the BEAM technique is intended to minimize subjective bias and provides precise quantification of clinical electrocortical abnormality. It should be recognized, however,

TABLE 10.5
Distribution of Small Supratentorial White Matter Lesions Identified by MRI in Six Cases of Spasmodic Dysphonia

Case No.	Total No. of Lesions	Left Side	Right Side
1	6	Corona radiata (2) External capsule (1) Occipito-parietal trigone (1)	Corona radiata (1) Posterior limb internal capsule (1)
2	2	Corona radiata (1)[a] Inferior basal ganglia (1)[b]	
3	10	Corona radiata (2) Frontal horn (1)	Corona radiata (4) Frontal horn (1) Occipito-parietal trigone (2)
4	3	Frontal horn (1)	Frontal horn (2)
5	8	Corona radiata (1) Frontal horn (1)[b] Occipito-parietal trigone (2)	Corona radiata (1) Frontal horn (2) Occipito-parietal trigone (1)
6	1	Parietal white matter (1)[b]	

Note. From *Extralaryngeal Functions in Spasmodic Dysphonia: Vocal Track and Manual Control* (unpublished doctoral dissertation, University of Texas at Dallas, 1986) by M. P. Cannito. Printed by permission.
[a]Adjacent to caudate body.
[b]Comparatively larger lesions.

that topographic brain mapping is highly experimental and that its clinical validity has yet to be established (American Academy of Neurology, 1989).

The SD subjects were compared to control subject data from the BEAM standardization sample (Duffy, Bartels, & Burchfield, 1981), which included subjects from the third, fourth, fifth, and sixth decades of life. The experimental subjects ranged in age from 33 to 65 years, with a mean of 48.2 ($SD = 8.97$). The sample included two males and eight females. Reported time postonset of SD ranged from 2 to 21 years. Results indicated abnormalities in excess of ± 3 standard deviations from normal in the classic EEG spectral bands in 50% of the patients, auditory cortical-evoked potential abnormalities in 90%, and visual cortical-evoked potential abnormalities in 60% of the patients. Sixty percent of the combined evoked potential abnormalities were bilaterally distributed, 30% left-lateralized, and 10% right-lateralized. Typical localiza-

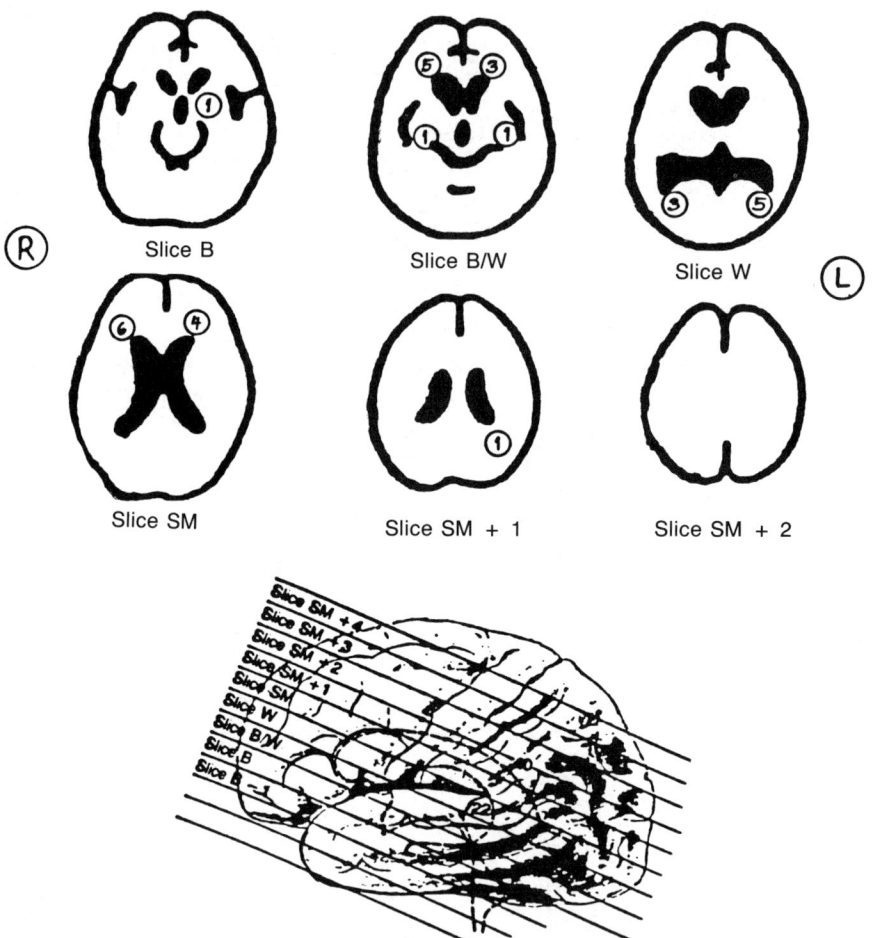

Figure 10.4 Neuroanatomic distribution of deep supratentorial white matter lesions identified in six cases of spasmodic dysphonia by MRI. From *Extralaryngeal Functions in Spasmodic Dysphonia: Vocal Tract and Manual Control* (unpublished doctoral dissertation, University of Texas at Dallas, 1986) by M. P. Cannito. Printed by permission. CT templates from "Lesion Localization in Aphasia with Cranial Computed Tomography and the Boston Diagnostic Aphasia Exam" by M. A. Naeser and R. W. Hayward, 1978, *Neurology, 28*, pp. 545–551. Reprinted by permission.

tions were left temporofrontal, medial frontal, and right parieto-occipital, pictured in Figure 10.5.

In addition to individual data, group effects were demonstrated for three electrodes during the 108–144 ms epoch following onset of the audi-

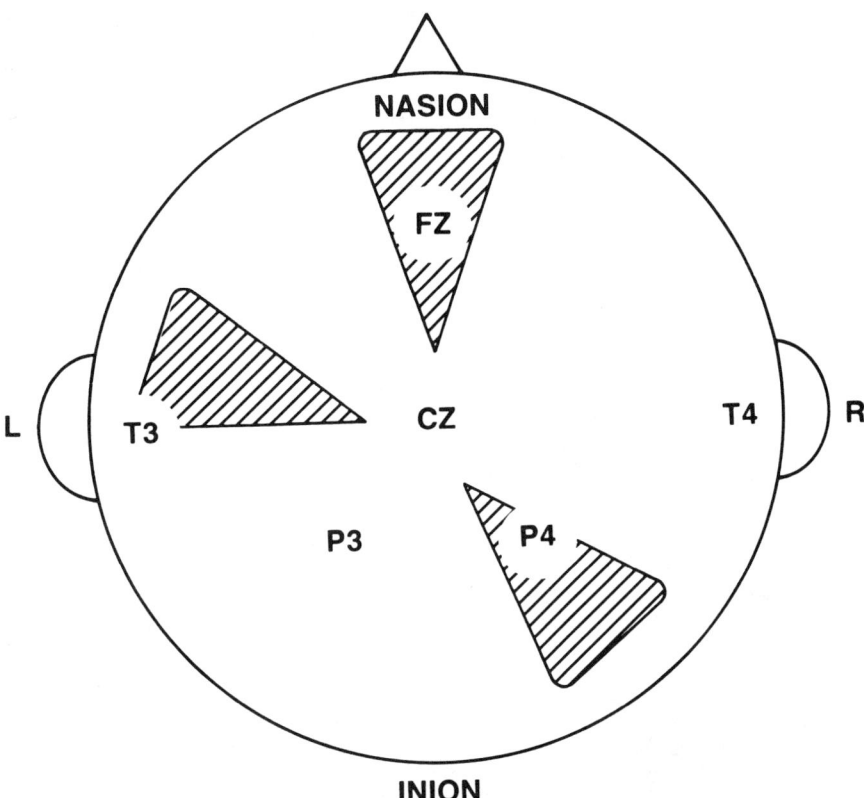

Figure 10.5 Composite diagram of the approximate scalp distributions of areas of overlapping electrocortical dysfunction in 10 cases of SD. From *Extralaryngeal Functions in Spasmodic Dysphonia: Vocal Tract and Manual Control* (unpublished doctoral dissertation, University of Texas at Dallas, 1986) by M. P. Cannito. Printed by permission.

tory tone stimulus. Electrode locations were left anterior temporal (T3), right anterior temporal (T4), and medial frontal (FZ). The raw amplitude data in microvolts from the SD subjects were compared with that of the normal controls, blocked by age in decades. The respective means and standard deviations are presented in Table 10.6. A between-subjects ANOVA was computed for each electrode by five subject groups. Resultant F-ratios were significant at the .001 level of probability. Paired means comparisons (Newman-Keuls) revealed significant differences between the SD subjects and all control groups for all three electrodes. Within the SD sample, abnormal activity from both the temporal lobe electrodes was highly correlated ($r = .71$), whereas the frontal activity

TABLE 10.6
Group Means, Standard Deviations, and Newman-Keuls Comparisons for Cortical Auditory Evoked Response at 108–144 ms

Group	x̄ (μV)	Standard Deviation	Degrees of Freedom	Significance
Electrode T3 by Groups ($F=8.03$, $p<.001$)				
Spasmodic dysphonics	−1.793	0.793		
30–39 yrs	+0.012	0.726	18	**
40–49 yrs	+0.353	0.421	12	**
50–59 yrs	+0.049	1.145	22	**
60–69 yrs	−0.181	0.787	19	**
Electrode FZ by Groups ($F=13.25$, $p<.001$)				
Spasmodic dysphonics	−3.384	1.800		
30–39 yrs	+1.307	1.707	18	**
40–49 yrs	+2.160	1.888	20	**
50–59 yrs	+0.509	2.276	22	**
60–69 yrs	−0.472	1.358	15	**
Electrode T4 by Groups ($F=5.59$, $p<.001$)				
Spasmodic dysphonics	−1.840	0.717		
30–39 yrs	−0.166	0.905	22	**
40–49 yrs	+0.228	0.917	22	**
50–59 yrs	−0.248	1.175	22	**
60–69 yrs	−0.879	0.981	22	*

Note. From *Extralaryngeal Functions in Spasmodic Dysphonia: Vocal Tract and Manual Control* (unpublished doctoral dissertation, University of Texas at Dallas, 1986) by M. P. Cannito. Printed by permission.
* Spasmodic dysphonics differed from normals with probability less than .05.
** Spasmodic dysphonics differed from normals with probability less than .01.

was uncorrelated with that of either temporal lobe. Significant interhemispheric asymmetry of the evoked potential abnormality, with greater left-sided difference, was demonstrated using a *t*-test for correlated samples with patient's *z* scores from the temporal lobe electrodes ($p = .016$).

These findings provide evidence of abnormal higher brain activity in the SD subjects. Localization of these differences tended to occur over the left and right central and medial frontal electrode placements. It is intriguing to speculate on a relationship between these scalp distributions and underlying brain topography. For example, medial frontal cortex is now regarded as a "starter mechanism" of vocalization for speech (Freedman et al., 1984). Left central cortex is of course the classical speech and language area. Recently, analogous functions for the processing of intonation have been hypothesized for the right central area (Ross, 1981). Despite all this, our present knowledge of the actual neural generators of so-called cortical EEG and evoked potential activity, as well as the localizing significance of such automated patient-to-normal comparisons (American Academy of Neurology, 1989), is limited, and we must acknowledge that attempts at such brain-behavior correlations in SD remain in the realm of speculation. Since the original study, abnormal BEAM findings in SD have been replicated using larger sample sizes and corroborated with regional cerebral blood flow (SPECT) imaging (Chapman et al., 1989).

CONCLUSION

While many neural explanations of SD have been proposed, it is apparent that some are less satisfactory than others on either logical or empirical grounds. Peripheral neuropathy is today generally rejected as an explanation for SD (Izdebski & Shipp, 1985). Bulbar-level explanations fail to account for the intermittent and speech-specific nature of the SD symptom complex, nor are SD symptoms similar to those exhibited by patients with documented bulbar disease. Although multiple cranially innervated structures frequently exhibit spasmodic abnormalities in SD, "cranial nerve spasmodic disorders cited are generally considered to be of supranuclear (basal ganglia) origin" (Hartman & Vishwanat, 1984, p. 403). The intactness of nonspeech, affective vocalization in SD appears to rule out limbic structures or the periaqueductal gray as primary lesion loci. Yet because the signs and symptoms that have been noted in association with SD are not exclusively basal gangliar, it is probably appropriate to hypothesize a more general type of supranuclear involvement. Specifically, abnormalities observed in structures innervated by the cranial motor neuron pool probably reflect deviant neuronal interactions conditioned by the descending, modulating influence of impaired structures projecting from higher levels within the CNS.

A variable supranuclear lesion locus appears appealing at this point in our understanding of SD. Premotor association cortex, pyramidal motor cortex, and the descending motor tracts lie in close proximity to the basal ganglia and share a common vascular supply. In addition, these structures interact as part of a single functional system during voluntary movement (Evarts, 1980; Kornhuber, 1984). A lesion variably affecting these structures might account for both spastic and dyskinetic vocal and nonvocal signs. These structures and their interactions are pictured schematically in Figure 10.6. Behavioral evidence from the dysarthrias, extralaryngeal motor findings in SD, and brain-imaging studies of SD are consistent with this view. Such an explanation is able to accommodate the apparent focality, function specificity, heterogeneity, intermit-

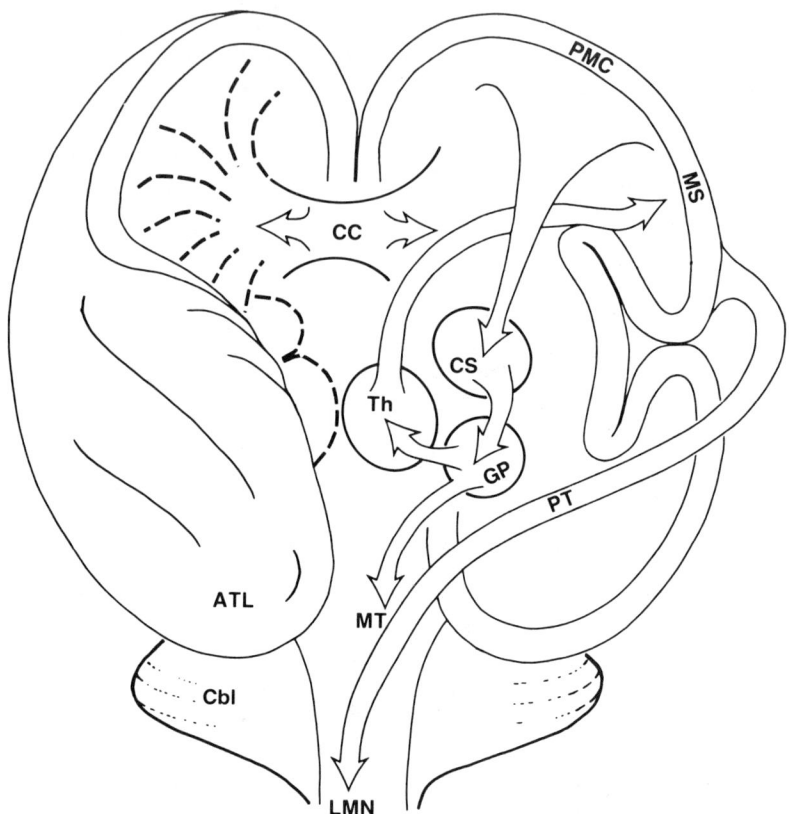

Figure 10.6 Semischematic diagram of proposed cerebral motor circuits that may be implicated in spasmodic dysphonia: *pmc*, premotor association cortex; *ms*, motor strip; *cc*, corpus callosum; *cs*, corpus striatum; *gp*, globus pallidus; *th*, thalamus; *mt*, midbrain tegmentum; *lmn*, lower motor neuron; *atl*, anterior temporal lobe; *cbl*, cerebellum.

tency and affect sensitivity of symptoms associated with this unusual voice disorder.

Implications for Management

It has been argued in this chapter that SD represents a supranuclear motor disturbance that predominantly affects the pathways for phonation for speech, but may variably involve pathways for other cranial and somatic motor functions. Such a view places SD squarely within the realm of neuromotor speech disorders, which also emcompasses the dysarthrias and apraxia of speech. Specifically, SD should be regarded as a family of focal, supranuclear dysarthrias. Whether SD represents a disorder of motor preprogramming or of execution and regulation of vocal motor commands remains unknown. Nevertheless, a supranuclear dysphonia of this type should probably be approached therapeutically somewhat differently from a voice disorder arising from either functional or peripheral vocal fold lesion etiologies. As Rosenbek and LaPointe (1985) have written: "Only if a dysarthric patient's nervous system returns to normal will speech return too. The return to normal—either because of natural or physiologic recovery or because of medical treatment—is a rare circumstance indeed. Therefore, the aim of all dysarthria treatment is compensated intelligibility. With professional guidance and by dint of individual effort, many dysarthric patients can learn to talk better. They can do so for two reasons: (1) physiologic support for a patient's speech can be enhanced; or (2) they can learn to make better use of whatever residual support is left to them" (p. 104).

These observations are germane to SD because the SD patient must recognize that the neural machinery is broken, the premorbid voice will never be achieved again, and that rather than normal voice the goal of therapy is the best compensatory voice possible. Thorough counseling in this regard is a critical prerequisite to progress in therapy. Many SD patients will resist the compensatory voice, stagnant in mourning for their premorbid one. Maximization of the physiologic substrate can be achieved in specific cases by fixation of one vocal fold, through surgery or botulinus toxin injection, or by pharmacologic treatment (Rosenfield, 1988). Compensated intelligibility can be achieved using a variety of dysarthria therapy techniques including reduced rate, exaggerated stress and articulation, phrasing, and airflow maintenance (cf. Darley et al., 1975; Yorkston, Beukelman, & Bell, 1988). Counseling is also important for helping patients deal with the negative impact of SD on their professional and personal lives. Using the *Self-rating of Depression Scale* (Zung, 1967) and the *State-Trait Anxiety Scale* (Spielberger et al., 1983), Cannito (1986) has demonstrated that over half of 18 spasmodic dysphonic females studied were clinically depressed or anxious. This is not to say that emotional problems cause SD in these patients any more than postmorbid depression would be regarded as causing an aphasia in a stroke patient. However, depression and anxiety may well exacerbate an affect-sensitive neuromotor problem (see Chapter 5 in this volume) and impede progress in therapy. These easy-to-administer paper and pencil scales serve well as a preliminary screening (in conjunction with patient interview) for potential professional counseling referral. The psychosocial impact of dysarthria and the importance of counseling for dysarthric individuals and their families are discussed at length in Chapter 6 of this volume.

The guiding principles of therapy for apraxia of speech as described by Rosenbek (1985) include "(1) efforts to improve the speech programmer by specific concentration on programmer function, and (2) efforts to reorganize speech function by systematically incorporating intact or relatively intact systems into the function of the speech programmer" (p. 270). These observations may be germane to SD in that retraining of phonatory programming may be possible by repetitive contrastive drill (see Chapter 9 of this volume). The well-established preservation of non-speech vocalizations provides a broad repertoire of "relatively intact systems" that may be brought, through therapy, under volitional control. The facilatory effects of speech produced in a context of vegetative vocalization (i.e., yawning or laughing) in SD have been demonstrated acoustically by Freeman et al. (1985a). It seems reasonable to believe that approaching SD therapy within the broader context of treatment for other neuromotor speech disorders may provide some useful general strategies that may be adapted to the unique needs of the patient with SD. It should also be clear that the management of SD patients is a multidisciplinary endeavor involving otolaryngology, neurology, and in many cases psychotherapy, in addition to speech pathology.

Neuromotor-oriented Treatment

SD has proven to be dramatically resistant to traditional voice therapy, leading some to question the wisdom of the speech pathologist even treating such individuals beyond, perhaps, a short trial course of laryngeal tension-reducing exercises. Implicit in this thinking has been the tenacious assumption that SD patients are crazy and could talk alright if they really wanted to! Approaching SD management within a motor speech disorders framework radically alters all phases of the clinical process—from diagnosis to selection of treatment goals, to counseling, to ongoing monitoring of treatment efficacy. The following case study, originally reported by Cannito, Louera, and Rosenfield (1989), describes an SD patient treated within a context of dysarthria management in which the focus was shifted away from traditional voice therapy techniques toward enhancement of the physiologic substrate and compensated intelligibility. It also points out the value of intelligibility testing in the assessment and ongoing management of more severe manifestations of SD.

CASE STUDY

M. M. is a 72-year-old retired businesswoman. Her voice disorder was originally diagnosed as a mixed (adductor-abductor) SD with voice tremor by an examining laryngologist in 1976. Tremors of the tongue and head were also noted. She began traditional voice therapy soon after and was treated for about a year. The dysphonia persisted. She subsequently tried periods of psychotherapy and biofeedback relaxation therapy without noticeable benefit. She was reinstated in voice therapy at the University of Texas Speech and Hearing Center in the summer of 1987, when she reported experiencing difficulty establishing new relationships following her retirement due to her voice disorder. Relaxation of the laryngeal area and loudness reduction were employed in treatment, in addition to the traditional voice therapy techniques of easy onset of phonation, tone focus, and control of breath support.

M. M. was seen by the author for evaluation in September 1987. Vocal quality was characterized by the presence of strained-strangled phonation and intermittent breathiness. Presence of frequent hard glottal attacks, intermittent breaks in phonation, glottal stops, vocal fry, and audible voice tremor were noted. She was unable to sustain a vowel for more than approximately 4 seconds. There was a ratio discrepancy of approximately 12 seconds between sustained /s/ and /z/. The timing of laryngospasms between syllables gave the perceptual impression of frequent omissions of initial consonants. Conversational speech was unintelligible and dysfluent.

M. M.'s phonation quality improved across a variety of nonspeech tasks including humming, paralanguage (e.g., "un-huh"), laughing, coughing, yawning, and grunting. Whispering was facilitory but not spasm-free. Better voice quality was noted for vowels sustained at high pitch, but duration remained dramatically curtailed, even in falsetto register. On examination oral structure and function were unremarkable, with the exception that velar spasms were noted to occur in synchrony with the laryngospasms. A case history revealed no prior neurological or psychiatric involvement (other than SD). She admitted "stammering" as a child, but said dysfluency resolved with speech therapy by age 12.

M. M. continued voice therapy, but the treatment approach was modified somewhat. Rather than focusing attention on traditional dimensions of voice quality, improved intelligibility was targeted as the treatment goal. A soft, breathy phonatory pattern, prolonged syllable duration, and light articulatory contacts were incorporated into the therapy techniques. After 22 sixty-minute, biweekly sessions, her speech intelligibility was evaluated using Yorkston and Beukelman's *Assessment of Intelligibility of Dysarthric Speech* (Yorkston & Beukelman, 1984). It was found that when not actively using her "speech controls," her connected utterances were only 17% intelligible; however, when controls were employed her intelligibility score increased to 77%. The patient reported the compensated speech was difficult and demanded excessively high levels of concentration.

In February 1988, while continuing the intelligibility-oriented speech therapy, M. M. was referred to Dr. David Rosenfield at Baylor College of Medicine in Houston for comprehensive neurological evaluation. Neurologic examination indicated severe intention tremor of the upper extremities and axial (head-neck) tremor as well as phonatory tremor. Fiberoptic examination of the larynx indicated constant movement of laryngeal musculature, with significant starts and stops and hyperfunctional laryngeal contraction on adduction with overrelaxation with which she attempted to compensate. MRI revealed supranuclear white matter lesions in the deep cerebral white matter (centrum semiovale and periventricular regions) of the cerebral hemispheres as well as small bilateral lesions in the pontine region of the brain stem. These were associated with biopsy-proved arteritis, but may or may not have been related to the laryngeal tremor disorder. Alcohol was reported to improve the condition, while stress worsened it. A diagnosis of spasmodic dysphonia secondary to underlying essential tremor was applied, and the patient was started on a regimen of 10 mg of oral propranolol (Inderal) three times daily for one month; the dosage was then increased to 20 mg three times daily for one month.

M. M.'s intelligibility score increased from a baseline level of 48%, 32%, and 57% (average of 46% across three successive AIDS administrations) to 75% and 80% (average of 78%) following 2 months of pharmacotherapy. In conjunction with pharmacotherapy, she was seen for speech therapy for 19 fifty-minute individual sessions biweekly. During this period M. M. reported using her controls successfully in various situations. She also became increasingly responsive during treatment and more cognizant of her vocal quality in therapy. Voice tremor on sustained phonation was noticeably reduced.

M. M. took a vacation from speech therapy in summer of 1988 to travel, but returned in September. At that time she revealed that she had discontinued the Inderal due to the inconvenience of returning to Houston for follow-up, and because in her opinion the medication was not responsible for her voice improvement. In September her baseline intelligibility score was 36% to 59% (average of 44%). In December 1988, following 17 more biweekly fifty-minute sessions of speech therapy without medication, her intelligibility score was at 40% to 57% (average of 50%). The patient reported that she was unable to maintain her controls outside of the therapy situation and in the therapy situation only for short periods and with great difficulty.

Spasmodic dysphonia is notoriously variable; however, results of the intelligibility assessment data indicate that M. M.'s intelligibility continues to fluctuate in a range from 36% to 59% without medication when she is not consciously applying therapy controls. The high intelligibility values noted during treatment with Inderal are striking because no instruction to use the therapy controls was employed during those administrations of the AIDS. Further, the generalized ease reported for using controls during that period, within and without the therapy room, is notable. It is likely that speech therapy targeting compensated intelligibility in conjunction with pharmacotherapy to enhance the underlying physiologic substrate for speech was an effective combination for this patient. At present counseling efforts have been aimed at educating M. M. in this regard, so that she will resume taking the Inderal as part of treatment. No negative side effects have been reported, yet the patient harbors some reservations about taking such medication on a routine basis. She is also considering the alternative of botulinum toxin injection through a research program of the National Institute of Neurologic Communication Disorders and Stroke.

REFERENCES

American Academy of Neurology. (1989). Assessment: EEG brain mapping. *Neurology, 39*, 1100-1101.

Aminoff, M. J., Dedo, H. H., & Izdebski, K. (1978). Clinical aspects of spasmodic dysphonia. *Journal of Neurology, Neurosurgery and Psychiatry, 41*, 361-365.

Aronson, A. E. (1973). *Audio seminars in speech pathology—psychogenic voice disorders*. Philadelphia: W. B. Saunders.

Aronson, A. E. (1978). Differential diagnosis of organic and psychogenic voice disorders. In F. L. Darley & D. C. Spriesterbach (Eds.), *Diagnostic methods is speech pathology* (pp. 535-560). New York: Harper & Row.

Aronson, A. E. (1985). *Clinical voice disorders. An interdisciplinary approach* (2nd ed.). New York: Thieme.

Aronson, A. E., Brown, J. R., Litin, M. E., & Pearson, J. S. (1968a). Spastic dysphonia: Part 1. Voice, neurologic, and psychiatric aspects. *Journal of Speech and Hearing Disorders, 33*, 203-218.

Aronson, A. E., Brown, J. R., Litin, M. E., & Pearson, J. S. (1968b). Spastic dysphonia: Part 2. Comparison with essential (voice) tremor and other neurologic and psychogenic dysphonias. *Journal of Speech and Hearing Disorders, 33*, 219-231.

Aronson, A. E., & DeSanto, L. W. (1983). Adductor spastic dysphonia: Three years after recurrent laryngeal nerve section. *Laryngoscope, 93*, 1-8.

Aronson, A. E., & Hartman, D. (1981). Adductor spastic dysphonia as a sign of essential (voice) tremor. *Journal of Speech and Hearing Disorders, 46*, 52-58.

Axelrod, J. (1974). Neurotransmitters. *Scientific American, 230*, 58-71.

Benson, D. F. (1979). *Aphasia, alexia and agraphia*. New York: Churchill Livingstone.

Blitzer, A., Lovelace, R., Brin, M., Fahn, S., & Fink, M. (1985). Electromyographic findings in focal laryngeal dystonia (spastic dysphonia). *Annals of Otology, Rhinology and Laryngology, 94*, 591-594.

Boccino, J. V., & Tucker, H. M. (1978). Recurrent laryngeal nerve pathology in spasmodic dysphonia. *Laryngoscope, 88*, 1274-1280.

Boone, D. R. (1977). *The voice and voice therapy.* Englewood Cliffs, NJ: Prentice-Hall.

Botez, M. I., & Barbeau, A. (1971). Role of subcortical structures and particularly of the thalamus, in the mechanisms of speech and language. *International Journal of Neurology, 8,* 300–320.

Bril, V., Sharpe, J. A., & Ashby, P. (1979). Midbrain asterixis. *Annals of Neurology, 6,* 362–364.

Brodnitz, F. S. (1976). Spastic dysphonia. *Annals of Otorhinolaryngology, 85,* 210–214.

Cannito, M. (1986). *Extralaryngeal functions in spasmodic dysphonia: Vocal tract and manual control.* Unpublished doctoral dissertation. University of Texas at Dallas.

Cannito, M. (1989). Vocal tract steadiness in spasmodic dysphonia. In K. Yorkston & D. Beukelman (Eds.), *Recent advances in clinical dysarthria* (pp. 243–262). Austin, TX: PRO-ED.

Cannito, M. P., Freeman, F. J., Kondraske, G. V., Pool, K. D., Schaefer, S., & Finitzo, T. (1986, October). *Spastic dysphonia: A dysarthria?* Paper presented at the Third Biennial Clinical Dysarthria Conference, Tuscon, AZ.

Cannito, M. P., Finitzo, T., Freeman, F. J., & Pool, K. D. (1985). Brain electrical activity mapping in adductor spasmodic dysphonia. *Journal of the Acoustical Society of America, 77*(Suppl. 87).

Cannito, M. P., & Johnson, J. P. (1981). Spastic dysphonia: A continuum disorder. *Journal of Communication Disorders, 14,* 215–223.

Cannito, M. P., & Kondraske, G. V. (1990). Rapid manual abilities in spasmodic dysphonic and normal female subjects. *Journal of Speech and Hearing Research, 33,* 123–133.

Cannito, M., Louera, B., & Rosenfield, D. (1989, March). *Neurogenic spasmodic dysphonia: A case for successful intervention.* Paper presented at the annual meeting of the Texas Speech and Hearing Association, El Paso, TX.

Carpenter, M. B. (1978). *Core text of neuroanatomy.* Baltimore, MD: Williams & Wilkins.

Chapman, S. D., Watson, B. C., Pool, K., Devous, M. D., Freeman, F., Schaefer, S. D., Kondraske, G. V., Mendelsohn, D. B., Close, L. G., Finitzo, T. (1989). Multifocal cortical dysfunction in spasmodic dysphonia. In K. Yorkston & D. Beukelman, *Recent advances in clinical dysarthria* (pp. 227–242). Austin, TX: PRO-ED.

Clark, R. G. (1975). *Essentials of clinical neuroanatomy and neurophysiology.* Philadelphia: F. A. Davis.

Cooper, I. S. (1976). Dystonia: Surgical approaches to treatment and physiologic implications. In M. D. Yahr (Ed.), *The basal ganglia* (pp. 369–383). New York: Raven Press.

Critchely, M. (1939). Spastic dysphonia ("inspiratory speech"). *Brain: A Journal of Neurology, 62,* 96–103.

Darley, F. L. (1978). Differential diagnosis of acquired motor speech disorders. In F. L. Darley & D. C. Spriestersbach (Eds.), *Diagnostic methods in speech pathology* (pp. 492–513). New York: Harper & Row.

Darley, F. L., Aronson, A. E., & Brown, J. R. (1975). *Motor speech disorders.* Philadelphia: W. B. Saunders.

Dedo, H. H., & Izdebski, K. (1983). Problems with surgical (RLN section) treatment of spastic dysphonia. *Laryngoscope, 93,* 268–271.

Dedo, H. H., Townsend, J. J., & Izdebski, K. (1978). Current evidence for the organic etiology of spastic dysphonia. *Otolaryngology, 86,* 875–880.

Diamond, I. T. (1979). The subdivisions of neocortex: A proposal to revise the traditional view of sensory, motor and association areas. *Progress in Psychobiology and Physiological Psychology, 8,* 1–43.

Dubner, R., Sessle, B. J., & Storey, A. T. (1978). *The neural basis of oral and facial function.* New York: Plenum Press.

Duffy, F. H., Bartels, P. H., & Burchfield, J. L. (1981). Significance probability mapping: An aid in the topographic analysis of brain electrical activity. *Electroencephalography and Clinical Neurophysiology, 51,* 455–462.

Evarts, E. V. (1980). Brain mechanisms in voluntary movement. In D. McFadden (Ed.), *Neural mechanisms in behavior* (pp. 223–252). New York: Springer-Verlag.

Feldman, M., Nixon, J. V., Finitzo-Hieber, T., & Freeman, F. J. (1984). Abnormal parasympathetic vagal function in patients with spasmodic dysphonia. *Annals of Internal Medicine, 100,* 401–495.

Finitzo, T., & Freeman, F. J. (1989). Spasmodic dysphonia, whether and where: Results of seven years of research. *Journal of Speech and Hearing Research, 32,* 541–555.

Finitzo-Hieber, T., Freeman, F. J., Gerling, I., Dodson, L., & Schaefer, S. (1981). Auditory brainstem response abnormalities in adductor spasmodic dysphonia. *Amerian Journal of Otolaryngology, 3,* 26–30.

Foltz, E. L., Knopp, L. M., & Ward, A. A. (1959). Experimental spasmodic torticollis. *Journal of Neurosurgery, 16,* 55–72.

Fox, D. (1969). Spastic dysphonia: A case presentation. *Journal of Speech and Hearing Disorders, 34,* 275–279.

Franzen, E. A., & Myers, R. E. (1973). Neural control of social behavior: Prefrontal and anterior temporal cortex. *Neuropsychologia, 11,* 141–157.

Freedman, M., Alexander, M. P., & Naeser, M. A. (1984). Anatomic basis of transcortical motor aphasia. *Neurology, 34,* 409–417.

Freeman, F., Cannito, M., Finitzo, T., & Schaefer, S. (1985). Disordered laryngeal control: Fiberoptic studies of spasmodic dysphonia. *Journal of the Acoustical Society of America, 77*(Suppl. 87).

Freeman, F. J., Cannito, M. P., & Finitzo-Hieber, T. (1985a). Classification of spasmodic dysphonia by perceptual-acoustic-visual means. In G. Gates (Ed.), *Spasmodic dysphonia: The state of the art, 1984* (pp. 5–18). New York: Voice Foundation.

Freeman, F. J., Cannito, M. P., & Finitzo-Hieber, T. (1985b). Getting to know spasmodic dysphonic patients. *Texas Journal of Audiology and Speech Pathology, 10,* 14–19.

Hall, J. W. (1981). Central auditory function in spasmodic dysphonia. *American Journal of Otolaryngology, 2,* 188–198.

Hall, J. W., & Jerger, J. (1976). Acoustic reflex characteristics in spasmodic dysphonia. *Archives of Otolaryngology, 102,* 411–415.

Hartman, D. E., & Vishwanat, B. (1984). Spasmodic dysphonia [Letter to the editor]. *Annals of Internal Medicine, 101,* 403.

Hast, M. H., Fischer, J. M., Wetzel, A. B., & Thompson, V. E. (1974). Cortical motor representation of the laryngeal muscles in macaca mulatta. *Brain Research, 73,* 229–240.

Hast, M. H., & Milojevic, B. (1967). The response of the vocal folds to electrical stimulation of the inferior frontal cortex of the squirrel monkey. *Actaotolaryngologica, 61,* 196–204.

House, E. L., Pansky, B., & Siegal, A. (1979). *A systematic approach to neuroscience.* New York: McGraw-Hill.

Izdebski, K., & Shipp, T. (1985). Model of spastic dysphonia. In G. A. Gates (Ed.), *Spastic dysphonia: The state of the art, 1984* (pp. 44–47). New York: Voice Foundation.

Jankovic, J. (1981). Drug-induced and other orofacial-cervical dyskinesias. *Annals of Internal Medicine, 94,* 788–793.

Jankovic, J. (1983). Brainstem origin of blepharospasm. *Neurology, 33,* 162.

Jankovic, J., & Fahn, S. (1980). Physiologic and pathologic tremors: Diagnosis, mechanisms and management. *Annals of Internal Medicine, 93,* 460–465.

Jankovic, J., & Ford, J. (1982). Blepharospasm and orofacial-cervical dystonia: Clinical and pharmacological findings in 100 patients. *Annals of Neurology, 13,* 402–411.

Jurgens, U. (1976). Projections from the cortical larynx area in the squirrel monkey. *Experimental Brain Research, 25,* 401–411.

Jurgens, U., & Ploog, D. (1970). Cerebral representation of vocalization in the squirrel monkey. *Experimental Brain Research, 10,* 532–554.

Jurgens, U., & Ploog, D. (1981). On the neural control of mammalian vocalization. *Trends in Neuroscience, 4,* 135–137.

Jurgens, U., & Pratt, R. (1979a). Role of the periaqueductal gray in the vocal expression of emotion. *Brain Research, 167,* 367–378.

Jurgens, U., & Pratt, R. (1979b). The cingular vocalization pathway in the squirrel monkey. *Experimental Brain Research, 34,* 499–570.

Kelley, A. H., Beaton, L. E., & Magoun, H. W. (1946). A midbrain mechanism for facio-vocal activity. *Journal of Neurophysiology, 9,* 181–189.

Kelso, J. A. S., & Tuller, B. (1981). Toward a theory of apractic syndromes. *Brain and Language, 12,* 224–245.

Kiml, P. J. (1965). Recherches experimentales de la dysphonie spastique. *Folia Phoniatrica, 17,* 241–301.

Kirzinger, A., & Jurgens, U. (1982). The effects of brainstem lesions on vocalization in the squirrel moneky. *Brain Research, 358,* 150–162.

Kornhuber, H. H. (1984). Mechanisms of voluntary movement. In W. Prinz and A. F. Sanders (Eds.), *Cognition and motor processes.* New York: Springer-Verlag.

Kuypers, H. A. (1982). A new look at the organization of the motor system. *Progress in Brain Research, 57,* 381–403.

Lang, A. E., & Marsden, C. D. (1983). Spasmodic dysphonia in Gilles de la Tourette's disease. *Archives of Neurology, 40,* 51–52.

Luchsinger, R., & Arnold, G. E. (1965). *Voice-speech-language clinical communicology: Its physiology and pathology.* Belmont, CA: Wadsworth.

Ludlow, C., & Connor, N. (1987). Dynamic aspects of phonatory control in spasmodic dysphonia. *Journal of Speech and Hearing Research, 30,* 197–206.

Maroun, F. B., Jacob, J. C., & Gowing, P. (1970). Dysphonia associated with cortical neoplasms. *Journal of Neurosurgery, 32,* 671–676.

Marsden, C. D. (1976). Dystonia: The spectrum of the disease. In M. D. Yahr (Ed.), *The basal ganglia.* New York: Raven Press.

Marsden, C. D., & Sheehy, M. P. (1982). Spastic dysphonia, Meige disease, and torsion dystonia [Letter to the editor]. *Neurology, 32,* 1202.

McCall, G. N. (1974). Spasmodic dysphonia and the stuttering block: Commonalities or possible connections. In L. M. Webster & L. C. Furst (Eds.), *Vocal tract dynamics and dysfluency* (pp. 124–151). New York: Speech and Hearing Institute.

Merson, R. M., & Ginsberg, A. P. (1979). Spasmodic dysphonia: Abductor type. A clinical report of acoustic, aerodynamic and perceptual characteristics. *Laryngoscope, 89,* 129–139.

Merzenich, M. M., & Kaas, J. H. (1980). Principles of organization of sensory-perceptual systems in mammals. *Progress in Psychobiology and Physiological Psychology, 9,* 1–42.

Meyers, R. (1976). Comparative neurology of vocalization and speech: Proof of a dichotomy. *Annals of New York Academy of Science, 280,* 745–757.

Murphy, A. T. (1964). *Functional voice disorders.* Englewood Cliffs, NJ: Prentice-Hall.

Naeser, M. A., & Hayward, R. W. (1978). Lesion localization in aphasia with computed tomography and the Boston Diagnostic Aphasia Exam. *Neurology, 28,* 545–551.

Pechadre, J. C., Larochelle, L., & Poirier, L. J. (1976). Parkinsonian akinesia, rigidity and tremor in the monkey: Histopathological and neuropharmacological study. *Journal of Neurological Science, 28,* 147–157.

Penfield, W., & Roberts, L. (1976). *Speech and brain mechanisms.* New York: Atheneum.

Ravits, J. M., Aronson, A. E., DeSanto, L. W., & Dyck, P. J. (1979). No morphometric abnormality of recurrent laryngeal nerve in spastic dysphonia. *Neurology, 29,* 1376–1382.

Reich, A., & Till, J. (1983). Phonatory and manual reaction times of women with idiopathic spasmodic dysphonia. *Journal of Speech and Hearing Research, 26,* 10–18.

Robe, E., Brumlik, J., & Moore, P. (1960). A study of spastic dysphonia: Neurologic and electroencephalographic abnormalities. *Laryngoscope, 70,* 219–245.

Rosenbek, J. C. (1985). Treating apraxia of speech. In D. F. Johns (Ed.), *Clinical management of neurogenic communicative disorders* (pp. 267–312). Austin, TX: PRO-ED.

Rosenbek, J. C., & LaPointe, L. L. (1985). The dysarthrias: Description, diagnosis, and treatment. In D. F. Johns (Ed.), *Clinical management of neurogenic communicative disorders* (pp. 97–152). Austin, TX: PRO-ED.

Rosenfield, D. B. (1982). The brain and the stutterer. *Journal of Fluency Disorders, 7*, 81–92.

Rosenfield, D. B. (1984). Stuttering. *CRC Critical Reviews in Clinical Neurobiology, 1*, 117–139.

Rosenfield, D. B. (1988). Spasmodic dysphonia. In J. Jankovic & E. Tolosa (Eds.), *Advances in neurology: Vol. 49. Facial dyskinesias* (pp. 317–327). New York: Raven Press.

Ross, E. D. (1980). Localization of the pyramidal tract in the internal capsule by whole brain dissection. *Neurology, 30*, 59–64.

Ross, E. D. (1981). The aprosodias. *Archives of Neurology, 38*, 561–569.

Rowland, L. P. (1982). Diseases of chemical transmission at the nerve-muscle synapse: Myasthenia gravis and related syndromes. In E. R. Kandel & J. H. Schwartz (Eds.), *Principles of neural science* (pp. 132–137). New York: Elsevier/North Holland.

Rubens, A. B., & Kertesz, A. (1983). The localization of lesions in transcortical aphasias. In A. Kertesz (Ed.), *Localization in neuropsychology* (pp. 245–268). New York: Academic Press.

Schaefer, S. D. (1983). Neuropathology of spasmodic dysphonia. *Laryngoscope, 93*, 1183–1204.

Schaefer, S. D., Finitzo-Hieber, T., Gerling, I. J., & Freeman, F. J. (1983). Brainstem conduction abnormalities in spasmodic dysphonia. *Annals of Otology, Rhinology and Laryngology, 92*, 59–63.

Schaefer, S., Freeman, F., Finitzo, T., Close, L., Cannito, M., Ross, E., Reisch, J., & Marivella, K. (1985). Magnetic resonance imaging findings and correlations in spasmodic dysphonia patients. *Annals of Otology, Rhinology and Laryngology, 94*, 595–601.

Sharbrough, F. W., Stockard, J. J., & Aronson, A. E. (1978). Brainstem auditory evoked responses in spastic dysphonia. *Transactions of the American Neurology Association, 103*, 198–201.

Shipp, T., Izdebski, K., Reed, C., & Morrissey, P. (1985). Intrinsic laryngeal muscle activity in a spastic dysphonia patient. *Journal of Speech and Hearing Disorders, 50*, 54–59.

Siegel, S. (1956). *Nonparametric statistics*. New York: McGraw-Hill.

Spielberger, C. D., Gorusch, R. L., Lushene, R., Vagg, P. R., & Jacobs, G. A. (1983). *Manual for the state-trait anxiety inventory*. Palo Alto, CA: Consulting Psychologists Press.

Stillman, R. (1980). Auditory evoked potentials. In P. Levinson & C. Sloan (Eds.), *Auditory processing and language* (pp. 19–34). New York: Grune & Stratton.

Sutton, D., Larson, C., & Lindeman, R. C. (1974). Neocortical and limbic lesion effects on primate phonation. *Brain Research, 71*, 61–75.

Traube, L. (1871). Spastische formder nervoeson heiserkeit. In L. Traube (Ed.), *Gesammelte beitrage zur pathalogie und physiologie* (Vol. 2, pp. 674–678). Berlin: Hirschwald.

Vogel, M., & von Cramon, D. (1982). Dysphonia after traumatic midbrain damage: A follow-up study. *Folia Phoniatrica, 34,* 150–159.

Volpe, B. T., Sidtis, J. J., Holzman, J. D., Wilson, D. H., & Gazzaniga, M. S. (1982). Cortical mechanisms involved in praxis: Observations following partial and complete section of the corpus callosum in man. *Neurology, 32,* 645–650.

von Cramon, D. (1981). Traumatic mutism and the subsequent reorganization of speech functions. *Neuropsychologia, 19,* 801–805.

Wolfe, V. I., & Bacon, M. (1976). Spectrographic comparison of two types of spastic dysphonia. *Journal of Speech and Hearing Disorders, 41,* 325–332.

Yorkston, K., & Beukelman, D. (1984). *Assessment of intelligibility of dysarthric speech.* Austin, TX: PRO-ED.

Yorkston, K., Beukelman, D., & Bell, K. (1988). *Clinical management of dysarthric speakers.* Austin, TX: PRO-ED.

Zung, W. W. K. (1967). *The measurement of depression.* Milwaukee: Lakeside Laboratories.

Zwitman, D. (1979). Bilateral cord dysfunctions: Abductor type spastic dysphonia. *Journal of Speech and Hearing Disorders, 44,* 373–378.

ACKNOWLEDGMENTS

This chapter is based in part on the author's doctoral dissertation, completed at the University of Texas at Dallas in 1986 and supported by NIH Grant NS 18276. Portions of this chapter have been presented at the Third Biennial Clinical Dysarthria Conference, Tucson, AZ, 1985; the 109th Meeting of the Acoustical Society of America, Austin, TX, 1985; and the 33rd Annual Conference of the Texas Speech and Hearing Association, El Paso, TX, 1989. This author acknowledges David B. Rosenfield, MD, and Barbara Louera, MS, for their contributions to the case study. Several scholars have contributed to the development of ideas presented in this chapter through personal interaction over a period of years. The author acknowledges intellectual indebtedness to the following individuals: Terese Finitzo, PhD, Frances Freeman, PhD, George Gerken, PhD, George Kondraske, PhD, Kenneth Pool, MD, Elliott Ross, MD, and Stephen Schaefer, MD

CHAPTER 11

Noninvasive Instrumentation in the Treatment of Stuttering

Ben C. Watson and Peter J. Alfonso

> *Watson and Alfonso present a rationale for incorporating noninvasive instrumentation into the clinical environment to identify and treat movement abnormalities in the respiratory and laryngeal systems as well as aerodynamic irregularities associated with stuttering and other disorders of speech motor control. Illustrative examples demonstrate the potential value of kinematic monitoring devices in identifying physiologic abnormalities and in facilitating training of therapeutic targets.*

1. Describe clinical and laboratory evidence that abnormalities in control of the respiratory and laryngeal systems may be associated with stuttering.
2. Summarize several practical advantages of incorporating noninvasive instrumentation into therapy procedures.
3. How can attainment of therapeutic goals be facilitated through use of noninvasive kinematic biofeedback?

To date, the use of noninvasive instrumentation for monitoring physiologic events during speech production has been confined primarily to the laboratory setting. One important application of this instrumentation has been to identify and characterize physiologic deficits associated with disruptions of speech motor control observed in clinical populations. Results of this research have begun to suggest meaningful applications of noninvasive instrumentation in clinical settings. The goal of this chapter is to present a rationale for clinical use of noninvasive instrumentation to identify, characterize, and remediate certain physiologic deficits associated with stuttering. We focus on deficits revealed in movements of the respiratory and laryngeal systems or as reflected in patterns of airflow through the vocal tract. We do not specifically address direct monitoring of movements of the supralaryngeal articulators because this instrumentation is complex, often invasive, and expensive. Airflow measures are less complex and can be used to infer movements of the supralaryngeal articulators. We also discuss some practical issues regarding clinical applications of instrumentation. Our discussion of these issues is not intended to provide a "cookbook" for therapy, but to highlight specific advantages and disadvantages. Finally, we present several illustrative examples of initial applications of noninvasive instrumentation in the treatment of two speech disorders: stuttering and spasmodic dysphonia. These examples highlight the general applicability of noninvasive instrumentation.

While we will show that noninvasive instrumentation is appropriate for the treatment of deficits presented in a variety of clinical populations, our rationale emerged from research findings and clinical observations taken from the stuttering literature. This rationale is based on several assumptions. First, we assume that speech characteristics of stutterers are associated with disruption of the normal coordination of events within and between the respiratory, laryngeal, and articulatory systems. Furthermore, certain characteristics of these disruptions are observable in kinematic and airflow signals. Second, we assume that certain physiologic (i.e., kinematic) disruptions may precede the perceived moment of stuttering. That is, by the time the moment of stuttering is manifested in the speech acoustic signal, the physiologic disruption has already occurred. Third, we assume that certain physiologic disruptions are not perceptually evident or clearly identifiable in the acoustic signal. In fact, stutterers' perceptually "fluent" speech may be different from the fluent speech of nonstutterers at some physiologic level(s). Consequently, feedback of the acoustic signal alone is inadequate for developing compensatory strategies designed to avoid or minimize these disruptions. Finally, we assume that certain characteristics of physiologic disruptions associated with the moment of stuttering can be detected, quantified, and displayed to clients, and that this process will facilitate the development of strategies for reducing the magnitude of the disruption and thereby improve fluency.

Use of biofeedback in the treatment of stuttering is not a new concept. Guitar (1975) described a therapy program in which output from surface electrodes modulated an acoustic signal presented to subjects. As the amplitude of muscle activity increased, the frequency of the acoustic signal increased. Biofeedback representing level of muscle activity was effective in helping subjects reduce activity levels (i.e., facilitated relaxation) and improve fluency. The approach proposed here differs from that used by Guitar. That is, we propose the use of biofeedback to change specific laryngeal and respiratory behaviors in order to facilitate the production of fluent speech.

We begin developing our rationale by reviewing clinical observations and research findings associating disruption of respiratory and laryngeal coordination with stuttering. The goal of this review is to highlight salient characteristics of these disruptions. In so doing, we may provide a rationale for appropriate clinical targets for therapeutic intervention.

RESPIRATORY DISRUPTIONS

During speech production, the respiratory system provides expiratory airflow and adequate driving pressure to support phonation. This function is realized by a rapid prephonatory increase in lung volume followed by maintenance of a relatively stable positive pressure across a decreasing lung volume. Maintenance of the relatively stable expiratory driving pressure is accomplished by a balance of nonmuscular forces (i.e., gravity) and forces generated by the contraction of inspiratory and expiratory muscles (cf. Zemlin, 1988). Clinical observations of respiratory abnormalities in stutterers include reduced tidal volume, marked delay between onset of expiratory airflow and onset of phonation, continued speech production at inappropriately low lung volumes, interruption of speech by inspiratory gasps, and speech production on inspiration (Van Riper, 1982). These observations suggest that certain stutterers have difficulty coordinating respiratory events for speech.

Laboratory investigations of respiratory kinematics in stutterers are consistent with clinical observations. For example, Travis (1927) reported both prolonged duration of inspiration relative to duration of expiration and tremor of the abdominal wall. Travis also described pronounced antagonistic movements of the thoracic and abdominal walls. However, oppositional movements of the rib cage and abdominal wall have been observed in normal speakers and reflect the relatively independent contributions of changes in volumes of the thoracic and abdominal cavities to changes in total lung volume (cf. Hixon et al., 1973). So, oppositional movements alone do not necessarily reflect abnormal respiratory kinematics. Murray (1932) observed (1) increased variability in both amplitude and duration of inspiratory and expiratory gestures in stutterers relative to nonstutterers during a silent reading task, and (2) greater variability in amplitude of stutterers' inspiratory gestures during silent reading than during resting breathing. Nonstutterers showed an opposite pattern; they reduced variability of the inspiratory gesture during the reading task. Thus stutterers were apparently unable to meet increased demands for stability of the respiratory system during the reading task. Seth (1934) described respiratory disruption during a stuttering block as characterized by "halts, interruptions, sudden releases, and complete reversals" of expiration and inspiration.

The respiratory deficits noted above were observed during the moment of stuttering by all the researchers mentioned except for Murray (1932). Consequently, it is not clear to what extent these phenomena precipitate the stuttering episode or reflect stutterers' attempts to restore control over speech production. In a recent study, Watson and Alfonso (1986) observed several respiratory deficits before and during stutterers' voice onset for production of a perceptually fluent vowel. First, severe stutterers—unlike a mild stutterer and nonstutterers—rarely used prephonatory preparation intervals to execute gestures associated with inflation of the respiratory system. Indeed, analysis of kinematic signals in terms of changes in relative lung volume revealed that significantly lower prephonatory increases in lung volume were achieved by severe stutterers than by the mild stutterer and nonstutterers. Severe stutterers also frequently began respiratory compression (expiratory gestures) for phonation onset well before the moment of vocal fold closure. This pattern suggests inefficient management of the expiratory airstream. Again, analysis of kinematic data in terms of relative changes in lung volume supported this finding. Severe stutterers showed significantly greater reduction in lung volume before voice onset than did the mild stutterer or nonstutterers. That is, severe stutterers waste pulmonic air before voicing begins.

Taken together, clinical observations and laboratory findings suggest that disruption of normal respiratory function is associated with, and may precipitate, the moment of stuttering. In addition, this review suggests several targets for a therapy program designed to minimize contributions of respiratory disruption to stuttering. For example, therapy might focus on (1) ensuring adequate prephonatory inflation; (2) establishing smooth, uninterrupted airflow; (3) eliminating attempts to phonate on inspiration; and (4) facilitating efficient airflow management through appropriate organization of respiratory and laryngeal events.

LARYNGEAL DISRUPTIONS

Wingate (1967) noted that smooth transitions between voiced and voiceless segments are critical for fluent speech. Therefore an important dimension of laryngeal control during connected speech is rapid onset and offset of vocal fold vibration for the production of contiguous voiced and voiceless segments. Vocal fold vibration is a consequence of the interaction of myoelastic properties of the vocal folds and aerodynamic phenomena (e.g., transglottal pressure) (van den Berg, 1958). Consequently rapid voice onset and offset adjustments require precise regulation of vocal fold tension, medial compression, and position as well as transglottal pressure (Stevens, 1977). Clinical observations suggest a relation between stuttering and disrupted control of voice onset and offset. For example, stuttering is more likely to occur in association with voice onset for the initial word of an utterance or phrase (Brown, 1938).

Stutterers' ability to initiate and terminate voicing has been investigated using a variety of experimental paradigms. For example, some investigations compare frequency of stuttering and/or amount of adaptation on passages containing only voiced segments with passages containing both voiced and voiceless segments (Adams & Reis, 1971, 1974; Adams, Riemenschneider, Metz, & Conture, 1975; Manning & Coufal, 1976; Hutchinson & Brown, 1978). Most of these studies report greater frequency of stuttering and less adaptation for passages containing both voiced and voiceless segments. The interpretation most often applied to this finding is that increased frequency of stuttering or failure to adapt or both reflect stutterers' difficulty executing rapid voice onsets and offsets.

The reaction time paradigm is used to assess vocal control in terms of stutterers' ability to rapidly initiate voicing. The measure of interest is stutterers' voice onset latency relative to presentation of an external reaction signal (e.g., a tone or a light). Specifying the phonetic nature of the response (i.e., isolated vowel or consonant-vowel syllable) minimizes specific contributions of the articulatory system to reaction time values. Consequently delays in voice onset are presumed to reflect primarily respiratory-laryngeal deficits. Results of reaction time studies suggest that stutterers as a group have difficulty rapidly initiating phonation (cf. Adams & Hayden, 1976; Cross & Luper, 1979; Cullinen & Springer, 1980; Reich, Till, & Goldsmith, 1981; Starkweather, Hirschman, & Tannenbaum, 1976; Watson & Alfonso, 1982, 1983, 1987).

Insights into physiologic events associated with stutterers' apparent difficulty controlling both the laryngeal system and interactions between the respiratory and laryngeal systems derive from studies of laryngeal and respiratory physiology during stutterers' perceptually fluent or dysfluent speech. Conture, McCall, and Brewer (1977), based on fiberoptic filming of the vocal folds during connected speech, described abnormal positioning of the vocal folds associated with moments of dysfluency. Freeman and Ushijima (1978), recording electromyographic (EMG) signals from intrinsic laryngeal muscles, observed abnormal levels of activity and inappropriate reciprocity in antagonistic laryngeal muscles during dysfluencies. Shapiro (1980) observed similar EMG abnormalities.

Using electroglottography (EGG), Borden, Baer, and Kenney (1985) investigated laryngeal events associated with stutterers' production of perceptually fluent and dysfluent words in a counting task. The EGG signal provides information regarding changes in vocal fold contact area during a cycle of vibration. Analysis of the rise-time of the amplitude envelope of the EGG signal yields information corresponding to abruptness of voice onset. For example, abrupt onset of voicing is associated with a rapid increase in the amplitude of the EGG signal. In addition, as shown in Figure 11.1, landmarks in the EGG signal can be identified that correspond to increasing vocal fold contact (glottal closing), decreasing vocal fold contact (glottal opening), peak contact (glottal closure), and minimum contact (open glottis).

Borden et al. (1985) reported several differences between EGG patterns produced by normal speakers and those associated with stutterers' dysfluencies or attempts to recover from a dysfluency. Following a dysfluency, stutterers often demonstrated a more gradually increasing amplitude envelope of the EGG signal. This pattern was interpreted as a physiological correlate of perceptual judgments of "easy onset of voicing." Indeed, the authors suggest that the EGG signal provides a more reliable index of easy onset than the acoustic signal because it is independent of filtering effects imposed by the supralaryngeal vocal tract. With respect to details of the vibratory cycle after a dysfluency, severe

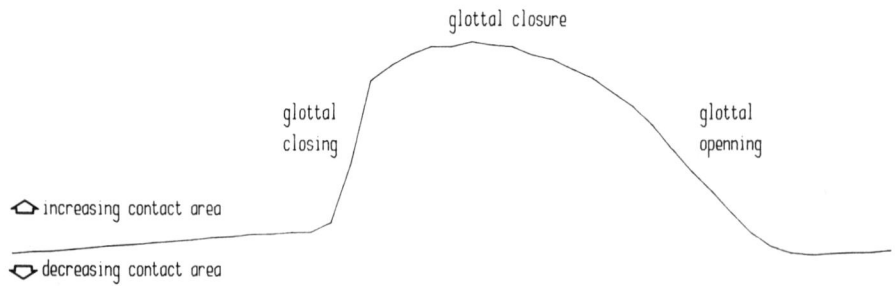

Figure 11.1 Electroglottographic signal corresponding to one cycle of vocal fold vibration. Important landmarks are indicated.

stutterers in particular demonstrated a pattern of rapid glottal opening and an open period of relatively short duration. Borden et al. (1985) suggest that this pattern reflects stiff vocal folds. This suggestion was confirmed by acoustic analyses that showed an increase in fundamental frequency when voicing was initiated after a block. The positive relationship between increases in vocal fold stiffness and increases in fundamental frequency in chest register is well documented (Gay, Hirose, Strome, & Sawashima, 1972). In summary, two aspects of the Borden et al. study are particularly relevant to our goal. First, this study demonstrates that the EGG signal can be a reliable indicator of easy onset of voicing and that changes in the fine structure of the EGG waveform can be used to infer vocal fold stiffness. Second, EGG biofeedback may facilitate establishment of fluency-enhancing techniques (clinical targets) and aid in reducing certain laryngeal abnormalities (such as increased vocal fold tension). These changes may in turn facilitate fluency.

Laboratory studies also reveal stutterers' deficits in organizing laryngeal and respiratory events. Watson and Alfonso (1987) reported abnormal delays in stutterers' onsets of vocal fold abduction and adduction gestures as well as evidence of inappropriate timing of vocal fold closure and onset of expiratory airflow associated with perceptually fluent onsets of isolated, voiced vowels. Peters and Hulstijn (1987), based on an analysis of patterns of prephonatory increases in subglottal pressure, also reported evidence of abnormalities in temporal coordination of respiratory and laryngeal events.

Taken together, studies of laryngeal function in stutterers highlight two classes of abnormality: (1) inappropriate levels of muscle activity that may be associated with increased vocal fold tension and laryngeal resistance to airflow; and (2) temporal disruption in the organization of laryngeal opening and closing gestures with respiratory inspiratory and expiratory gestures.

AERODYNAMIC DISRUPTIONS

The consequence of appropriate organization of respiratory and laryngeal events leading to voice onset is the generation of expiratory airflow that is modulated at the level of the larynx and then further modulated and filtered by altering the shape of supralaryngeal cavities. Hutchinson (1974) recorded airflow through the vocal tract and intra-oral air pressure in an attempt to characterize aerodynamic patterns produced by stutterers and to relate these patterns to dysfluency type. He identified seven distinct aerodynamic patterns associated with stuttering. While many of these patterns primarily reflected abnormalities in intra-oral air pressure, some of them were characterized by abnormal patterns of airflow. For example, the most frequently observed dysfluency ("abbreviated vowel element") was associated with abrupt cessation of airflow. Another example, "prolonged silent blocks," was associated with an absence of airflow. Hutchinson was able to simulate abnormal patterns associated with abbreviated vowel element dysfluencies by executing a glottal stop gesture. The pattern associated with prolonged silent blocks was simulated by "very stable posturing of the articulators with no variations in respiratory driving force." Further, he reported the sensation being "locked into one articulatory gesture" during the simulation. This sensation parallels that reported by stutterers during tonic blocks. The suggestion that specific dysfluency types may be associated with specific aerodynamic patterns implies that monitoring airflow during the production of phonetically specified utterances may be informative in identifying salient aerodynamic characteristics of a stutterer's dysfluencies and may aid in developing a strategy for modifying these patterns to facilitate fluency.

In sum, there is ample evidence—derived from both clinical observation and laboratory investigation—to conclude that abnormalities in respiratory and laryngeal function and in patterns of airflow through the vocal tract are associated with stutterers' dysfluencies. Furthermore, the evidence suggests that specific aspects of respiratory and laryngeal function may be amenable to modification by providing clients with biofeedback of kinematic (i.e., respiratory and laryngeal) and aerodynamic signals. For example, clinical targets that may be achieved through biofeedback of kinematic and aerodynamic signals include the following:

1. Adequate respiratory inflation before attempted speech onset
2. Maintenance of a smooth expiratory gesture during speech production
3. Appropriate organization of laryngeal opening and closing gestures with respiratory inspiration and expiration gestures
4. Appropriate levels of vocal fold resistance (i.e., stiffness)
5. Phonetically appropriate patterns of airflow through the vocal tract

CLINICAL APPLICATIONS: ADVANTAGES AND DISADVANTAGES

The next step in the development of a rationale for therapeutic application of noninvasive instrumentation is to consider advantages and disadvantages of an instrumented biofeedback approach as an adjunct to traditional approaches. The important consideration here is adjunct. We do not advocate replacing current therapy techniques with a purely instrumented approach. Instead, instrumentation provides additional information that can facilitate development of therapy goals and implementation of therapy procedures. Advantages of an instrumented approach include objectivity, quantifiability, real-time visual feedback, and long-term data storage. Disadvantages include the obvious expense of the instrumentation (monitoring, display, and storage devices), possible generalization difficulties, and clients' possible negative reactions to the instrumentation.

Objectivity and quantification are valuable in identification and treatment of deficits associated with any speech disorder. The ability to identify salient characteristics of physiologic deficits in particular should aid in focusing therapeutic efforts to match deficits presented by the client. For example, Watson (1983) found that delays in voice onset for a group of stutterers were associated with two different patterns of respiratory-laryngeal organization. The first pattern was characterized by significant delays between the moment of vocal fold closure and the onset of respiratory compression gestures. The second pattern was characterized by significant delays between the onset of compression gestures and the moment of vocal fold closure. Idiosyncratic differences in temporal sequencing of prephonatory respiratory and laryngeal events may be important in developing appropriate therapeutic strategies. While therapy emphasizing easy voice onset (i.e., onset of exhalation before the moment of vocal fold closure) may be appropriate for a stutterer who demonstrates the first pattern described above, this approach may not be appropriate for a stutterer who demonstrates the second pattern. Instead, this client may benefit from therapy designed to minimize the delay between onset of respiratory compression (i.e., exhalation) and the moment of vocal fold closure.

Apart from the ability to clearly characterize physiologic deficits contributing to an individual's stuttering behavior, quantification of deficits has practical benefits for both clinician and client. In the current atmosphere of increased demands for accountability in health care professions, documentation of both baseline abnormality and changes over time is important in establishing a clear strategy and goals for therapy and in documenting benefits of therapy.

Real-time visual feedback of kinematic signals is advantageous for other reasons. First, clients can more clearly appreciate the nature of physiologic disruptions and what steps can be taken in therapy to minimize their impact on speech production. This appreciation can increase motivation. Second, the process of minimizing these disruptions is facilitated because both client and clinician receive immediate feedback regarding the success of attempted strategies. Immediate feedback assists the clinician in tailoring therapy strategies and assessing their viability. Immediate feedback assists the client in mastering these strategies and incorporating them into a new pattern of speech production.

Advantages of long-term data storage parallel those of quantification. The ability to maintain records of baseline measures and periodic assessments of progress during therapy is important in meeting demands for accountability and for providing clients with a tangible chronology of their progress. In addition, periodic review of these data may aid clinicians in identifying the strategies most successful in facilitating improvement in a subgroup of clients. This process will in turn assist in the development of more efficient and effective treatment programs.

Potential limitations associated with clinical application of instrumentation arise from the interaction of client with equipment. For example, Borden and Watson (1987), in their discussion of laboratory use of instrumentation, noted that attaching monitoring devices to subjects seems to produce a decline in the frequency and severity of stuttering behaviors. That is, there is a novelty effect associated with the instrumentation. Clients who experience this effect may not produce stuttering behaviors. As a consequence, certain subtle physiologic deficits may not be identified. However, repeated experience with the instrumentation will lessen the novelty effect. Indeed the novelty effect can be used to great advantage to document physiologic events associated with this "artificial fluency."

The following discussion describes noninvasive instrumentation currently used in many speech science laboratories. These devices may be effectively integrated into a biofeedback therapy program designed to address the aspects of respiratory and laryngeal function described above.

RESPIRATORY MONITORING

With respect to respiratory kinematics, research and clinical observations suggest that stutterers may benefit from feedback regarding coordination of thoracic and abdominal movements during inspiration and expiration as well as coordination between movements of the respiratory and laryngeal systems.

Respiratory kinematics can be evaluated by monitoring changes in the chest wall in several dimensions. For example, Hixon, Goldman, and Mead (1973) describe a magnetometer system for monitoring changes in rib cage diameter and in abdominal diameter. Baken (1977) describes a mercury strain-gauge system for monitoring changes in the anterior hemicircumference of the thorax and abdomen. Finally, Cohn, Watson, Weisshaut, Stott, and Sackner (1975) describe an inductance-coil plethysmograph system (Respitrace) for monitoring changes in the total circumference of the rib cage and abdomen. Although differing with respect to specific principles of operation, all three systems provide information regarding coordination between the thoracic and abdominal cavities. All three systems can also be calibrated to reveal changes in relative or absolute lung volume.

LARYNGEAL MONITORING

The above review of laryngeal behavior associated with stuttering suggests that certain stutterers may benefit from increased control over several aspects of vocal fold vibration as well as coordination of laryngeal and respiratory movements. Noninvasive monitoring of vocal fold activity may be achieved using electroglottography (for a comprehensive review of electroglottography, see Childers and Krishnamurthy, 1985). An electroglottograph (EGG) is sensitive to changes in vocal fold contact area. Briefly, this device detects changes in resistance to a high-frequency, low-amplitude signal transmitted between surface electrodes attached superficially to the laminae of the thyroid cartilage (Baken, 1987). Increased vocal fold contact decreases resistance while decreased contact increases resistance.

Resistance changes detected by the EGG may reflect relatively slow articulatory adjustments of the vocal folds (i.e., abduction and adduction) or rapid changes in contact area during each cycle of vibration. Most commercially available EGG devices provide separate output of both a slow signal (associated with postural adjustments) and a fast signal (associated with vibratory details). However, caution must be used in inferring abductory and adductory vocal fold movements since the slow signal is affected by changes in structures remote from the glottis (e.g., jaw movements or tension in strap muscles) as well as vertical displacement of the larynx. For this reason, the most widely accepted use of EGG is to infer vibratory characteristics of the vocal folds.

Baken (1987) summarizes the primary threats to the validity of the EGG signal. In general, many of these threats are reduced if the electrodes are secured in place at the level of the vocal folds and head movements are kept to a minimum. An additional method of minimizing movement artifacts in the fast EGG signal is to route the EGG output signal through a highpass filter. This eliminates low-frequency components associated with head movements, contraction of strap muscles, and abduction-adduction movements.

AERODYNAMIC MONITORING

In addition to monitoring respiratory and laryngeal kinematics, treatment of dysfluencies may be aided by use of aerodynamic measures. Airflow is monitored by channeling the expiratory airstream through a flow transducer coupled to a face mask (Baken, 1987). When respiratory driving pressure is held constant and laryngeal resistance is known, airflow measures can be used to infer the degree of vocal tract constriction. That is, as the degree of constriction increases, aerodynamic resistance increases and airflow decreases. In addition, several transducers (e.g., pneumotachygraph) differentiate between egressive and ingressive airflow (Baken, 1987). Thus an airflow monitoring system may serve as an important supplement to feedback of respiratory kinematic information to document continuity of expiratory airflow during speech.

CLINICAL EXAMPLES

As noted in the Introduction, clinical examples will illustrate the potential value of noninvasive instrumentation in the identification and treatment of patients with two respiratory and laryngeal abnormalities: stuttering and spasmodic dysphonia. These patients share the characteristic of disordered vocal motor control (McCall, 1974). Consequently they are appropriate for illustrating clinical use of respiratory and laryngeal kinematic monitoring devices. Figure 11.2 illustrates the placement of respiratory and laryngeal monitoring devices. In the following examples, respiratory kinematics were transduced using a Respitrace inductance plethysmograph (Ambulatory Monitoring Systems, Inc.). A single inductance coil was placed around the subject's chest wall and provided a gross measure of respiratory system displacement. This is a nonstandard recording procedure. Use of one inductance coil does not permit unambiguous identification of the unique contributions of rib cage and abdominal wall displacements to changes in lung volume during respiration. In many clinical applications, use of separate rib cage and abdominal coils will be more informative. Laryngeal kinematics were transduced using an electroglottograph (Synchrovoice, Inc.). Electroglottographic signals were routed through a highpass filter (Glottal Enterprises, Inc., model LPHP-2A) to eliminate low-frequency artifact. The resulting signal reveals changes in vocal fold contact area during the vibratory cycle.

Identification of Abnormalities

The first example illustrates an application of the EGG signal to identify physiological disruption associated with stuttering. Figure 11.3 shows EGG and acoustic signals recorded from an adult male stutterer during two readings of a short passage. Upward deflection of the EGG signal corresponds to increasing vocal fold contact area, or the closing phase of a vibratory cycle. Downward deflection corresponds to decreas-

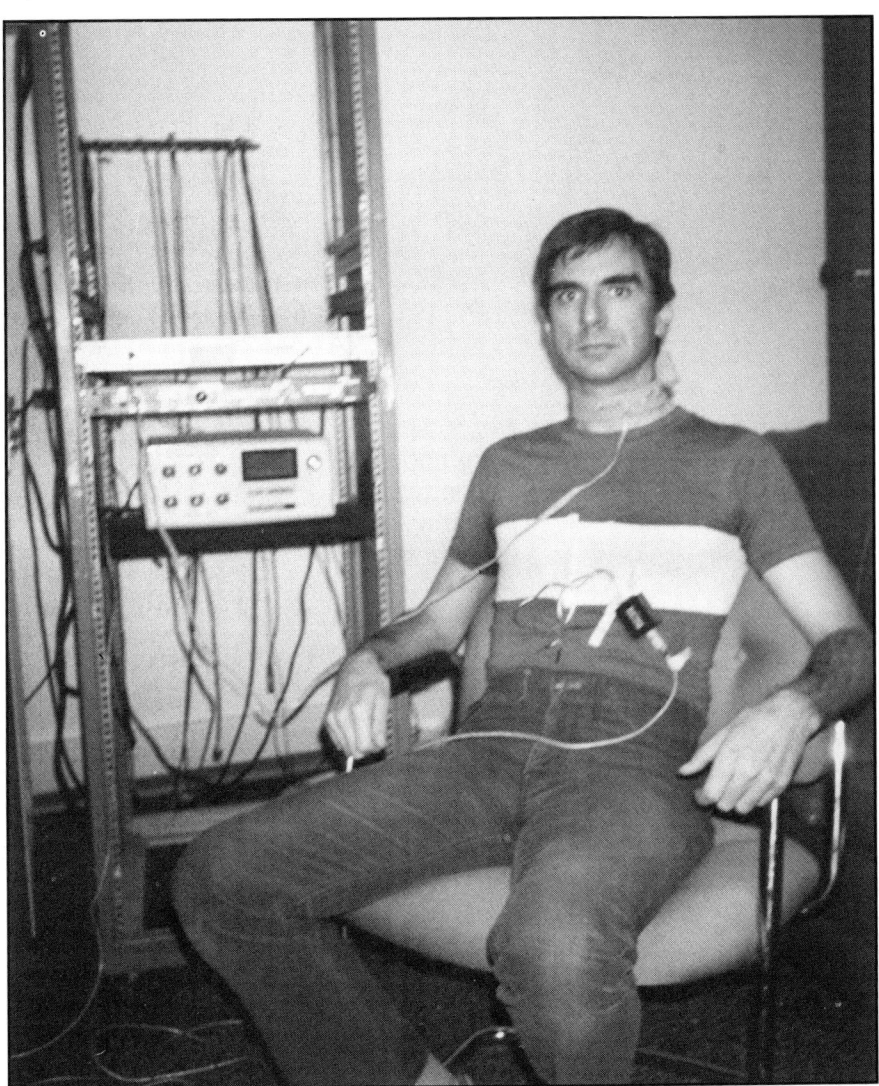

Figure 11.2 Placement of the electroglottograph and a single Respitrace band for clinical applications.

ing vocal fold contact area, or the opening phase of the cycle. Positive peaks in the EGG signal represent the closed phase and negative peaks represent the open phase of a cycle.

The top set of traces was recorded as the subject produced a double-unit repetition of the initial /s/ in "sister." The EGG signal shows no

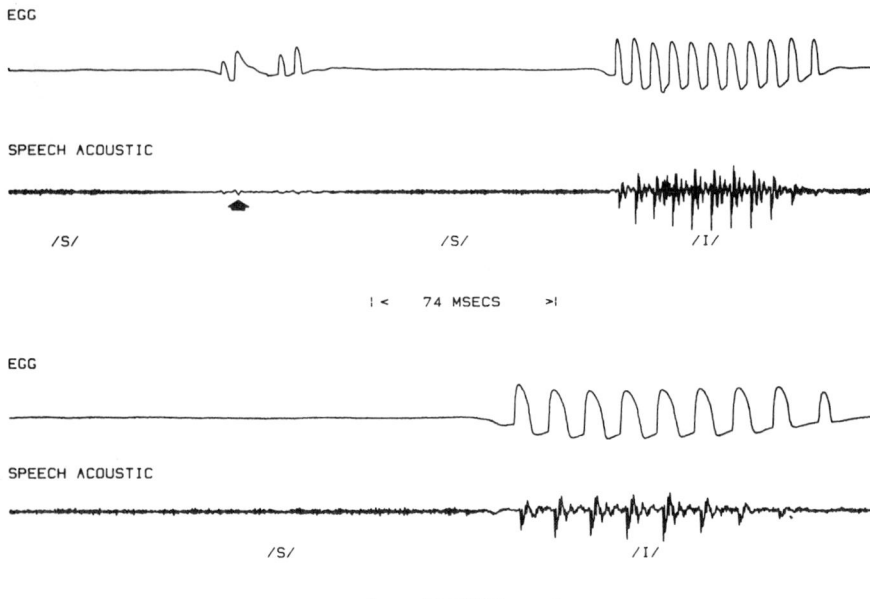

Figure 11.3 Simultaneous electroglottographic and acoustic signals recorded during a stutterer's perceptually dysfluent and fluent productions of the word "sister." EGG signal reveals that repetition of voiceless /s/ in the dysfluent production is associated with inappropriate laryngeal activity.

changes in vocal fold contact area during the initial period of frication seen in the acoustic signal (corresponding to the initial /s/). Next, the EGG signal shows multiple changes in vocal fold contact area that, although appearing as low amplitude pulses in the acoustic signal (indicated by the arrow), are not perceptually evident. Finally, the EGG signal shows no change in vocal fold contact area during production of the second /s/. Perceptually, this was a voiceless repetition. The acoustic signal shows no obvious evidence of voicing during the repetition. The EGG signal, however, shows *multiple changes in vocal fold contact during the dysfluency*. These changes in contact area appear to represent an aborted attempt to initiate voicing. That is, this perceptually voiceless dysfluency is associated with inappropriate laryngeal activity.

The bottom set of traces was recorded during this client's perceptually fluent production of the same material. Note that the EGG signal shows no changes in vocal fold contact area during fluent production of the voiceless /s/. Finally, apparent differences in fundamental frequency for the vowel /I/ in the two acoustic traces reflect the different time scales used in this figure and do not appear to be related to differences in the fluency of these productions.

In this example, the EGG signal permitted identification of an inaudible laryngeal abnormality associated with a voiceless dysfluency. Inappropriate laryngeal activity during voiceless dysfluencies has been documented in laboratory settings through analysis of electromyographic signals (Freeman & Ushijima, 1978) and fiberoptic films (Conture, McCall, & Brewer, 1977). This example illustrates, however, that inappropriately organized laryngeal-articulatory activity can be documented in the clinical setting using noninvasive instrumentation. With this information, therapy can focus on eliminating inappropriate laryngeal gestures by instructing the subject to keep the EGG signal at a "neutral" position during voiceless consonants.

The next example illustrates an application of the Respitrace signal. Figure 11.4 shows speech acoustic and Respitrace signals recorded from a stutterer during production of a multiunit syllable repetition. Upward deflection of the Respitrace signal corresponds to expansion of the respiratory system; downward deflection corresponds to compression. The dashed line shows the shape of the predicted, normal respiratory compression gesture for this utterance. In this example, the dysfluency is associated with a disruption in the normal continuity of the compression gesture. Specifically, each repetition unit is preceded by expansion of the chest wall. These cyclic expansion gestures interrupt the compression gesture. Identification of this abnormality motivates implementation of therapy procedures designed to increase the continuity of expiratory gestures during speech. This may provide a foundation for improved fluency.

The preceding examples show that certain characteristics of the physiologic disruption associated with a stutterer's dysfluency can be identified when noninvasive, kinematic instrumentation is used in conjunction with traditional acoustic recordings. These examples also illustrate that much of the clinically valuable information associated with dysfluencies may occur during silent periods. That is, kinematic records can be important in obtaining sufficiently detailed descriptions of dysfluent speech for design of appropriate therapy goals.

Treatment

The next example illustrates a therapeutic application of the EGG signal. Figure 11.5 shows acoustic and EGG signals recorded as a stutterer attempted to use continuous voicing. The top set of traces illustrates an unsuccessful attempt. Note the clear discontinuity in the EGG signal. The bottom set of traces shows a successful attempt. Here the EGG signal and voicing, as indicated in the acoustic signal by continuation of the vertical pulses (waveform), are continuous. This figure also illustrates the advantage of using EGG signals as evidence of continuous

SPEECH ACOUSTIC

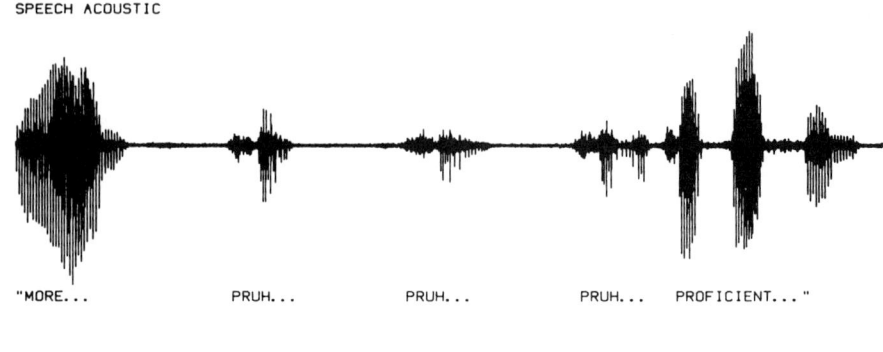

CHEST WALL DISPLACEMENT

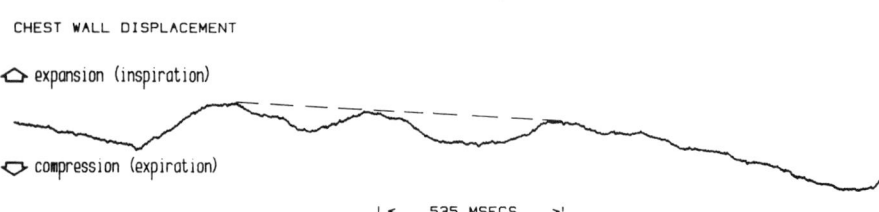

Figure 11.4 Simultaneous Respitrace and acoustic signals recorded during a stutterer's perceptually dysfluent production of the word "production." The dashed line indicates the predicted normal respiratory pattern. Repetitions are associated with inspiratory chest wall gestures that interrupt exhalation.

voicing. Specifically, amplitude of the acoustic signal is markedly reduced during the period of oral closure for /n/ in /man/. The EGG signal, however, displays a constant amplitude, since it is not subjected to damping properties of the vocal tract. Consequently the EGG signal provides a more stable and reliable index of the activity of the vocal folds than does the acoustic signal.

This example also illustrates a procedural issue regarding visual feedback of kinematic signals. At issue is the duration of the window over which immediate feedback is provided. The temporal window in Figure 11.5 is 500 msec. This window is too long to provide meaningful feedback to the client. That is, too much information is presented. Figure 11.6 shows the effect of decreasing the duration of the window. A portion of the EGG signal shown in the top half of Figure 11.5 is repeated here in a 100 msec window. The discontinuity in vocal fold vibration is more pronounced when shown in this shorter window. Clients report little difficulty monitoring the EGG signal when the window is relatively short (i.e., 50–100 msec). However, longer windows (i.e., 2–5 sec) are useful in providing clearer feedback of the slower-moving respiratory kinematic signal.

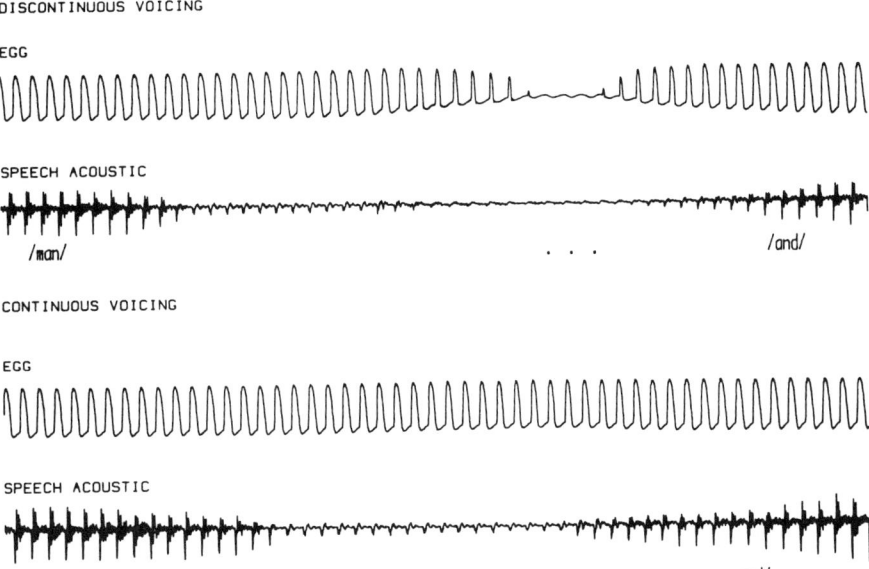

Figure 11.5 Simultaneous electroglottographic and acoustic signals recorded during a stutterer's unsuccessful (top) and successful (bottom) attempts to produce an all-voiced passage using continuous phonation. Note the obvious discontinuity in the EGG signal during the unsuccessful attempt.

The final example illustrates use of EGG signals to document change as a function of therapy and the applicability of noninvasive instrumentation in assessing and treating a variety of motor speech disorders. Figure 11.7 shows pre- and post-therapy recordings of acoustic and EGG signals recorded from a client with spasmodic dysphonia. Both sets of tracings show this client's attempts to initiate the isolated, voiced vowel /a/. Pretherapy tracings, shown in the top half of the figure, reveal multiple interruptions in the attempt to initiate voicing. Note that the initial, aborted attempt is associated with a short rise-time in the EGG signal. Rise-time refers to the interval between onset of the acoustic signal and the point of maximum signal amplitude. This pattern is consistent with high levels of medial compression likely to be associated with the laryngospasm.

A brief trial therapy was conducted to (1) identify and stabilize an optimal vocal pitch, and (2) establish soft voice onsets. Therapy procedures involved visual feedback of acoustic and EGG signals using a Visi-Pitch (Kay Elemetrics) installed on a personal computer. Optimal pitch was stabilized by instructing the client to either increase or decrease

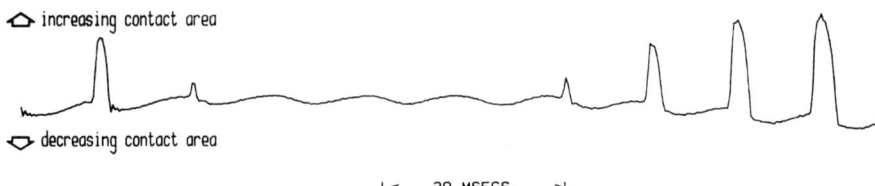

Figure 11.6 Expanded version of the discontinuity in the EGG signal shown in Figure 11.5. The shorter time window shown here facilitates client use of visual feedback of the EGG signal.

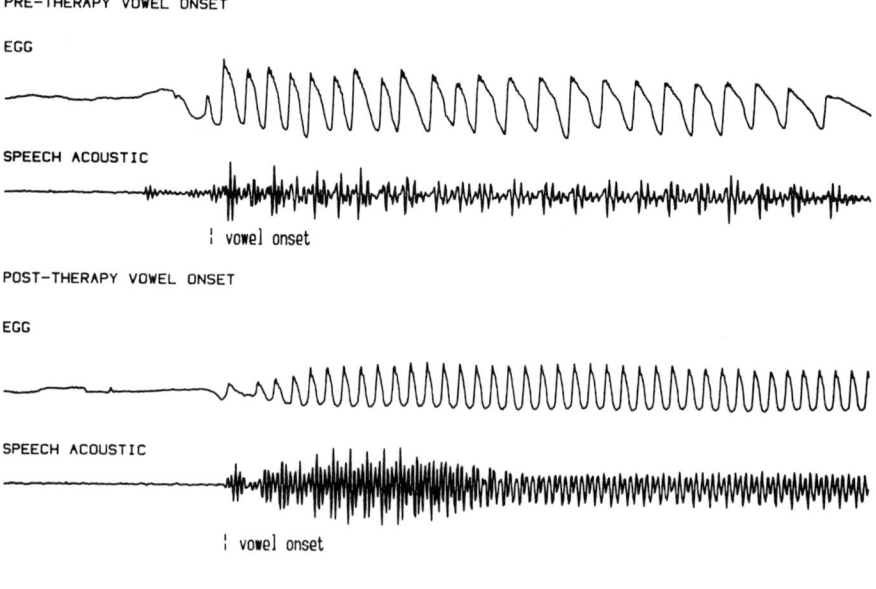

Figure 11.7 Simultaneous electroglottographic and acoustic signals recorded during pre- and posttherapy attempts by a patient with spasmodic dysphonia to initiate an isolated voiced vowel. Pretherapy EGG signal shows abrupt amplitude rise-time and asymmetrical pattern of changes in vocal fold contact. Posttherapy EGG signal shows more gradual amplitude rise-time and more symmetrical pattern of changes in vocal fold contact.

the number of cycles of vocal fold vibration (as shown in the EGG waveform) displayed on the Visi-Pitch screen. A slightly breathy vocal quality was established and stabilized by instructing the client to increase the duration of the open phase of the vibratory cycle as revealed in the EGG signal. Finally, soft voice onset was trained by instructing the client to increase the rise-time of the amplitude envelope of the acoustic signal (i.e., the interval from onset of the acoustic signal to maximum amplitude).

After one 20-min therapy session, the client produced the vowel onset shown in the bottom half of Figure 11.7. Note that voicing was initiated without interruption. Also note the gradual rise in the overall amplitude of the EGG signal. Finally, note the increased consistency in the shape of the EGG waveform. Gradual rise-time of the posttherapy acoustic signal suggests that the client was using a softer mode of vocal attack. Greater periodicity of vocal fold vibration is also evident in the EGG signal. In sum, this example illustrates an application of laryngeal kinematic information in documenting change in vocal control as a direct result of therapy. In addition, therapy techniques used to produce the documented change relied heavily on visual feedback of information obtained using noninvasive kinematic instrumentation.

SUMMARY AND CONCLUSIONS

We have presented a rationale for incorporating noninvasive kinematic and aerodynamic instrumentation in the clinical setting to facilitate identification and treatment of deficits associated with disordered speech motor control. Several examples illustrated the potential benefits of this approach. To date, we have used visual feedback from noninvasive instrumentation, particularly the EGG signal, to treat vocal symptoms associated with stuttering, spasmodic dysphonia, and head trauma.

Our observations and clients' comments support the potential value of clinical applications of this instrumentation. For example, insights gained into the nature of physiologic events associated with perceptual symptoms facilitate the development of relevant therapeutic goals. Realization of therapy goals is also facilitated. Clients can "see" the underlying abnormal physiological gesture and the correct physiological gesture. This information helps clients to understand the rationale for therapy techniques. Finally, the visual display can be explained to clients at different levels of cognitive complexity. For example, simple descriptions of shapes and patterns may be appropriate for many children and cognitively impaired adults, while more complex descriptions of the physiologic mechanism(s) producing the display may be appropriate for other clients. We have successfully applied this approach with a cognitively impaired, post-head-trauma patient and believe programs can be developed for young children.

Finally, clinical application of noninvasive instrumentation will facilitate an exchange of ideas and information between clinics and laboratories. Often the most interesting and rewarding research has its origins in clinical observations. Increasing the precision and sensitivity of these observations will no doubt generate important research questions. On the other hand, clinicians often correctly question the clinical applicability of laboratory findings. A shared technology between clinic and laboratory can facilitate the transfer of laboratory findings to clinical efforts. In the final analysis, more meaningful interaction between clinic and laboratory permitted by a shared technology will benefit client, clinician, and researcher.

REFERENCES

Adams, M. R., & Hayden, P. (1976). The ability of stutterers and normal speakers to initiate and terminate phonation during production of an isolated vowel. *Journal of Speech and Hearing Research, 19,* 290–296.

Adams, M. R., Riemenschneider, S., Metz, D., & Conture, E. (1975). Voice onset and articulatory constriction requirements in a speech segment and their relation to the amount of stuttering adaptation. *Journal of Fluency Disorders, 1,* 24–31.

Adams, M. R., & Reis, R. (1971). The influence of the onset of phonation on the frequency of stuttering. *Journal of Speech and Hearing Research, 14,* 639–644.

Adams, M. R., & Reis, R. (1974). Influence of the onset of phonation on the frequency of stuttering: A replication and re-evaluation. *Journal of Speech and Hearing Research, 17,* 748–755.

Baken, R. J. (1977). Estimation of lung volume change from torso hemicircumpherences. *Journal of Speech and Hearing Research, 20,* 808–812.

Baken, R. J. (1987). *Clinical measurement of speech and voice.* Austin, TX: PRO-ED.

Borden, G. J., Baer, T., & Kenney, M. K. (1985). Onset of voicing in stuttered and fluent utterances. *Journal of Speech and Hearing Research, 28,* 363–372.

Borden, G. J. & Watson, B. C. (1987). Methodological aspects of simultaneous measurements: Limitations and possibilities. In H. F. M. Peters & W. Hulstijn (Eds.), *Speech motor dynamics in stuttering* (pp. 83–96). New York: Springer-Verlag Press.

Brown, S. (1938). The theoretical importance of certain factors influencing the incidence of stuttering. *Journal of Speech Disorders, 3,* 223–230.

Childers, D. G., & Krishnamurthy, A. K. (1985). A critical review of electroglottography. *CRC Critical Reviews in Biomedical Engineering, 12,* 131–161.

Cohn, M., Watson, H., Weisshaut, R., Stott, F., & Sackner, M. (1975). A transducer for non-invasive monitoring of respiration. In F. Stott, E. Rafferty, P. Sleigh, & L. Gouldring (Eds.), *Proceedings of the Second International Symposium on Ambulatory Monitoring* (pp. 119–128). New York: Academic Press.

Conture, E. G., McCall, G. N., & Brewer, D. W. (1977). Laryngeal behavior during stuttering. *Journal of Speech and Hearing Research, 20,* 661–668.

Cross, D. E., & Luper, H. L. (1979). Voice reaction time of stuttering and nonstuttering children and adults. *Journal of Fluency Disorders, 4,* 59–77.

Cullinen, W. L., & Springer, M. T. (1980). Voice initiation and termination times in stuttering and nonstuttering children. *Journal of Speech and Hearing Research, 23,* 344–360.

Freeman, F. J., & Ushijima, T. (1978). Laryngeal muscle activity during stuttering. *Journal of Speech and Hearing Research, 21,* 533–562.

Gay, T., Hirose, H., Strome, M., & Sawashima, M. (1972). Electromyography of the intrinsic laryngeal muscles during phonation. *Annals of Otolaryngology, 81,* 401–409.

Guitar, B. (1975). Reduction of stuttering frequency using analog electromyographic feedback. *Journal of Speech and Hearing Research, 18,* 672–685.

Hixon, T. J., Goldman, M. D., & Mead, J. (1973). Kinematics of the chest wall during speech production: Volume displacement of the rib cage, abdomen, and lung. *Journal of Speech and Hearing Research, 16,* 78–115.

Hutchinson, J. M. (1974). Aerodynamic patterns of stuttered speech. In L. M. Webster & L. C. Furst (Eds.), *Vocal tract dynamics and dysfluency: Proceedings of the First Annual Hayes Martin Conference on Vocal Tract Dynamics* (pp. 71–123). New York: Speech and Hearing Institute.

Hutchinson, J. M., & Brown, D. (1978). The Adams and Reis observations revisited. *Journal of Fluency Disorders, 3,* 149–154.

Manning, W. H., & Coufal, K. J. (1976). The frequency of dysfluencies during phonatory transitions in stuttered and nonstuttered speech. *Journal of Communication Disorders, 9,* 75–81.

McCall, G. (1974). Spasmodic dysphonia and the stuttering block: Commonalities and possible connections. In L. M. Webster & L. C. Furst (Eds.), *Vocal tract dynamics and dysfluency: Proceedings of the First Annual Hayes Martin Conference on Vocal Tract Dynamics* (pp. 124–151). New York: Speech and Hearing Institute.

Murray, E. (1932). Dysintegration of breathing and eye movements in stutterers during silent reading and reasoning. *Psychological Monographs, 43,* 218–275.

Peters, H. F. M., & Hulstijn, W. (1987). Aerodynamic functions in fluent speech utterances of stutterers and nonstutterers in different speech conditions. In H. F. M. Peters & W. Hulstijn (Eds.), *Speech motor dynamics in stuttering* (pp. 229–244). New York: Springer-Verlag.

Reich, A., Till, J., & Goldsmith, H. (1981). Laryngeal and manual reaction times of stuttering and nonstuttering adults. *Journal of Speech and Hearing Research, 24,* 192–196.

Seth, G. (1934). An experimental study of the control of the mechanism of speech, and in particular of that of respiration, in stuttering subjects. *British Journal of Psychology, 24,* 375–388.

Shapiro, A. (1980). An electromyographic analysis of the fluent and dysfluent utterances of several types of stutterers. *Journal of Fluency Disorders, 5,* 203–231.

Starkweather, C. W., Hirschman, P., & Tannenbaum, R. S. (1976). Latency of vocalization onset: Stutterers vs. nonstutterers. *Journal of Speech and Hearing Research, 19,* 481–492.

Stevens, K. N. (1977). Physics of laryngeal behavior and larynx modes. *Phonetica, 34,* 264–279.

Travis, L. E. (1927). Studies in stuttering. Part 1: Disintegration of the breathing movements during stuttering. *Archives of Neurology and Psychiatry, 18,* 673–690.

van den Berg, J. (1958). Myoelastic-aerodynamic theory of voice production. *Journal of Speech and Hearing Research, 1,* 227–244.

Van Riper, C. (1982). *The nature of stuttering* (2nd ed.). Englewood Cliffs, NJ: Prentice-Hall.

Watson, B. C. (1983). *Simultaneous fiberoptic, transillumination, Respitrace, and acoustic analysis of laryngeal reaction time in stutterers and nonstutterers.* Unpublished doctoral dissertation. University of Connecticut, Storrs.

Watson, B. C., & Alfonso, P. J. (1982). A comparison of LRT and VOT values between stutterers and nonstutterers. *Journal of Fluency Disorders, 7,* 219–241.

Watson, B. C., & Alfonso, P. J. (1983). Foreperiod and stuttering severity effects on acoustic laryngeal reaction time. *Journal of Fluency Disorders, 8,* 183–205.

Watson, B. C., & Alfonso, P. J. (1986, November). *Prephonatory respiratory activity in stutterers and nonstutterers.* Paper presented at the annual convention of the American Speech-Language-Hearing Association, Detroit, MI.

Watson, B. C., & Alfonso, P. J. (1987). Physiological bases of acoustic LRT in nonstutterers, mild stutterers, and severe stutterers. *Journal of Speech and Hearing Research, 30,* 434–447.

Wingate, M. E. (1967). Stuttering as a phonetic transition defect. *Journal of Speech and Hearing Disorders, 34,* 107–108.

Zemlin, W. (1988). *Speech and hearing science: Anatomy and physiology* (3rd ed.). Englewood Cliffs, NJ: Prentice-Hall.

CHAPTER 12

Developmental Apraxia of Speech: Theory and Practice

Thomas P. Marquardt and Harvey M. Sussman

> *Marquardt and Sussman provide a neural dysmorphology theory to account for developmental apraxia of speech and suggest that the model may be helpful in explaining some of the disparate characteristics that have been proposed. They note that differential diagnosis of the disorder is difficult due to overlapping characteristics with phonological disorders and childhood aphasia, and that treatment for the disorder is based on approaches for children with articulation disorders.*
>
> 1. *Why should a theory of neural dysmorphology be employed to account for developmental apraxia of speech? What evidence is available to support this theory?*
> 2. *What group of behavioral characteristics serve as the basis for differential diagnosis of the disorder? Is any single feature sufficient to make the diagnosis?*
> 3. *Describe the range of therapy approaches available for treatment of developmental apraxia of speech. Why must treatment for each child be highly individualized?*

Developmental apraxia of speech (DAS) is defined as a neurologically based disorder in the ability to carry out coordinative movements of the speech production apparatus for articulation in the absence of impaired neuromuscular function. Although the disorder has been defined in similar terms for more than 30 years, there is little harmony in the description in terms of the neurological basis for the observed deficits, the characteristics of the disorder, or the most appropriate assessment and treatment regimens. The lack of harmony arises from two major paradoxes. First, neurological insult and maturational dysfunction are the only proposed etiologies, but studies have not found clear evidence of neurological deficits. Evidence for a neurological basis then rests on behavioral symptomatology and the argument for brain dysfunction becomes tautological: developmental apraxia is ascribed to neurological origins on the basis of apractic symptoms, which in turn are assigned to the brain dysfunction. Obviously, there will be little advance in our understanding of the disorder without a coherent neurological construct to account for the disorder. This will be one of our tasks in this chapter.

A second but less compelling paradox is the apparent lack of unique characteristics of the disorder. If there are no unique characteristics or valued treatment regimens specific to the disorder, then it can be argued that classification of children with DAS lacks diagnostic legitimacy (Guyette & Diedrich, 1981). This appears to be more a question of definition than of fact. It has long been a practice in classifying neurological disorders to assign the disorders to categories on the basis of the relative prominence of disordered behaviors such as naming, fluency, or agrammatism. No effort is made to search for behaviors that can be found only in a single type of aphasia or dysarthria. For example, adults with anterior left hemisphere damage typically have reduced fluency, but this feature is also common to global aphasia. The disorders are uniquely assigned to categories on the basis of additional criteria such as the relative involvement of auditory comprehension, naming, and so on. This framework for classification, although helpful in setting apart a group of children with similar features, also brings with it nomenclature problems as major as those observed in adult aphasia, because the group of symptoms used for classification has not been consistently applied. It is not surprising then that the disorder we are discussing has variously been labeled developmental verbal dyspraxia, childhood verbal dyspraxia, apraxic dysarthria, cortical dysarthria, and developmental apraxia of speech. A second task therefore will be to outline as carefully as possible the primary features of developmental apraxia and assessment procedures we view as requirements for reliable diagnosis.

Perhaps one of the most striking proposed features of DAS is the lack of progress in treatment. It is an unfortunate observation relative to the disorder, because the effect of therapeutic success is to negate the diagnosis. Given the lack of neurological evidence to cement an etiology, the inconsistency of selection criteria for diagnostic assignment, and the expected lack of progress, the large variation in approaches to treatment is fully expectable. Our task will be to review and evaluate the relative merits of these regimens, not because we are able to calibrate fully their worth but because their relative effectiveness is a necessary prerequisite to the selection of an approach. As part of our discussion of treatment, we will provide a case study to exemplify the diversity of therapy approaches for children with DAS.

Etiology

An implicit assumption in DAS is that the disorder is the result of brain dysfunction. Two not necessarily mutually exclusive forms of nervous system deficit may underlie the disorder. First, there may be diffuse or focal brain damage arising from birth trauma or nervous system pathology incurred early in life. Evidence supportive of this etiology is neural imaging data and historical reports of head trauma accompanied by neurological examination findings. A second possible etiology is a disturbance in normal neurological maturation—perhaps specific to cortical areas responsible for speech and language functions. Supportive data for this etiology are features similar to the first proposed etiology but with no history of head trauma or neurologically based disorders (e.g., cerebral palsy). Three studies of DAS will be examined to evaluate these observations.

Rosenbek and Wertz (1972) studied 50 children with DAS selected on the basis of diagnosis by a neurologist and a speech-language pathologist. No other exclusionary criteria were employed. Neurological examinations for 22 of 36 children from the group were normal with the exception of apraxia; the remaining 14 subjects demonstrated apraxia with associated neurological deficits including muscle weakness, hyperreflexia, spasticity, and hyperkinesis. EEG findings for 15 of 26 children were abnormal with cases of focal and generalized disturbance of the right or left hemispheres or both. Although it cannot be determined from the report what percentage of the children with abnormal EEG findings demonstrated neurological deficits in addition to apraxia, the data can be interpreted as indicating normal EEG results in at least 42% of the children and normal neurological examinations in 61% of the subjects with the exception of apraxia. Data from neural imaging might have increased the number of children diagnosed as having specific brain damage, but the exclusion of children with associated deficits consistent with cerebral palsy or other disorders would have left approximately half of the children with apraxia as the only definitive evidence of nervous system pathology.

Horwitz (1984) investigated 10 children with apraxia who did not have a history of perinatal hypoxia or acquired neurological disease. Diagnosis of apraxia was based on examinations by a pediatric neurologist and a speech-language pathologist following administration of a battery of tests. Results of the neurological examination, an EEG, a CT scan, and amino acid studies were reported. Eight of 10 subjects had abnormal neurological examination findings, but for 4 of the children the findings were restricted to ocular function. Nine of 10 EEG records were normal with the exception being that of a child with a nonverbal intelligence quotient below 80 who subsequently developed seizures. Similarly, 7 of 9 CT scans were normal with the 2 abnormal scans showing ventricular or cistern enlargement, and all 7 of the amino acids studies performed were normal. Horwitz observed that the study "failed to demonstrate consistent neurological findings or a specific localizing anatomical basis for the clinical manifestation of [DAS]" and that "the underlying nervous system abnormalities remain undefined" (pp. 116–117). He concluded by observing that the speech problem might represent a functionally circumscribed component of a larger brain dysfunction not likely to be attributable to isolated biochemical or neurotransmitter defects.

Yoss and Darley (1974a) studied 30 children with moderate to severe articulation disorders excluding those with an apparent organic basis. Dividing the group in two at the median of scores from a task of isolated volitional movements yielded a subgroup with characteristics indicative of developmental apraxia of speech. Fifteen of the 16 children of this apraxic subgroup demonstrated soft neurological signs such as difficulty with gait and coordination; only 4 of the 14 children from the residual subgroup showed neurological signs. The authors concluded that the neurological findings of the apraxic children were not ascribable to pathological dysfunction of the central nervous system but instead were consistent with developmental immaturity.

We have undertaken this brief review of three DAS studies because they point out an obvious fact about the neurological basis of DAS. Groups of children selected according to widely differing DAS criteria each include a large percentage who have no clear-cut evidence of specific neurological impairment. In fact, Williams, Ingham, and Rosenthal (1981), in a partial replication of the Yoss and Darley (1974a) study, found that their two groups of articulation-impaired subjects were not differentiated on the basis of neurological ratings. We would not argue that brain damage in children does not produce significant deficits in speech production, since it has been shown (Vargha-Khadem, Watters, & O'Gorman, 1985) that severe bilateral frontal pathology incurred at an early age produces profound speech programming disorders that preclude the development of intelligible speech and that are not mediated by structurally intact cortical regions outside the speech zones. Clearly, however, a hypothesis of specific brain damage as the etiological basis for DAS is insufficient for many children with the disorder. Following a review of the primary characteristics of DAS, we will propose a specific neurobiological hypothesis for etiologies typically encompassed under the rubric of neurological immaturity.

Characteristics

The complex of symptoms indicative of DAS is not universally agreed upon and includes nonspeech as well as speech characteristics. Guyette and Diedrich (1981), in a major review of the literature, concluded that there was little agreement on the behaviors or symptoms necessary and sufficient for diagnosis of DAS, that there was little empirical evidence to support conclusions even when agreement was found, and that there was no precise description of how these data could be used as diagnostic indicators. However, it is possible to provide the major characteristics identified from studies of children assigned the DAS diagnostic label. Later we will deal with the issue of assessment and diagnostic classification.

Speech. A key feature of DAS is a severe articulation deficit characterized by a restricted phonemic repertoire (Chappell, 1973; Edwards, 1973); speech sounds are limited to those that occur early in development and that contain simple combinations of distinctive features. Crary (1984b), for example, found that the DAS children of his study consistently scored 2 standard deviations below their age level on the *Templin-Darley Screening Test of Articulation* (Templin & Darley, 1969). Plosives and nasals are observed, but there is an absence of fricatives and affricates. There is a predominance of omission errors (Rosenbek & Wertz, 1972), and vowel errors are observed that are not seen in children with functional articulation deficits (Rosenbek & Wertz, 1972; Smartt, LaLance, Gray, & Hibbett, 1976). DAS children demonstrate metathetic, perseverative, and anticipatory assimilative errors (Smartt et al., 1976) that may be related to the sequencing of sound elements and to reductions in the complexity of word shapes. In the children we have studied, there appears to be a significant reduction in word shapes with a predominant use of CV, CVC, CVCV, and VC forms. Although not fully explored, restricted use of canonical forms is an expected finding in a child with difficulty in the sequencing of articulatory movements. In a phonological process study of imitative and spontaneous speech, Crary (1984b) found that the most frequent errors included omissions, cluster simplification, prevocalic voicing, and metathetic and assimilation errors.

Speech production deficits are most obvious in longer units of speech output. Initiation of utterances is difficult and speech may be accompanied by articulatory groping in the form of sound prolongations, repetitions, or silent posturings preceding or interrupting imitative utterances (Chappell, 1984). Increases in output length are accompanied by increases in errors and reductions in intelligibility, and these children demonstrate difficulty in the production of syllables on diadochokinetic tasks (Nicolosi, Harryman, & Kresheck, 1978).

Rosenbek, Hansen, Baughman, and Lemme (1974) suggested that the errors of DAS children are inconsistent. Inconsistency in terms of speech sound production errors needs to be defined. One would expect to observe variations in speech sound production as a function of phonetic context or length. The increased performance demands associated with particular phonetic contexts and expanded length of the phrase to be repeated or produced have the effect of increasing the difficulty of the task. Inconsistency might better be evaluated by examining repeated production of the same items. Figure 12.1 shows the mean percentage of errors produced by a DAS child on three productions of three 10-item word lists made up of CVC, disyllabic, and polysyllabic words, respectively. Errors were computed as a percentage of total occurrence of the speech sounds on the lists. It is obvious that the effect of increasing length was to produce an increase in the mean percentage of omissions and a corresponding decrease in the frequency of substitution errors. More important, however, is the finding (Figure 12.2) that in repeated productions of the same words, there is a higher frequency of productions changed from correct to incorrect than from incorrect to correct. Clearly, speech sound productions of these children are inconsistent when the effects of both length and context are removed. This finding is not in agreement with the results of a study by Bowman, Parsons, and Morris (1984) who reevaluated the data on children of the Williams et al. (1981) study. Based on an analysis of phonological process rankings, Bowman and colleagues found that children with DAS use consistent types and frequency of phonological processes in the production of spontaneous speech, restricted spontaneous speech, and imitation of specific words from a restricted speech sample. We would suggest that repeated productions of the same words and phrases are a more sensitive indication of consistency than phonological process rankings.

Prosody. There are no experimental data on prosody in DAS and it is not possible to determine at this point whether observed prosodic disturbances are an intrinsic part of the disorder or a compensatory strategy employed in response to motor programming problems. McClumpha and Logue (1972) observed an increase in prosodic disturbances with increasing utterance length, noting longer than normal segmental duration,

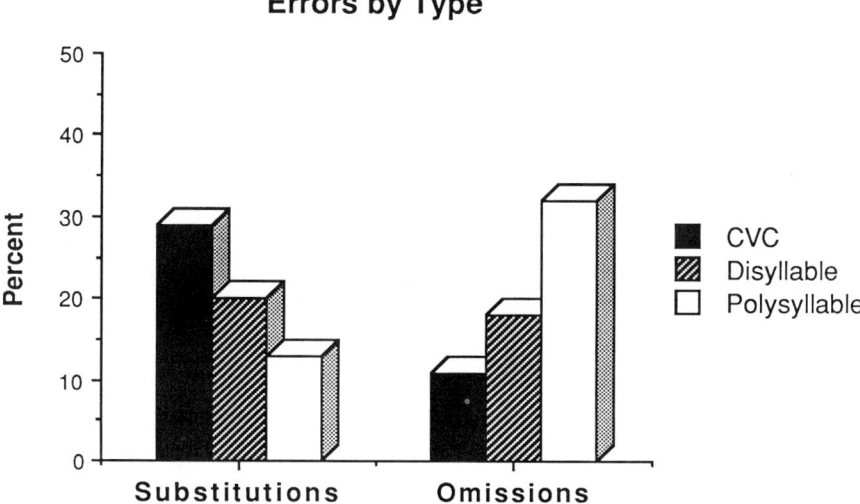

Figure 12.1 Mean percentage of errors for CVC, disyllable, and polysyllable word productions by DAS child.

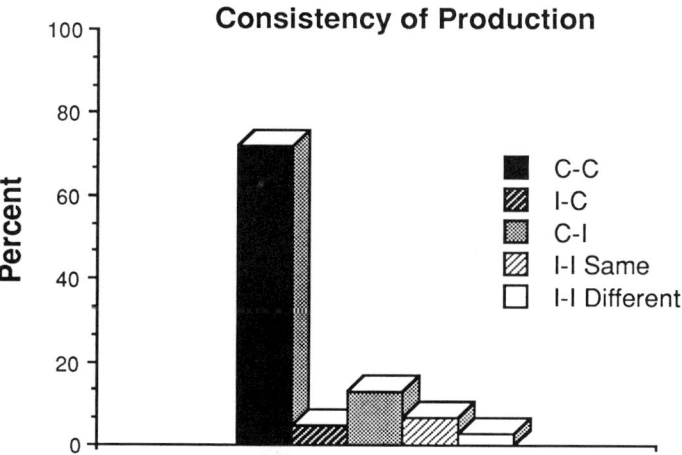

Figure 12.2 Consistency of speech sound production by a DAS child. *C*, correct; *I*, incorrect.

unsteady pitch, and reduced sound blending. Yoss and Darley (1974a) described an overall reduction in speech rate and a monotony of stress patterning, particularly for older children.

In DAS there is an increase in speech sound errors with increases in length. A higher incidence of errors coupled with syllable omissions and transpositions have the cumulative effect of altering the intonational contour of the child's utterance. Durational lengthening, monotony of stress, and lack of speech sound blending can be explained as attempts to compensate for severe speech production problems.

Volitional nonspeech movements. Children with DAS demonstrate impaired ability to produce volitional movements of the speech production structures for nonverbal tasks such as rounding and retraction of the lips and protrusion of the tongue (Rosenbek & Wertz, 1972). Vegetative activities such as chewing and swallowing, in contrast, are unimpaired. This feature of DAS is viewed as so pervasive by some investigators (Smartt et al., 1976; Yoss & Darley, 1974a) that impaired ability to volitionally program nonspeech movements has been a primary selection criterion for subjects. This finding, however, is not universal, and Court and Harris (1965) and Morely and Fox (1969) found normal volitional oral movements in some DAS children.

There are few data relative to volitional programming of limb movement in DAS children. Gubbay, Ellis, Walton, and Court (1965) noted fine coordination problems in their sample of children, and Logue and McClumpha (1970) concluded that DAS children may have difficulty in planning sequential movement patterns. Kools and Tweedie (1975), however, did not find a strong relationship within any age interval between articulatory ability and oral and limb praxis in a group of normal children. Similarly Kornse, Manni, Rubenstein, and Graziani (1981) found no significant differences in the manual dexterity of normal and DAS children, although DAS females showed impaired motor skills while the female control group did not. The data at this point are simply insufficient to determine whether programmed movements other than of the speech production apparatus are impaired in DAS children.

Cognition. The incidence of DAS in retarded children appears to be higher than in children with intellectual abilities appropriate for their age. So are a host of other disorders. DAS has been identified in both nonretarded (Yoss & Darley, 1974a) and retarded children (Ferry, Hall, & Hicks, 1975). In terms of qualitative differences in intellectual abilities, Gubbay et al. (1965) and Walton, Ellis, and Court (1962) found verbal IQ scores markedly superior to performance IQ scores. Decreased intellectual functioning does not appear to be a characteristic distinctive to DAS and may not even serve as a valuable selection criterion for subjects.

Language. Children with apraxia frequently present with delayed development of language (Aram, 1979; Edwards, 1973), particularly for expressive skills (Ekelman & Aram, 1983; Crary, 1984a; Bowman et al., 1984). Rosenbek and Wertz (1972) proposed that the delay is characterized by receptive language skills that are superior to expressive skills. Snyder, Marquardt, and Peterson (1977) found significantly higher receptive than expressive scores on the *Northwestern Syntax Screening Test* (Lee, 1971) for DAS children and children with functional articulation disorders but not for normal children.

The effect of a limited repertoire of phonemic elements as found in DAS is the production of language deficits at multiple levels. Bowman et al. (1984) found a significant increase in final consonant deletion in the three-syllable words and spontaneous speech of their subjects. Final consonant deletion appeared to be more sensitive to increased word and sentence complexity and had the effect of producing morphological errors—in effect changing the meaning of a word or an entire utterance. Crary (1984a, 1984b) suggested that syntactic deficits observed in DAS children were, for the most part, a result of phonological (phonemic) limitations. Crary and Towne (1984) viewed DAS as an "asynergistic" disorder in which syntactic and phonological systems do not work together, which causes specific deficits in expressive syntax and phonology rather than simply a delay in expressive language ability. They proposed that syntactic errors are produced by phonological limitations, thus supporting the concept of bottom-up interference in expressive language.

Ekelman and Aram (1983) found that DAS children demonstrated many specific syntactic errors even though mean length of utterance was greater than that associated with Brown's Stage V of syntactic development. Subjects in their study demonstrated difficulty with Stage V and more complex markers, and several subjects had difficulty using Stage II markers. Developmental sentence scores were well below what would be expected for their chronological ages. Phonological limitations could be related to some of the errors observed, such as omission of regular past tense, plural and present progressive markers, and substitutions for irregular past tense. Errors such as omission of "in," incorrect use of regular and irregular third-person-singular markers, omission of articles, incorrect use of contractible and uncontractible copula and auxillary, and errors in constructing yes-no and *wh* questions, however, could not be assigned to phonological deficits. Ekelman and Aram concluded that an expressive syntactic disorder rather than simply a delay in expressive language was characteristic of their subjects.

Neurological dysfunction sufficient to preclude the development of a full complement of phonemic elements would be expected to produce a multilevel language deficit characterized by deficits in phonological, morphological, and syntactic organization. Coupled with these bottom-up language deficits might be other specific grammatical errors secondary to neurological damage or maldevelopment. Results from standardized tests of language would show a more prominent deficit in expression compared to comprehension.

Sensory deficits. Chappell (1973) and Macaluso-Haynes (1978) included orosensory deficits (2-point discrimination, oral sterognosis) as characteristics of DAS. Aram and Horwitz (1983) found significantly reduced auditory-sequencing ability in DAS children on the *Denver Auditory Phoneme Sequencing Test* (Aten, 1979) and the Auditory Sequential subtest of the *Illinois Test of Psycholinguistic Abilities* (Kirk, McCarthy, & Kirk, 1968). However, sensory deficits of this type are common to developmental speech and language disorders and do not appear to be a unique feature of DAS.

Prognosis. Poor treatment effects cannot be viewed fruitfully as a characteristic of DAS from the standpoint of diagnosis, because prognosis is dependent on the appropriateness of the treatment regimen, the competency of the clinician, and the motivation of the child. However, it has been noted (Rosenbek et al., 1974; Yoss & Darley, 1973; Blakeley, 1983) that DAS children have a poor prognosis for improvement even with intensive treatment intervention.

Summary. Both speech and nonspeech characteristics must be used to reach diagnostic decisions regarding DAS. The overlap of features of DAS with childhood aphasia, functional articulation disorders, and mental retardation requires that the relative prominence of deficits in speech, language, cognition, and motor and sensory functioning be used to guide diagnosis of the disorder. There are several potentially salient speech characteristics that may lead to more efficient decision making (e.g., high frequency of vowel errors, inconsistency in repeated production of the same words), but these features must await further study. Following presentation of a neurologically based explanatory construct for understanding DAS, we will return to procedures for differential diagnosis of the disorder.

THEORETICAL FRAMEWORK TO EXPLAIN DEVELOPMENTAL APRAXIA OF SPEECH

A major lacuna in DAS research is a viable neurologically based etiological construct to account for the diverse behavioral symptoms of the disorder. To date, only vague generalizations have been offered in an attempt to come to grips with this elusive disorder. Crary (1984b), for example, explained DAS as a "motor linguistic disorder of the developing phonological system with the underlying etiology being deficits in spatial-temporal control of the speech mechanism" (p. 80). Such output-oriented explanations of DAS fail to capture the wide scope of the disorder and the resultant deficiencies in all aspects of linguistic development. Our position is that the two domains of phonological organization —input segmental representation/categorization and articulatory motor output—do not operate in development in a mutually exclusive fashion. Nor can phonological development be dissociated from morphological and syntactic language components. In our view of the neurogenesis of the phonological component of grammar, perceptually established neural substrates—isomorphic to phonemic units—operate as prerequisites for normal language development. The sine qua non of phonological rule systems for any natural language is the utilization of a finite set of segments (the phonemes) juxtaposed in syllable-bound phonotactic strings to contrast distinctive features that cue meaning. Without the neurological hard-wired establishment of phonemic units, lexical construction would be severely compromised. Anomalous or faulty development of brain areas subserving this function would necessitate learning a language without minimal pairs and thus each lexical item would "phonetically be a Gestalt lacking any systematic physical relation to any other" (Lindblom, MacNeilage, & Studdert-Kennedy, 1988, p. 1). While some form of brain dysfunction is implicitly assumed in DAS, the most likely source appears to lie at a microscopic rather than a gross morphological level (Galaburda, Sherman, Rosen, Aboitiz, & Geschwind, 1985; Cohen, Campbell, Elmore, & Yaghmai, 1988; Jernigan, Tallal, & Bellugi, 1988).

Previous work (Sussman, 1986, 1988) based on applications of the "combination-sensitive" neuron found in the auditory cortex of the moustached bat (Suga, O'Neill, Kujirai, & Manabe, 1983) to language acquisition has provided a speculative model of how normal prototypical segmental and syllabic development might form in the child. Substantive contributions to our understanding of what constitutes the hard-wiring underlying the "innateness notion" can be made if findings from animal neurophysiology, especially in species biologically specialized for hearing, are incorporated into human models of language structure.

Recent case studies utilizing both postmortem microscopic examination of cerebral tissue and magnetic resonance imaging (Cohen, Campbell, Elmore, & Yaghmai, 1988; Jernigan et al., 1988; Plante, 1988) have revealed cortical anomalies thought to underlie the etiology of developmental dysphasia. As stated by Jernigan et al. (1988), "Preliminary studies suggest that specific cerebral subsystems develop in anomalous ways in these children and that anomalies of development are reflected in gross cerebral dysmorphologies" (p. 19). A child forced to operate with impoverished or deficient neural substrates destined, in the normal brain, to derive and signal invariant phonemic categories would be expected to be seriously compromised in all aspects of language function.

DAS is stereotypically regarded as an output speech disorder, even though sensory and language deficits have been reported. Our perspective is that speech perception, speech production, and language will be adversely affected, to some degree, by structurally and operationally deficient neural substrates mediating phonemic identity and categorization. The extent of differential impairment of these interrelated components will not be uniform or linearly predictable, but rather will vary for each individual case. Speech-related motor and sensory processes develop from the very beginning as early infant sounds and babbling are processed. The motor and sensory systems are intricately interwoven throughout language development so that a level of isomorphism or automatism is created between the two. At the very core of a developing language system, there must exist an internal representation of the phonemic units (i.e., "spectrotopically" mapped fields as described in Sussman, 1989) needed to structure the morphological and lexical output units of language structure. Such internal representations must, by necessity, form from sensory input experience. Experimental work in the discrimination of nonnative speech contrasts has shown that an initial discrimination ability declines during ontogeny in the absence of language experience with phonemic contrasts (Werker, Gilbert, Humphrey, & Tees, 1981; Werker & Tees, 1984). Thus there is evidence for selective phonological tuning during the first year of life, from an initially broad sensitivity to any natural language stimulus contrast to specific sounds comprising the phonemic system being acquired by the child.

Our position on the underlying etiology of DAS is that the child may not have the basic perceptual processing and internal representation mechanisms that must concurrently develop with speech motor output skills. Deficits in skilled motor articulations can be viewed as stemming from a deficient internal target representation of phonemic elements that are needed to guide or serve as the phonological intent for the motor output algorithms of speech production. The two do not operate as mutually exclusive domains, nor do they function independently from the grammatical rule systems whose syntactic frames must guide phonetic output.

The proposed speculative theory does not take into account pragmatic assumptions underlying recent psycholinguistic models of language acquisition. Each of these models has at its core, however, the assumption of an innate predisposition for the development of grammar. By focusing on sensory-related language processes, the proposed theory provides a missing, brain-based link enabling the innateness notion to become more meaningful and applicable to developmental language disorders, such as DAS, that lack a lesion-specific etiology.

The theory does not uniquely account for deficits in DAS. The symptom complex of DAS is best viewed, as we noted earlier, by the severity of deficits rather than by characteristics specific to the disorder alone. DAS has been defined in terms of motoric deficits mainly because input perceptual processes, with few exceptions, have not been explored experimentally. In the few instances where input processes have been investigated (Aram & Horwitz, 1983), deficits in auditory processing have been identified. In effect, we would argue that DAS is a subtype of disorders typically subsumed under the rubric of developmental aphasia, a topic we will return to in the section on differential diagnosis.

Rhyming

An experimental paradigm that can effectively assess the productive integrity of a phonological system driven by internal "target" representations is the ability both to generate and to recognize rhyme. Four DAS children, ages 5–7, were compared to age-matched normal controls on four rhyming tasks (Marion, Marquardt, & Sussman, 1988). A comprehensive battery of clinical tests and procedures, including the *Screening Test for Developmental Apraxia of Speech* (Blakeley, 1983), the *Test for Auditory Comprehension of Language* (Carrow-Woolfolk, 1985), the *Peabody Picture Vocabulary Test* (Dunn & Dunn, 1981), and the *Templin-Darley Screening Test of Articulation* (Templin & Darley, 1969) were used to assign children to a DAS group. Subjects were tested on four rhyming tasks; three involved judging the appropriateness of a rhyme, and one involved generating rhyming words from a target word.

Experiment 1: Production of rhyme. Twelve target words were used from which children were asked to generate rhyming words. After each target word was presented, children had 30 sec to produce as many words as they could that they thought rhymed with the referent word (e.g., "pot," "bit," "sad"). Examples of rhyming words were given as practice. The number of correct rhyming words was the dependent variable. The mean number of rhyming words produced by the four normal children was 45 compared to a mean of 2 words by the DAS children. Nonrhyming responses (viz., words that began with the same consonant) constituted the largest type of responses obtained from the DAS children.

Experiment 2: Forced choice rhyming pairs. To assess the child's intuitive grasp and relative ability to judge a rhyme, a forced choice situation was created in which the child was presented with a target word (e.g., "ball") and asked to indicate which of two choices best rhymed with the target (e.g., "bought" or "fall"). Besides legitimate rhymes, six conditions constituting a continuum of partial rhymes were used that allowed us to make a differential analysis of the child's ability to focus on various combinations of CVC foils: agreement on C_1 only, C_2 only, C_1V, VC_2, C_1-C_2, V only. The percentage of correct scores for the normal children ranged from 95% to 100% for all conditions except vowel-only similarities, which produced a 75% correct level. In sharp contrast, the DAS children ranged from 32% to 58%, with a mean correct response level of 44.6%.

Experiment 3: Rhyme memory. One explicit prediction from the neurogenesis of phonology theory is that an impoverished internal representation system of a phonological unit will result in an elusive target storage with which to compare on-line stimuli. In this experiment a target word was pronounced and followed by 10 words, 4 rhymed (agreement in vowel nucleus + final consonant) and 6 did not. The child had to indicate yes or no as each of the 10 foils was produced and to indicate, at the end of the 10-trial block, what the initial target word was. Normal children performed this task almost perfectly with a hit rate of 97%. DAS children had enormous difficulty with the task (hit rate = 55%) with the majority of erroneous responses being false positives in which the similarity was the same initial consonants. Sixteen of the 20 trial blocks were not completed with the DAS children, as they were unable to provide the target word at the end of each set of 10 words. Only 3 (of 20) trial blocks were not completed by the normal subjects.

Experiment 4: Vowel similarity. This task focused on the ability of DAS children to judge acoustic similarity across vowels in a forced choice arrangement. A CVC word with a target vowel was followed by two CVC foils contrasting the medial vowel; one vowel of the choice pair was always closer to the target in vowel distance. The percentage of correct scores was then tabulated. DAS children exhibited gross insensitivity to auditory agreement of vocalic sounds with a mean group score of 35.6% compared to 80% for the normal subjects. Two DAS subjects had scores of 25% and 22.5% correct, which was significantly below chance, and the other two had 55% and 40% correct. The individual scores for the four normal subjects were 80%, 80%, 87.5%, and 72.5% correct.

In sum, the four DAS children studied showed extreme inability to (*a*) recognize proper rhymes, (*b*) maintain a target word representation in short-term auditory memory, (*c*) judge vocalic similarities and dissimilarities, and (*d*) spontaneously generate rhyming words in output. Control subjects matched for age and sex were very capable of performing all the above tasks in almost perfect fashion, indicating they had a well-formed internalized phonological system that could be accessed to provide a comparison with on-line input stimuli.

Though lacking full experimental support, we believe the neurogenesis of phonology theory holds great promise of providing an explanatory construct for the neurobiological bases of DAS. At the moment it provides a guide for further exploration of the disorder, but direct benefits relative to clinical diagnosis and treatment must await further research.

Assessment

The use of a group of prominent speech- and language-related characteristics appears to be the most effective means of reliably assigning a diagnosis of DAS. We will begin by describing the types of test instruments for determining the level of functioning in each of the major characteristic areas and will follow this description with some comments on differential diagnosis. A case study is included to serve as an example of the type of child diagnosed as having DAS.

Screening. There is one screening tool specifically constructed as an aid to establishing a diagnosis of DAS. Data obtained are not sufficient to fully detail important features of DAS or to plan therapy, but it is at least an initial step in selecting children for additional testing. The *Screening Test for Developmental Apraxia of Speech* (Blakeley, 1983) is composed of eight subtests. The subtests investigate the discrepancy between expressive and receptive language ability, production of vowels and diphthongs in words, oral motor movements, production of three-syllable sequences, imitation of multisyllabic motorically complex words, production of words presented three at a time, transpositions in the imitation of words, and prosody in connected speech. Weighted scores are used to determine the likelihood of correct assignment to the diagnostic category of DAS. The Blakeley test is not without theoretical and methodological problems (Guyette & Diedrich, 1983), but it has been shown to reliably differentiate children with DAS from children with functional articulation disorders (Weeks & Madison, 1985).

Additional testing is carried out to explore the most important diagnostic criteria in more detail. A single test seldom will be sufficient in each area of assessment and the instruments selected are conditioned by the age of the child.

Articulation. Tests of articulation are chosen to determine the developmental level of the child, to investigate the frequency and type of speech sound errors, to assess the consistency of production in repeated productions of the same stimuli, and to explore differences in production between single words and connected speech. Typically a norm-based instrument such as the *Templin-Darley Articulation Test* (Templin & Darley, 1969) or the *Goldman-Fristoe Test of Articulation* (Goldman &

Fristoe, 1969) is administered. Items from the test can be elicited several times in sequence to determine consistency. A speech sample should be obtained to establish a phonetic inventory and distribution, to carry out analyses of consonant and vowel errors, phonologic process and phonotactic structure use, prosody, intelligibility, and severity (Shriberg & Kwiatowski, 1980).

Language. Two important purposes are served by administration of language measures: examining whether a discrepancy between receptive and expressive language skills is apparent and obtaining a qualitative description of language use. Qualitative expressive language information such as mean length of utterance, grammatic morphemes used, complex sentence analysis, and structural development is available from the language sample (Miller, 1981). The choice of additional tests will depend on the age of the child. For young children (less than age 4) it may include the *Sequenced Inventory of Communicative Development* (Hedrick, Prather, & Tobin, 1975). Tests that provide expressive and receptive age scores (e.g., *Reynell Developmental Language Scales,* 1977) are particularly helpful for the older child. Regardless of which combination of measures is chosen, the *Peabody Picture Vocabulary Test* (Dunn & Dunn, 1981) will be administered, since it is the recommended test for determining a receptive vocabulary score for use on the *Blakeley Screening Test for Developmental Apraxia.*

Cognition. Multiple areas of functioning are explored in the psychological examination. A potentially important, but by no means necessary, result for use in the diagnosis of DAS is a discrepancy between performance and verbal IQ scores. The *Wechsler Intelligence Scales for Children–Revised* (Wechsler, 1975) provide verbal, performance, and full-scale scores and are perhaps the tests of choice when investigating children of a wide age range. In our experience, DAS children typically demonstrate performance scores at least 10 points higher than verbal scores on tests of intelligence.

Sensory and motor functioning. Audiometric testing is used to rule out hearing loss as a potential etiology for observed symptomatology. Although verbal sequential deficits are not unique to children with apraxia, use of a measure such as the *Denver Auditory Phoneme Sequencing Test* (Aten, 1979) may provide additional information relative to the verbal-sequencing abilities of these children (Aram & Horwitz, 1983). The oral-peripheral examination evaluates the strength, range of motion, and speed of movement of the speech production structures and may be used to determine if a neuromuscular disorder is responsible for observed deficits. Kent, Kent, and Rosenbek (1988) have provided a review of maximum diadochokinetic rates expected for children of different age levels that can serve as a normative reference in examining the reduced rates for DAS children expected as part of this examination. Both verbal and nonverbal diadochokinetic rates should be determined, but there are as yet no mathematically derived criteria for expected performance by DAS children. Additional testing of volitional oral movements can be obtained by administration of the adaptation (Kools, Williams, Vickers, & Caell, 1971) of the DeRenzi, Pieczuro, and Vignolo (1966) measure for adults with apraxia. Fine and gross motor skills also should be examined with age-appropriate assessment tools such as the *Bruininks-Oseretsky Test of Motor Proficiency* (Bruininks, 1978).

Differential diagnosis. Determining whether a child demonstrates DAS is dependent on careful consideration of information obtained from neurologic, psychologic, and communicative assessment. As noted earlier, there is no assurance that the neurologic examination, even when it includes neural imaging, will reveal specific neurologic damage or dysfunction. The examination, however, may provide evidence of related symptoms—for example, limb apraxia, delayed motor development, or a significant history of head injury—that can support a diagnosis of neural dysfunction. Co-occurring neuropathology has been reported with sufficient frequency to warrant routine neurologic referral of DAS children. The psychological examination is important in determining the presence or absence of mental retardation, may allow emotional disorders to be ruled out as a causal basis for observed symptoms, and is important in establishing a possible significant discrepancy between performance and verbal intelligence scores.

Neurological and psychological examinations should rule out neuromuscular disorders, emotional disturbance, and auditory impairment as the basis for observed deficits. Evaluation of communicative functioning should further refine the diagnosis to exclude phonological disorders and childhood aphasia. The typical DAS child will demonstrate auditory language comprehension abilities that are near or within normal limits while expressive language is delayed, which is the key differentiating distinction between DAS and childhood aphasia. Children with aphasia typically will show language impairment in both comprehension and expression. The presence of a reduced repertoire of phonemes, restricted use of word shapes, inconsistency of production with repetition of the same items, reduced volitional oral movement and verbal diadochokinetic rates, prosodic abnormalities, and a very high incidence of omission errors are the key factors or group of symptoms that will allow DAS to be distinguished from phonological disorders. However, it must be remembered that apraxia may be evident in other disorders such as cerebral palsy and mental retardation as well as independently and is best viewed both as a symptom and as a constellation of deficits. We would argue that when the group of symptoms appears independent of other disorders it deserves a diagnostic categorization that we have chosen to call developmental apraxia of speech.

THERAPY

The suggested treatment regimens for DAS are based primarily on approaches developed for children with phonological disorders (see Table 12.1). These approaches are particularly relevant because little is known about the most effective treatment for DAS, both DAS and phonological disorders occur during the emergence of speech and language, and deficits in syntax are frequently observed in both groups.

A major distinction between the two types of disorders is the relatively poor prognosis for improved articulation in DAS. Even when intensive stimulation using tactual, kinesthetic, auditory, and visual modalities is employed in conjunction with facilitating contexts, transfer of correct production to other words and linguistic contexts frequently is difficult. The diversity of symptoms in DAS demands that treatment be eclectically developed. Following a discussion of therapy principles and procedures for DAS, we will review treatment approaches adapted specifically for children with the disorder.

Therapy Principles and Procedures for DAS

There is relatively little documentation of the efficacy of treatment for DAS based on retrospective reviews of progress. Even when this information is available, the diversity of children described makes it difficult to capture the underlying principles of the therapy used. The following discussion, based on a review of therapy for DAS (Marquardt, Dunn, & Davis, 1985), will look at therapy principles from the standpoint of (1) treatment goals, (2) structure of the treatment sessions, (3) sound stimuli, (4) teaching hierarchy, and (5) treatment strategies.

Goals of treatment. Primary problems of children with DAS are the failure to develop normally the full repertoire of phonemes of the language and the inability to produce combinations of sounds for words and sentences of increasing length and complexity. Frequently there is a breakdown between the production of single sounds in isolation and the use of these sounds in longer units of speech output. The primary goals of treatment are to establish the complex, volitional sensorimotor production patterns that the child has failed to develop, as we have noted, because of dysmorphologies of the underlying neural substrates for phonemes.

TABLE 12.1
Therapy Approaches for Phonological and Articulation Disorders

Phonetic Placement (Scripture & Jackson, 1927)	A highly pragmatic technique that utilizes phonetic placement to correct production of phonemes in error by directions for articulatory points of contact, kinesthetic patterns, airstream dynamics, etc.
Moto-kinesthetic Speech Training (Young & Hawk, 1955)	Tactual cues and auditory stimulation are used in conjunction with manual manipulation to elicit correct production of target sounds. For example, in the production of /p/, the clinician places the thumb and forefinger on the jaw and moves it upward to contact the lower and upper lips. The jaw is then quickly brought downward to provide the jaw motion and lip abduction requisite for release of the bilabial plosive.
Traditional Articulation Therapy (Van Riper, 1978)	This approach is characterized by a sequence of activities for identifying the standard sound, discriminating it from its error, varying and correcting productions until they are produced correctly, and stabilizing and strengthening correct production in various contexts and speaking situations.
Multiple Phoneme Approach (McCabe & Bradley, 1975)	A modification of the traditional approach, multiple phoneme therapy addresses several error sounds at the same time. It is recommended for children who exhibit several sound errors that reflect a common underlying pattern.
Sensory-Motor Approach (McDonald, 1964)	This treatment is based on the rationale that improved articulatory performance can be gained by heightening the auditory, tactile, and proprioceptive feedback of motor patterns. The objectives of treatment are to increase responsiveness to motor productions in connected speech, to reinforce correct production of error sounds, and to facilitate correct production of the sound in systematically varied phonetic contexts. Contexts first are investigated to determine which facilitate correct production of the error sound. Stress and rate then are used as transfer mechanisms to elicit correct production in contexts where the sound previously was produced in error.

TABLE 12.1. Continued

Integral Stimulation (Milisen, 1954)	Auditory, visual, and tactile cues are used to evoke correct production of target sounds. This "watch me and listen" imitative instruction is carried through several levels of complexity (e.g., isolation, syllables) beginning at the highest level at which correct production is achieved.
Contextual Facilitation (Kent, 1982)	The underlying rationale is that certain contexts will facilitate correct production of the target sound and that this is the beginning point for production training. Contextual facilitation is a critical feature of sensory motor training.
Contrast Therapy (Costello & Onstine, 1976)	Treatment to address systematic simplifications of sound classes or word structures is the intent of this approach. Minimal word pairs are presented to the child, who is required to produce correctly the target sound. If the child does not, the resulting communicative breakdown due to uncertainty forces the child to become aware of the error and to change the underlying concept. The approach may be effective in helping children to more readily identify the critical elements to be learned.
Paired Stimuli (Irwin & Weston, 1971)	Like McDonald's sensory motor approach, paired stimuli begin with the identification of a context that facilitates correct production of the target sound. The underlying rationale is that pairing the word in which the target is produced correctly (key word) with another word in which the target appears in the same word position has the effect of transferring correct production to the new context.
Successive Approximation (Nemoy & Davis, 1954)	This is a shaping technique in which the child is guided through a series of transitional movements to the correct production of the target sound.
Speech Pattern Remediation (Hodson, 1982)	This treatment approach is predicated on the assumption that a sound may be within the child's repertoire, but is not used correctly. Since phonological processes do not operate at the level of the single sound, the training unit is generally the syllable or word. Other approaches (e.g., contrast ther-

TABLE 12.1. Continued

apy, multiple phoneme approach) may be used within this therapy technique to achieve the goal of developing contrasts in the child's phonological system.

Note. Citations are intended to serve as example sources for obtaining information on the treatment approaches described in the table.

Structure of treatment sessions. Children with DAS appear to improve slowly and only after a great expenditure of time and effort. Yoss and Darley (1973), for example, found that only 1 of 10 children enrolled in therapy had been discharged 12 to 16 months later, and then only after 139 hours of intensive treatment. Intensive, systematic, drill-oriented sessions on a daily basis (Blakeley, 1983; Morely & Fox, 1969) are most successful because they provide practice for the motor patterns of the sounds selected for training.

Stimuli. Children with DAS frequently demonstrate vowel errors. If vowels are not produced accurately, it is recommended that correct production of these speech sounds precede work with consonants (Blakeley, 1983; Chappell, 1973). Chappell (1973) recommended beginning with the vowels /o/, /a/, /i/, and /ae/ because they represent highly contrastive tongue positions. It also is apparent that they are acoustically dissimilar and may be easier for the child to distinguish.

The consonants selected for treatment should be those that occur early in development (Blakeley, 1983) and that are highly visible (Macaluso-Haynes, 1978; Rosenbek et al., 1974; Smartt et al., 1976; Yoss & Darley, 1974b). Chappell (1973), however, recommended that treatment begin using consonants that offer maximal contrasts in terms of point of articulation and pattern of movement (/p/, /t/, /k/, /f/, /s/). His rationale was that these sounds are highly distinguishable and, once established, are available for shaping, modifying, and combining for the production of other consonants.

In summary, the initial point of treatment is the stabilizing of consonants and vowels already in the child's repertoire. Selection of additional targets should be based on choosing sounds that occur early in development, are highly visible, and offer maximal articulatory and acoustic contrasts.

Teaching hierarchy. In the case of the severely impaired child, it may be necessary to begin treatment at the sound level to gain and maintain production of the speech sounds in isolation. The beginning of treatment, however, typically is at a nonsense syllable level using simple CV combinations. Gradually reduplicated CVCV combinations are taught followed by monosyllabic words that are very salient (meaningful) to the child and that contain the sounds taught at the single syllable level. Chappell (1973) suggested that backward chaining be employed to facilitate the transition from isolated sounds to syllables. This technique involves the production of the new sound at the beginning of the syllable. For example, in the word "cat" the child is first requested to produce /t/, then /at/, and finally the entire word "cat." Multisyllabic words are introduced to increase the length and complexity of speech output followed by the production of the trained words in phrases and sentences.

Treatment strategies. Treatment for the DAS child is marked by the cuing strategies used for establishing movement patterns. In working with children with functional articulation problems, the auditory modality is most important for establishing speech sound production. Children with DAS, however, have difficulty learning sensorimotor patterns through auditory cues alone, so visual and tactual inputs must be used as well. Visual cues include visual monitoring in front of a mirror to see articulatory placements and pairing written symbols with the sound. Tactual cues include stimulation of the articulators by application of various textures or pressure and swabbing or probing the lips and tongue at the site of desired contact.

The use of rhythm, stress, and intonation paired with movement patterns has been recommended to facilitate treatment (Rosenbek et al., 1974). For children who can produce phrases and sentences, rhymes and songs are paired with physical movements such as beating time with the hand or squeezing a beanbag for each syllable. Children are urged to slow their rate of speech in order to maintain an even stress pattern, which is necessary for maintaining the sounds in the target sequences.

A major problem in working with DAS children is the retention of movement patterns so that they can be used in longer and more complex contexts. Chappell (1973) recommended that the time used to practice movement patterns be increased so that accuracy can be maintained for the duration of the task. He also suggested that the time between practice of patterns be gradually increased to aid the child in establishing the memory for particular movement sequences. Finally, he recognized the need to develop self-monitoring skills so that the child can identify and correct errors.

Additional considerations in treatment. Several other factors may bear on treatment. Rosenbek and Wertz (1972) recommended that for older children, meaningful words, phrases, and sentences be used as stimuli and that self-monitoring and compensatory strategies (pauses, equal stress on syllables, intrusive schwa in consonant clusters) be taught. Crary (1984b) proposed that differential approaches be used as a function of severity based on the identification of three subgroups of apraxic children. Syllable structure errors were characteristic of the most severely impaired group; sound class errors characterized the middle group; and specific sound errors were the primary feature of the least impaired group. He noted that an increase in sound substitutions corresponded to a decrease in errors related to sequential constraints and syllable shape alterations. This shift occurred not only as a result of the child's replacing omitted segments with substituted phonemes, but also as a result of "grammatical trade-off." By trade-off he meant incorrect production of previously correct segments as other segments previously produced in error are corrected. Accordingly, he opposed sound-by-sound remediation and instead advocated approaches that facilitated correct production of various syllable shapes at the word level, with careful attention paid to performance load (effects on sound sequencing due to increases in length) and grammatical trade-off during intervention. Finally, Ekelman and Aram (1984) documented syntactic deficits in children with DAS and suggested that remediation of syntactic deficits be integrated with therapy procedures directed toward improved motor planning and phonological development.

Summary. Therapy principles for DAS clearly are in keeping with the definition of the disorder as an inability to carry out preplanned speech movements in the absence of neuromuscular impairment. Treatment focuses on the production of individual speech sounds in isolation or in longer units of output depending on the entry-level skills of the child. Intensive, systematic drill is required, because movement sequences are gained only through repeated long-term practice utilizing a maximum of speech-related sensory input. If the underlying basis for the disorder is a failure to develop neural substrates for phonemic representation, however, the future direction of treatment lies as much on input types of remedial procedures as it does on the ability to plan and execute speech movements.

Adapted Therapy Approaches for DAS

Several approaches for treating communication disorders have been adapted for use in DAS. To a large extent they incorporate the therapy principles marked as important to remediation of children with the disorder. Their unique feature is the sequencing of series of tasks within a defined theoretical umbrella.

Prompts for Restructuring Oral Muscular Phonetic Targets (PROMPT). The PROMPT system (Chumpelik, 1984) is constructed to treat DAS as a movement disorder with possible disruptions in planning, sequencing, or executing speech movements. In contrast to other therapy approaches that use imitation or perceptual comparisons, PROMPT imposes a target position or sequence on the child and utilizes a tactile-based method for reshaping articulatory positions and sequences by providing externally applied cues to the face, the chin, structures associated with voicing and nasality, and jaw opening. A different set of prompts is provided for each English phoneme. The timing of the prompts is important in moving from relatively static segments to transitional-coarticulatory movements in phrases and sentences. These transitional effects are facilitated and controlled by the duration of the prompt, the degree of pressure on particular muscle groups, and the tension placed on these muscle groups, and are intended to provide feed-forward information to aid the child in carrying out the preprogrammed sequence as the child is guided toward articulatory targets and transitions. The assumption is that "the system may help provide the lacking and essential kinesthetic feedback (closed-loop) while providing the feed-forward of sequential information (open-loop) that the system needs for transforming conscious motor control into automatic sequences" (p. 152).

The PROMPT system requires that the therapist cue each target or target sequence at a syllable, word, or phrase level. Prompts are strung together in a sequence or administered selectively for specified targets (e.g., final consonants). Timing of prompts for transitive movements and stress is accomplished by altering the duration of individual prompts, the overall speed of combined prompts, and the selection of key prompts over others. Transfer is gained through practice of each phoneme in various contexts.

Touch-Cue Method. This method (Bashir, Grahamjones, & Bostwick, 1984) is an adaptation of cued speech for the deaf and is intended to address phonemic sequencing and patterning deficits in DAS children. Touch cues are the tactile topographic indicators presented in conjunction with auditory and visual cues during initial phases of therapy for consonant sounds. In three discrete stages of treatment, the child progresses from simple CV and CVC syllable shapes to the production of multisyllabic sequences and finally to production of utterances in spontaneous speech. Stage I uses nonsense syllable drill to teach the topographical cues, to improve sequencing, and to develop self-monitoring accuracy. Bashir et al. indicated that it is critical to the success of the program at this stage that the touch cue elicit the articulatory movements represented by the cue and that accurate self-monitoring of production be established. Stage II is composed of drills that utilize previously learned sequential movements to produce nonsense and meaningful monosyllabic and polysyllabic words. In Stage III, tasks are employed to carry learned sequencing and self-monitoring skills into elicited utterances and spontaneous speech.

Melodic Intonation Therapy (MIT). MIT was initially developed to provide a vehicle for establishing propositional phrases in adults with apraxia or Broca's aphasia (e.g., Sparks & Holland, 1976). It utilizes stereotypical intonation, exaggerated stress, and lengthened tempo in conjunction with hand tapping to capitalize on intact abilities of the nondominant hemisphere in the production of a series of phrases selected on the basis of grammatical simplicity. The program moves through a series of stages from maximum aid from the clinician to increased independence on the part of the patient for the production of the phrase. MIT was adapted for children with DAS by Helfrich-Miller (1984). Candidacy criteria for MIT include those children 7 to 8 years old with a mean length of utterance of 3 to 4 words, poor repetition skills, and an attention span of 15 to 20 min. Helfrich-Miller indicated that it takes children who are scheduled for therapy three to four times per week approximately 10 to 12 months to complete the program.

The adapted MIT program includes three stages. Perhaps the major adaptation is the substitution of signed English for the hand tapping that is included for adults. In progressing through the three stages, output length and phonemic complexity are increased and dependency on the clinician and reliance on intonation are reduced. Phrases in Stage I are two to three words in length, composed of vowels and bilabial stops, and contain a minimum of grammatical morphemes. By Stage III, maximum phonological, morphological, and syntactic complexity is evident in the phrases chosen as stimuli with high priority given to the functional content of the phrases.

Summary and conclusions. It is not possible to create a fail-safe cookbook for providing appropriate and efficient treatment for the child with DAS. What has been offered is a review of techniques for functional articulation disorders that are adaptable for DAS and several organized systems of therapy that have evolved from other disorders but that appear to have value for working with DAS children. What they have in common is a set of principles for treatment including:

1. Use of developmental norms for determining the sequence of speech sounds to be taught
2. Maximum utilization of multimodal inputs (auditory, visual, tactual) to build articulatory movement patterns
3. Recognition of the facilitating effects of context in establishing target productions
4. Early introduction of self-monitoring skills to facilitate self-correction
5. Intensive, systematic drill that provides repetition of sound patterns
6. Emphasis on facilitatory effects of rhythm, stress, intonation, and motor activity in the production of sequences of speech sounds

7. A hierarchical sequence of treatments proceeding from relatively simple canonical forms to more complex sequences with greater emphasis on movement sequences and syllabic integrity than on production of individual speech sounds
8. Recognition of the necessity for guiding treatment based on the child's entry-level skills and responsiveness to different treatment approaches

The following case study is presented to provide cohesion to our discussion of appraisal, diagnosis, and treatment procedures for a child with DAS.

CASE STUDY

The purpose of this case study presentation is to provide an example of test findings and primary symptomology in a child with DAS. It is common for these children to undergo testing for an extensive period of time before a diagnosis is made, and frequently treatment is initiated before testing is complete. Therefore treatment effects may color test findings during the course of assessment. We will present an overview of some of the more important test results for a child with DAS over a 3-year period (see Table 12.2) and then will focus on features of the disorder after 3 years of treatment.

Appraisal and Diagnosis

N. was first evaluated at 3 years of age. Motor developmental milestones were within normal limits, although speech development was characterized as slow. His mother reported that he talked infrequently, was seldom intelligible, and had an oral vocabulary of approximately 35 words.

Administration of the *Sequenced Inventory of Communication Development* (Hedrick, Prather, & Tobin, 1975) yielded a receptive age of 32 months and an expressive age of 16 months. N.'s phonetic inventory was limited to vowels, stops, nasals, and glides. Phonological processes noted included final consonant deletion, cluster reduction, stopping, velar fronting, and unstressed syllable reduction. Although all English vowels were represented in his phonetic repertoire, they frequently did not approximate their phonemic target. Regardless of context, /d/ was typically substituted for target consonants. The most frequently used word shape was CV, which also was used when more complex canonical shapes were attempted.

Conversational speech was severely reduced in intelligibility and attempted communication was accompanied by a well-developed gestural

TABLE 12.2
DAS Child N. Test Performance from CA 3-0 to 6-6

Age	Articulation	Language	Motor	Cognition	Other
		SEMESTER 1			
CA 3-0 to 3-4	I. *Goldman Fristoe Test of Articulation*	*Sequenced Inventory of Communicative Development*	Oral-peripheral examination		Pure tone audiometric screening results within normal limits
	Vowels present [ae, e, i, ɛ, aɪ, I, o, ɔ, u, ʊ, ʌ, ɜ, aʊ]	Receptive language age = 32 months	Structures within normal limits but tongue movement limited and speed reduced		Normal middle ear function based on impedance testing
	Consonants present Initial [d, w, n, m] Medial [d, b] Final [ʧ, p]	Expressive language age = 16 months			
	II. Phonological process analysis				
	Processes observed: cluster reduction, stopping, velar fronting, final consonant deletion, initial consonant deletion, unstressed syllable deletion				

TABLE 12.2. Continued

Age	Articulation	Language	Motor	Cognition	Other
		SEMESTER 2			
CA 3-5 to 3-9	I. Phonetic inventory Initial [d, b, w, h, m] Medial [None] Final [m, t, p, s]	*Peabody Picture Vocabulary Test* Raw score = 40 CA = 3-7 Age score = 3-11 Percentile = 68	I. *Developmental Test of Visual Motor Integration* CA = 3-7 Age score = 3-2 II. Oral-peripheral examination/ apraxia measures Difficulty performing more complex oral apraxia tasks (e.g., pucker-up-to-smile sequence, licking lips)	*Leiter Performance Scales* CA = 3-7 MA = 4-5 Ratio IQ = 123	
	II. Syllable shapes CV, VC				
		SEMESTER 3			
CA 3-10 to 4-1	I. Phonetic inventory Initial [m, b, k, h, w] Medial [d, k] Final [m, s]				
	II. Syllable shapes CV, VC, CVCV				

TABLE 12.2. Continued

Age	Articulation	Language	Motor	Cognition	Other
		SEMESTER 4			

CA 4-2 to 4-5	I. *Assessment of Phonological Processes*
	
	Syllable reduction = 0%
	Cluster reduction = 100%
	Standard deletion = 75%
	Obstruent omissions
	  Prevocalic = 87%
	  Postvocalic = 16%
	Omission of /l/ and /r/
	Prevocalic consonants deleted in medial position
	
	II. Phonetic inventory
	Initial [m, p, b, t, d, k, g, s, t, w, j]
	Medial [None]
	Final [m, n]
	
	III. Syllable shapes
	CV, VC, CVCV, VCVC
		Analysis of speech sample (92 utterances)
		
		MLU = 3.08
			Screening Test for Developmental Apraxia
			
			Oral Movement subtest: Performed tasks but could not position tongue behind upper teeth. Unable to complete three-syllable sequences.		

TABLE 12.2. Continued

Age	Articulation	Language	Motor	Cognition	Other
		SEMESTER 5			
CA 4-5 to 4-9	I. *Templin-Darley Test of Articulation*	I. *Test of Auditory Comprehension of Language*			
	Score Norm Diagnostic 32 106.4 Screening 5 34.7	Score = 69 CA = 4-6			
	II. *Assessment of Phonological Processes*	Age score = 4-3 to 4-7 Percentile rank = 74			

	Syllable reduction 0%
	    Cluster reduction 88%
	    Stridency deletion 89%
	    Velar deviation 62%
	    Obstruent
	      omission
	      Prevocalic 81%
	      Postvocalic 10%
	    Liquid deviation
	      /l/ 54%
	      /r/ 58%
	    Nasal Omissions 58%
		II. *Carrow Elicited Language Inventory*
		CA = 4-8
		Total errors = 116
		Articles = 21
		Nouns = 5
		Plurals = 6
		Pronouns = 18
		Verbs = 51
		Negatives = 8
		Prepositions = 3
		Demonstratives = 1
		Conjunctions = 3			

	III. Syllable shapes CV, VC, CVCV, CVC				
	IV. Conversational speech sample simplifications				

	Cluster reduction
	    Stridency deletion
	    Final consonant deletion				

TABLE 12.2. Continued

Age	Articulation	Language	Motor	Cognition	Other
			SEMESTER 6		

CA 4-10 to 5-1	I. Assessment of Phonological Processes
	
	Cluster reduction = 50%
	Stridency deletion = 66%
	Velar deviation = 50%
	Final obstruent omission = 73%
	Liquid deviation /l/ = 100%
	Nasal omissions = 20%
	
	II. Phonetic inventory
	Initial [m, n, p, b, t, d, k, g, f*, r*, w, j, h]
	Medial [m, n, p, b*, t*, d, k*, w, j, ʔ]
	Final [m, n, p, t*, d*, r*, f]
	*newly acquired
	
	III. Syllable shapes CV, VC, CVCV, CCV, CVC
		Peabody Picture Vocabulary Test
		
		Raw score = 68
		CA = 5-0
		Age score = 5-10
		Percentile = 77
			I. Bruininks-Oseretsky Test of Motor Proficiency within normal limits
			
			II. Modified DeRenzi et al., Tests of Apraxia
			
			Limb apraxia 5/10 correct
			Oral apraxia 5/10 correct
			
			III. Boston Diagnostic Aphasia Examination
			A. Verbal agility = 8/14
			B. Nonverbal agility = 6/12
				McCarthy Scales of Children's Abilities
				
				CA = 5-1
				
				General Cognitive Index = 90
				
				          Scale Index
				Verbal 43
				Perceptual-
				  Performance 48
				Quantitative 44
				Memory 38
				Motor 48
					Prosody on longer utterances marked by inappropriate use of stress, most noticeably the overemphasis of stressed syllables

			SEMESTER 7		
CA 5-2 to 5-4	No testing completed				

TABLE 12.2. Continued

Age	Articulation	Language	Motor	Cognition	Other
		SEMESTER 8			
CA 5-5 to 5-8	I. Assessment of Phonological Processes Final consonant deletion = 63% Cluster reduction = 86% Stridency deletion = 48% Velar deviation = 29% Liquid deviation /l/ = 85% /r/ = 73% Nasal omissions = 5% II. Phonetic inventory Initial [m, p, t, d, k, f, dʒ, w] Medial [m, n, p, t, d, k, ʔ, s, ʃ] Final [m, n, p, t, ʔ, s, ʃ] III. Syllable shapes CV, VC, CVCV, CVC, CCV, CVCC, CVCVC	*Carrow Elicited Language Inventory* CA = 5-6 Total errors = 101 Score *Percentile* Articles 28 <1 Nouns 3 <1 Pronouns 17 <2 Verbs 38 <1 Negatives 8 <1 Prepositions 1 14 Demonstratives 2 1 Conjunctions 3 1 (Speech characterized by final morpheme deletion as well as word omissions and difficulty with complex sentences)			Pure tone audiometric screening within normal limits bilaterally Impedance testing: middle ear function normal

TABLE 12.2. Continued

Age	Articulation	Language	Motor	Cognition	Other
		SEMESTER 9			

CA 5-9 to 6-1	I. *Assessment of Phonological Processes*
	
	Final consonant deletion = 40%
	Cluster reduction = 48%
	Stridency deletion = 36%
	
	II. Phonetic inventory
	
	Elements missing
	
	Initial [ð, z, r, l]
	Medial [v, θ, ð, z, ʒ, dʒ]
	Final [v, θ, ð, z, ʒ, l]
	
	III. Syllable shapes
	V, CV, VC, VCV, CVCV, CVC, CCVC, CVCC, CCVCVC
		Conversational speech marked by final morpheme deletions (plural, past, present, progressive) and word omissions (articles, verbs, conjunctions, negatives, pronouns)	*Kaufman Assessment Battery for Children*
			
			CA = 6.1
			
			                         Per-
			                     Score *centile*
			Sequential
			  Processing 85 16
			Simultaneous
			  Processing 109 73
			Mental
			  Processing
			  Composite 100 50
			Achievement 97 42
					Intelligibility in connected speech increased with reduced rate.

TABLE 12.2. Continued

Age	Articulation	Language	Motor	Cognition	Other
		SEMESTER 10			
CA 6-2 to 6-6	I. *Assessment of Phonological Processes* Final consonant deletion = 35% Cluster reduction = 52% Stridency deletion = 34% II. Phonetic inventory Elements missing Initial [ð, r, l] Medial [v, ð, ɵ, l, ʒ] Final [v, ð, ɵ, l, ʒ]	Language sample analysis Problems with grammar (grammatical morphemes and complex sentences). Deletes -ing, plurals, possessives, regular past tense, and irregular third-person singular. Omits articles and contractive forms of "is" and "are," in complex sentences.			

system. Oral-peripheral examination of the speech mechanism revealed normal structures. However, alternate movement sequences of the tongue and lips and diadochokinetic rates for stop-vowel syllables were performed slowly and some multisyllabic sequences could not be imitated. Performance on the *Arthur Adaptation of the Leiter Performance Scales* (Arthur, 1952) yielded an intelligence quotient of 123, which was in the high average to superior range. Receptive vocabulary and visual motor integration were within normal limits.

At age 5, additional testing was completed to provide qualitative information on language expression. Results from the *McCarthy Scales of Children's Abilities* (McCarthy, 1972) were within the average range. Frequent omissions of articles, pronouns, verbs, negatives, and conjunctions were found on the *Carrow Elicited Language Inventory* (Carrow, 1974). Adjectives, adverbs, and nouns, however, were almost always retained.

Production of sentences from the *Carrow Inventory* was marked by inconsistent, context-dependent speech sound errors. Variability in sound production was reduced on more complex sentences, with frequent substitution of /d/, /b/, and /w/ for target sounds. Word shapes were primarily CV combinations, and longer utterances were highly unintelligible due to sound and syllable omissions and transpositions. A score of 32 was obtained on the *Templin-Darley Diagnostic Articulation Test* (Templin & Darley, 1969). The mean for male children at this age is 106, indicating a severe delay and a disorder in articulatory development. Phonological process analysis results were similar to performance at age 3. The most frequent processes were consonant deletion, cluster reduction, and stridency deletion. N.'s phonetic inventory was limited to vowels, stops, nasals, glides, and infrequently liquids. No fricatives or affricates were noted. Avoidance behavior in conversational speech was noted on words containing fricatives, and prosody was characterized by inappropriate loudness dynamics on longer utterances.

Additional measures were used to explore possible limb and oral apraxia. The probability of N.'s correct assignment to an apraxic diagnostic category was greater than 99% based on the results of the *Screening Test for Developmental Apraxia of Speech* (Blakeley, 1980). Perseveration, avoidance, and groping behaviors were noted during testing. On the Boston Verbal Agility subtest (Goodglass & Kaplan, 1972), N.'s productions of multisyllabic stimuli were characterized by transpositions of sounds and syllables and reductions in word complexity. Six of the 10 items of the Kools et al. (1971) adaptation of the DeRenzi et al. (1966) test of oral apraxia were scored as incorrect based on defective amplitude, accuracy, and force. N. also demonstrated difficulty in rapidly producing six of the seven tasks from the Boston Oral Agility subtest (Goodglass & Kaplan, 1972). N. produced only 5 of the 10 items of the

Kools et al. (1971) adaptation of the DeRenzi et al. (1966) test of limb apraxia, but non-oral fine and gross motor skills were within normal limits based on the results of the *Bruininks-Oseretsky Test of Motor Proficiency* (Bruininks, 1978).

At 6 years and 5 months of age, a detailed analysis of speech and expressive language functioning was completed. Included in the assessment was the analysis of a speech sample and the administration of the *Carrow Elicited Language Inventory* (Carrow, 1974), the *Assessment of Phonological Processes* (Hodson, 1980), and the *Templin-Darley Diagnostic Test of Articulation* (Templin & Darley, 1969). Results are shown in Table 12.3.

N.'s phonetic inventory contained all sound classes including vowels. Frequently occurring phonological processes included cluster reduction, liquid simplification, and stridency deletion. Consonants were correct 78% of the time, and vowels were correct 87% of the time. Word and syllable shapes were predominantly simple; however, more difficult canonical shapes were used including initial, medial, and final clusters. The most frequently used word shapes were V, VC, CV, VCV, CVC, CVCV, and CVCVC.

Analysis of the speech sample and *Carrow Inventory* revealed variable context-dependent errors. As word and sentence length increased, the number of errors increased and word shapes and the complexity of phonemic features were reduced. Intelligibility was reduced due to frequently omitted motorically complex speech sounds, vowel distortions, variable productions of the same word, and the combining of multiword utterances into a single word.

On the *Carrow Inventory*, articles, verbs, and conjunctions frequently were omitted, but not adjectives, adverbs, prepositions, pronouns, and nouns. The spontaneous speech sample analysis yielded a mean length of utterance of 6.4 and a limited number of grammatical morphemes (deVilliers & deVilliers, 1973) and complex sentence types, given N.'s age. Grammatical morphemes observed included "-ing," "in," "on," "a," "the," plurals, and possessives.

In summary, N. demonstrated a severe articulation disorder characterized by vowel errors, inconsistent productions, severely reduced intelligibility, prosodic abnormalities, and reduced use of complex canonical shapes. There also was evidence of oral and limb apraxia in the presence of normal fine and gross motor skills. Although cognitive functioning and receptive language were within normal limits, specific deficits and delays were apparent in expressive language. No evidence of specific neurological damage was reported, but we believe the characteristics demonstrated by N. are consistent with our description of the symptom complex that uniquely sets apart a group categorized as children with DAS.

TABLE 12.3
Summary of Speech and Language Assessment Following 10 Semesters of Treatment for Client N.

	Speech

Sound Classes[a]	Nasals: /m/IMF,/n/ImF,/ŋ/F
	Stops: /p/IMF,/b/IMF*,/t/IMF,/d/IMF,
	  /k/IMF,/g/IF
	Glides: /j/IM,/w/IM
	Liquids: /l/IM*F,/r/MF
	Fricatives: /f/IF,/v/I*F*,/s/IMF/z/F,/h/I,
	  /ʃ/I,/ð/I
	Affricates: /tʃ/IF*,/d,ʒ/I

Consonant error analysis (by %)[b]	n = 12 ŋ = 50 t = 43 d = 20 k = 16 g = 43 w = 10 j = 67 l = 17 r = 44 f = 12 v = 86 s = 19 z = 33
Vowel error analysis (by %)[c]	i = 7 u = 30 I = 10 ɔ = 11 æ = 8 a = 10
Phonological processes (used more than 40% of the time)	Cluster reduction
Templin-Darley Test of Articulation	Raw score = 95 Mean = 117
Predominant word shapes (used more than 10% of the time)	V VC CV CVC VCV CVCV CVCVC
	Language
Mean length of utterance	6.4
Grammatical morphemes	<50% >50% -ing -plurals -in -possessives -on -the -a

TABLE 12.3. Continued

Complex sentences	Conjoined sentences
	wh infinitive clauses
	Simple infinitive clauses with equivalent subjects
	Noninfinitive *wh* clause

[a] Asterisks indicate sounds produced two or fewer times.
[b] Total percentage of errors = 22.
[c] Total percentage of errors = 13.

Treatment

Retrospective views of treatment effects have inherent limitations. They do not allow control over relevant variables such as clinician training and pre- and posttesting instruments. Of greater importance over long periods of treatment is the reduced ability to separate out treatment effects from expected development of articulation skills in children with developmental apraxia. These shortcomings notwithstanding, we will review therapy for N. over a 10-semester period. Since the main thrust of treatment was on phonology and articulation, an estimate of improved performance can be made from a review of assessment results in the articulation category shown in Table 12.2 and from Table 12.3. Treatment approaches for each semester are shown in Table 12.4.

Semesters 1 and 2. Recommendations for management based on initial test results were (1) to establish use of final consonants, beginning with /p/ and /t/; (2) to introduce frication, beginning with /s/ in the final position; (3) to increase use of CVC or CVCV canonical shapes by using target words with these shapes while working on other goals; (4) to establish consistent initial production beginning with /h/ or /w/; and (5) to establish correct vowel production, based on further probing of specific vowels. A modified phonological approach based on Hodson and Paden (1982) was used with several error sounds targeted in each session. Instruction focused on contrast drill in CV and VC syllables and words. A multiple baselines design was implemented because it provided a means of detecting small changes in behavior over time. Clinical techniques included auditory bombardment and auditory-visual stimulation. Every 3 weeks, N.'s parents received a list of one-syllable words containing target phonemes to practice at home.

Progress was slow and carryover was seldom observed. Levels of self-monitoring obtained in CV and VC sequences were not demonstrated in connected speech, and performance on sounds previously mastered

TABLE 12.4
Treatment Approaches by Semester for DAS Child N.

Semester	Treatment Approach
1	Hodson's phonological process remediation
2	Hodson's phonological process remediation
3	McDonald's sensory-motor Multiple phoneme approach
4	McDonald's sensory-motor Multiple phoneme approach
5	McDonald's sensory-motor Contrast therapy Traditional approach
6	McDonald's sensory-motor Contrast therapy Melodic intonation
7	McDonald's sensory-motor Contrast therapy Melodic intonation
8	Hodson's phonological process remediation
9	Hodson's phonological process remediation
10	Hodson's phonological process remediation

deteriorated markedly between semester intervals. By the end of Semester 2, N. evidenced only three additional sounds in his phonetic inventory. Contrastive use of sounds was limited. The absence of medial consonants and the reduced number of sounds occurring in final position indicated that N. was unable to maintain syllable structure. His inability to produce sounds in a variety of word structures, variability in production, and reduced ability to perform speech-related movements mandated increased attention to movement sequences. Only two goals of treatment were achieved at the levels of expected accuracy during these first two semesters of treatment.

Semester 3. Remediation shifted in focus to a modified sensory-motor approach (McDonald, 1964) with utilization of nonsense bisyllabic drills (reduplicated CVCV syllables in which consonants and vowels were the same at first but later systematically varied according to consonant and vowel selection) to teach overlapping sequences of articulatory movements. Imitation of bisyllable combinations beginning with sounds already established in N.'s repertoire afforded a transition to more complex canonical shapes emphasizing slow rate, even stress, and careful self-monitoring. Occasional use of meaningful words was incorporated to illustrate the salience of newly learned movement sequences.

Phonological and linguistic elements also were incorporated into the treatment program. Included in the program were (1) selection of CV words at the basic level of production training; (2) acceptance of sound approximations that fell within the same sound class; (3) selection of target sounds (e.g., /k/ as representative of the velar class of sounds); (4) formulation of treatment goals that simultaneously considered phonology and syntax, and incorporated structures that were pragmatically useful (e.g., training of sounds at the sentence level using a cloze procedure such as "Give me the _____"); and (5) use of an auditory trainer to amplify production of specific target sounds and increase awareness of correct production.

Specific objectives included spontaneous production of initial /k/ in words and initial /h/ and /m/ in sentences. Consonants trained in final position included /s/, /d/, and /m/ at the sentence level. Projected goals at a 90% criterion level were not achieved. However, by the end of the semester N. produced six new sounds with greater than 50% accuracy, the velar class of sounds was added to his phonological system, and the /s/ was emerging. Treatment methods appeared successful in accomplishing objectives, although to a lesser degree than expected.

Semester 4. At this point N. produced all consonant manner classes except liquids, but labiodental, interdental, and palatal place features were absent. Six new sounds were added to his phonetic inventory and a total of 11 sounds appeared in initial position and 2 in final. Several other phones occurred less than three times in the sample and may have been emerging.

A modified McDonald sensory-motor approach was used to drill on sequencing of sounds already produced (/k/ and /p/) and to incorporate new sounds (/s/ and /f/) that he appeared to be acquiring. Additional goals included spontaneous production of monosyllabic words with final /p/, /s/, and /k/. Auditory, visual, and tactile cues were used to establish target production and then were faded to auditory or visual cues or both. The auditory trainer was used to heighten awareness of target phonemes. Chappell's backward chaining procedure was used in the elicitation of final consonants.

Only one of the projected therapy goals was achieved. While 90% accuracy was demonstrated in imitation of /k/ and /p/ in bisyllables with varied vowels, N. was unable to maintain /s/ in CVCV and VCVC sequences. He could not produce /f/ in combination with a vowel. Final consonants were produced with increased accuracy in imitation after training with backward chaining, but levels of accuracy were not maintained in spontaneous speech. Transfer into conversational speech did not occur.

The McDonald sensory-motor approach appeared effective in establishing productions of /k/ and /p/ in initial and medial word positions, but was not successful with either /s/ or /f/. Perhaps N. did not have sufficient control over production of these latter sounds to use them in bisyllables. Alternatively, since fricatives first emerge in final position, they should have been targeted in final rather than in initial and medial positions.

Semester 5. A substitution analysis was completed comparing N.'s phonological system with that of an adult. Only 7 consonants were produced more often correctly than incorrectly. All were produced in initial position. Stoel-Gammon and Dunn (1985) indicate that 4-year-old children customarily produce 21 consonants. They also list 11 consonants that are correctly produced by 90% of normal 4-year-old children—N. consistently produced only 7 consonants with 80% accuracy in initial position.

A child has eliminated most phonological processes by age 4 (Hodson & Paden, 1981). However, inspection of frequency of occurrence of processes (Table 12.2) shows that N.'s consonant production clearly was below age level. Stoel-Gammon and Dunn (1985) indicated that by age 4, errors of normal children occur in isolated sounds and not classes of sounds or word structures. N. had five processes that occurred more than 40% of the time. Finally, Templin (1957) indicated that many consonant clusters are produced consistently by 4-year-old children in initial and final positions. However, N. attempted only two words with clusters—both resulted in substition of /pw/ for /pl/. Obviously N. demonstrated substitution processes that accounted for many of his errors and, with the exception of /d/ and /r/, could be attributed to assimilation processes.

Intervention efforts continued to address imitation of bisyllable structures with systematic variation of consonants N. could produce correctly in combination with varying vowels. Integration of additional sounds (/b,d,m,n/) into the CVCV patterns with varying vowels was accomplished with 90% to 100% accuracy. Producing transitional patterns with systematic variation of the second consonant was achieved with greater than 50% accuracy for stop-nasal (e.g., p-m) and nasal-stop (e.g., m-k) combinations. A traditional approach was used to establish production of the strident phonemes /f/ and /s/ in the final position of monosyllabic words. Efforts to generalize production of these sounds consisted of activities in which N. used target words in meaningful situations.

Greater accuracy was demonstrated in imitation of /s/ and /f/ in CVC words and in spontaneous production. Spontaneous production of final /t,k,m/ and /p/ in CVC words was not achieved; however, contrast therapy was effective in establishing production in final position of /p/ (100%), /m/ (80%), and /t/ (40%).

By the end of the semester, N. had added six more sounds to his inventory, although these newly acquired phonemes occurred less than three times in the speech sample. He also demonstrated spontaneous use of the first-person pronoun "I" over half the time in conversational speech.

Advances were made during the semester using all three therapy approaches. Contrast therapy afforded a transition to more complex syllable shapes, using meaningful linguistic activities with phonemes N. was capable of producing. Phonemes that required more complex articulatory sequencing appeared sensitive to traditional therapy training. Carryover to the following semester was demonstrated on those sounds that received training using contrast therapy and sensory-motor bisyllabic drill. However, success with all three approaches was limited to imitative production.

Semester 6. Drill on CVCV patterns with varied vowels and consonants was continued. Stress patterns were systematically varied in this drill to reduce overemphasis on stressed syllables and to reduce steeper than normal intonational contours. Other tasks were directed toward improved rhythmic flow of speech and included (1) the production of two-, three-, and four-syllable words with appropriate stress patterns; and (2) practice on simple syllable frames and familiar nursery rhymes accompanied by body movements. The purpose of these drills was to increase awareness of the rhythmic aspects of spoken language. Rhythm was used as a technique to facilitate inclusion of sounds that N. had difficulty producing in connected speech (Rosenbek et al., 1974; Blakeley, 1983). At the beginning of the semester, N. could not clap in rhythm to a nursery rhyme, but this behavior reached 50% accuracy by the end of the 3-month period. Stress patterns were practiced in a hierarchical fashion based on difficulty. Once N. could distinguish between loud and soft auditory stimuli, activities shifted to clapping or tapping out two-part rhythm patterns in imitation. Stimulus words contained consonants that could be produced with the qualification that initially any medial consonant was acceptable. Cues included written stimuli showing the stressed syllables in larger physical movements such as hitting the table with the appropriate rhythm and auditory stimuli distinguishing between loud and soft. Initially N. could not produce a distinction between soft and loud CV syllables, but by the end of the semester he could produce the appropriate stress pattern with 60% accuracy on trisyllables. Prosody seemed more appropriate by the end of the treatment period.

A second major goal was spontaneous production of final stops and nasals in CVC words. Using contrast therapy, 100% accuracy was obtained in imitation of all final consonants, but these sounds were not consistently produced in spontaneous speech. A third goal was spontaneous production of strident phonemes in all word positions to increase intelligibility. An auditory trainer was used to provide auditory stimulation of words with initial /s/ blends and medial fricatives. N. reached the goal on /s/ and /f/ in final position, but could not imitate either of these sounds in initial position. Spontaneous production of final /s/ and /f/ was not accomplished.

Semester 7. Therapy activities focused on a more meaningful level as nursery rhyme and bisyllable drills were assigned to a home program. Goals included correct production of final /p,t,k,m/ and /n/ in CVC words, carrier phrases, and sentences. The language master was used along with verbal cuing to increase self-monitoring skills. The /s/ blends also were included for training at the single word and sentence level. Posttesting indicated a 22% increase in final consonant inclusion and improved self-monitoring. In a spontaneous speech sample, nasals and liquids were the most consistently included final consonants, followed by plosives. For the first time, other sound classes in final position—particularly the velar /k/—were noted in spontaneous speech.

Semester 8. The emergence of target sounds was the focus of remediation. Intervention was based on successive cycles (Hodson & Paden, 1982). Goals for cycling included production of the strident phoneme /s/ in final word position and in several final clusters, production of final /ʃ/ and /tʃ/ at the sentence level, and production of velars in words. Activities consisted of minimally paired contrast words, the language master, and card games. An auditory trainer was used to provide stimulation of words ending in final /s/, but was discontinued because N. consistently repeated target words incorrectly. At the end of the semester, imitation of final clusters /ts/ and /ps/ and final production of /ʃ/ and /tʃ/ were improved. However, no progress was demonstrated in spontaneous production. Velar consonants were imitated with 100% accuracy except for /ŋ/. Significant decreases were observed in cluster reduction, final consonant deletion, velar deviation, and liquid deviation and the phoneme /ʃ/ was added to the phonetic inventory.

The separate cycling of clusters, fricatives, and velars allowed N. to establish these manner classes by focusing attention on representatives from the classes in isolated time periods. (In Semester 4, N. had been confused when several manner classes were targeted in a single session.) The increased spacing between drills produced by the separate cycling periods facilitated production of target sounds.

Semester 9. Informal analysis at this point in treatment revealed spontaneous speech characterized primarily by nasals, stops, and glides. Word shapes were simple and no instances of abutting consonants were found. Goals were targeted in units lasting for approximately 4 weeks. Included were productions of initial and final /s/ and /f/, initial /s/ clusters, and final /g/. A generalization goal was implemented to provide transfer of targeted sounds to new environments, rhyming activities were continued, and self-monitoring was emphasized.

N. made excellent progress during the semester. He added nine sounds to his phonetic inventory, and phonological processes were substantially reduced and included only cluster reduction, final consonant deletion, and stridency deletion. Canonical forms added included CCVC and CCVCVC. Spontaneous use of correct sound production and generalization to new environments were observed, although continued difficulty was noted in rhyming.

Semester 10. A substitution analysis indicated that many of N.'s errors were related to the substitution of one sound for another (e.g., /w/ for /l/) rather than to classes of sounds. Goals built into 6-week units included production of initial and final /θ/ in spontaneous speech and production of /l/. A third goal was the production of /s/ and /z/ plural forms. Progress in production of the targeted speech sounds was fair—75% accuracy was obtained in the production of plural markers when pictures containing more than one person or object were described. Rhyming was combined with sound-symbol association and the mastery of 20 sight words in a reading readiness task. Good progress was shown in sound-symbol association and sight words, but poor progress was noted in rhyming. Recommendations for further management included implementation of self-monitoring and carryover activities, continued development of a home program, and increased attention to expressive language and reading skills.

Conclusions

Retrospective reviews of treatment have inherent limitations, as we noted earlier, due to the inability to control relevant variables or to accurately factor treatment effects from developmental progression. However, several observations about treatment for DAS resulted from this in-depth examination.

1. The production phase of a traditional approach to treatment may be effective in dealing with residual error sounds. The traditional

approach is less useful in early stages of treatment due to the focus on single consonants.
2. The multiple phoneme approach and auditory bombardment were successful in establishing initial productions of target sounds in CV and VC sequences. The McDonald sensory-motor drill helped to establish seven sounds in medial position and to stabilize a number of transitions from varying consonants. Bisyllable drills were effective when used with contrast techniques.
3. Greater progress was demonstrated with minimal pair contrasts when therapy goals were restricted to stabilizing the production of two pairs of sounds containing similar place features such as /m/ and /n/.
4. Semesters during which both bisyllable drill and contrast techniques were utilized resulted in the greatest number of additional sounds appearing in the child's inventory.
5. Nursery rhymes accompanied by movement, production of two-, three-, and four-syllable words with appropriate stress patterns, and bisyllabic drills with varied stress were successful in reducing prosodic abnormalities.
6. Auditory and visual stimulation, provided in the form of look and listen cues related to oral posturing and written stimuli, were more effective than auditory stimuli alone.

Quite obviously, another child with DAS may have required a different series of treatment approaches based on practical considerations. There is no preset idealized series of treatment steps and no treatment approaches so potent that they exclude others from consideration. Only when additional treatment data have been obtained will it be possible to determine what approaches are most efficacious for various aspects of the disorder.

SUMMARY

Developmental apraxia of speech (DAS) is a severe deficit in the ability to volitionally program speech movements. The disorder has a neurogenic etiology, but evidence of brain damage or dysfunction has not consistently been demonstrated in children diagnosed as having DAS on the basis of widely varying criteria. We have proposed a neurologically based model that effectively accounts for important observed behavioral characteristics of the disorder. Review of speech, language, cognitive, sensory, and motor characteristics provided a framework for appraisal and differential diagnosis of the disorder. Evidence relative to the effectiveness of treatment approaches for DAS is lacking, but a descriptive case study provides direction for therapy intervention.

REFERENCES

Aram, D. (1979, November). *Developmental apraxia of speech.* Paper presented at the annual convention of the American Speech and Hearing Association, Atlanta.

Aram, D., & Horwitz, S. (1983). Sequential and non-speech praxic abilities in developmental verbal apraxia. *Developmental Medicine and Child Neurology, 25,* 197–206.

Arthur, G. (1952). *The Arthur adaptation of the Leiter international performance scale.* Washington, DC: Psychological Service Center Press.

Aten, J. (1979). Denver auditory phoneme sequencing test. Austin, TX: PRO-ED.

Bashir, A., Grahamjones, F., & Bostwick, R. (1984). A touch-cue method of therapy for developmental verbal apraxia. *Seminars in Speech and Language, 5,* 127–138.

Blakeley, R. W. (1980). *Screening test for developomental apraxia of speech.* Austin, TX: PRO-ED.

Blakeley, R. (1983). Treatment of developmental apraxia of speech. In W. Perkins (Ed.), *Dysarthria and apraxia* (pp. 23–33). New York: Thieme-Stratton.

Bowman, S. N., Parsons, C. L., & Mowis, D. A. (1984). Inconsistency of phonological errors in developmental verbal dyspraxia children as a factor of linguistic task and performance load. *Australian Journal of Human Communication Disorders, 12,* 109–119.

Bruininks, R. (1978). *Bruininks-Oseretsky test of motor proficiency.* Circle Pines, MN: American Guidance Service.

Carrow, E. (1974). *Carrow elicited language inventory.* Lamar, TX: Learning Concepts.

Carrow-Woolfolk, E. (1985). *Test for auditory comprehension of language— Revised.* Allen, TX: DLM Teaching Resources.

Chappell, G. E. (1973). Childhood verbal apraxia and its treatment. *Journal of Speech and Hearing Disorders, 38,* 362–368.

Chappell, G. E. (1984). Developmental verbal dyspraxia: The expectant pattern. *Australian Journal of Human Communication Disorders, 23,* 15–25.

Chumpelik, D. (1984). The prompt system of therapy: Theoretical framework and applications for developmental apraxia of speech. *Seminars in Speech and Language, 5,* 139–153.

Cohen, M. J., Campbell, L. R., Elmore, J. A., & Yaghmai, F. (1988). Neuropathological abnormalities in developmental dysphasia: A case study. *Journal of Clinical and Experimental Neuropsychology, 10,* 56.

Costello, J., & Onstine, J. (1976). The modification of multiple articulation errors based on distinctive features theory. *Journal of Speech and Hearing Disorders, 42,* 199–215.

Court, D., & Harris, M. (1965). Speech disorders in children. Part 2. *British Medical Journal, 11,* 409–411.

Crary, M. A. (1984a). A neurolinguistic perspective on developmental verbal dyspraxia. *Communicative Disorders, 9,* 33–49.

Crary, M. A. (1984b). Phonological characteristics of developmental verbal dyspraxia. *Seminars in Speech and Language, 5,* 71–83.

Crary, M. A., & Towne, R. L. (1984). The asynergistic nature of developmental verbal dyspraxia. *Australian Journal of Human Communication Disorders, 12,* 27–37.

DeRenzi, E., Pieczuro, A., & Vignolo, L. A. (1966). Oral apraxia and aphasia. *Cortex, 2,* 50–73.

de Villiers, J., & de Villiers, P. (1973). A cross-sectional study of the acquisition of grammatical morphemes in child speech. *Journal of Psycholinguistic Research, 2,* 267–268.

Dunn, L. M., & Dunn, L. M. (1981). *Peabody picture vocabulary test–revised.* Circle Pines, MN: American Guidance Service.

Edwards, M. (1973). Developmental verbal dyspraxia. *British Journal of Disorders of Communication, 8,* 64–70.

Ekelman, B. L., & Aram, D. M. (1983). Syntactic findings in developmental verbal apraxia. *Journal of Communication Disorders, 16,* 237–250.

Ekelman, B. L., & Aram, D. (1984). Spoken syntax in children with developmental verbal apraxia. *Seminars in speech and language, 5,* 97–109.

Ferry, P., Hall, S., & Hicks, J. (1975). Delapidated speech: Developmental verbal apraxia. *Developmental Medicine and Child Neurology, 17,* 749–756.

Galaburda, A., Sherman, G., Rosen, G., Aboitiz, F., & Geschwind, N. (1985). Developmental dyslexia: Four consecutive patients with cortical anomalies. *Annals of Neurology, 18,* 222–233.

Goldman, R., & Fristoe, M. (1969). *Goldman-Fristoe Test of Articulation.* Circle Pines, MN: American Guidance Service.

Goodglass, H., & Kaplan, E. (1972). *The assessment of aphasia and related disorders.* Philadelphia: Lea & Febiger.

Gubbay, S., Ellis, E., Walton, J., & Court, S. (1965). Clumsy children: A study of apraxic and agnosic defects in 21 children. *Brain, 88,* 295–312.

Guyette, T., & Diedrich, W. (1981). A critical review of developmental apraxia of speech. In N. J. Lass (Ed.), *Speech and language: Advances in basic research and practice* (Vol. 5, pp. 1–49). New York: Academic Press.

Guyette, T., & Diedrich, W. (1983). A review of *Test for developmental apraxia of speech. Speech, Language, Hearing in Schools, 14,* 202–209.

Hedrick, D., Prather, E., & Tobin, A. (1975). *Sequenced inventory of communication development.* Seattle: University of Washington Press.

Helfrich-Miller, K. R. (1984). Melodic intonation therapy with developmentally apraxic children. *Seminars in Speech and Language, 5,* 119–125.

Hodson, B. (1980). *The assessment of phonological processes.* Austin, TX: PRO-ED.

Hodson, B. (1982). Remediation of speech patterns associated with low levels of phonological performance. In M. Crary (Ed.), *Phonological intervention: Concepts and procedures.* Austin, TX: PRO-ED.

Hodson, B., & Paden, E. (1981). Phonological processes which characterize unintelligible and intelligible speech in early childhood. *Journal of Speech and Hearing Disorders, 46,* 369–373.

Hodson, B., & Paden, E. (1982). *Targeting intelligible speech: A phonological approach to remediation.* Austin, TX: PRO-ED.

Horwitz, S. J. (1984). Neurological findings in developmental verbal apraxia. *Seminars in Speech and Language, 5,* 111–118.

Irwin, J., & Weston, A. (1971). *A manual for the clinical utilization of the paired-stimuli technique.* Memphis: National Education Services.

Jernigan, T. L., Tallal, P., & Bellugi, U. (1988). Cerebral morphology on magnetic resonance (MR) in developmental cognitive disorders. *Journal of Clinical and Experimental Neuropsychology, 10,* 19.

Kent, R., (1982). Contextual facilitation of correct production. *Language, Speech and Hearing Services in the Schools, 23,* 66–76.

Kent, R., Kent, J., & Rosenbek, J. C. (1988). Maximum performance tests of speech production. *Journal of Speech and Hearing Disorders, 52,* 367–387.

Kirk, S., McCarthy, J., & Kirk, W. (1968). *Illinois test of psycholinguistic abilities.* Urbana: University of Illinois Press.

Kools, J. A., & Tweedie, D. (1975). Development of praxis in children. *Perceptual and Motor Skills, 40,* 11–19.

Kools, J., Williams, A., Vickers, M., & Caell, A. (1971). Oral and limb apraxia in mentally retarded children with deviant articulation. *Cortex, 7,* 387–400.

Kornse, D. D., Manni, J. L., Rubenstein, H., & Graziani, L. J. (1981). Developmental apraxia of speech and manual dexterity. *Journal of Communication Disorders, 14,* 321–330.

Lee, L. (1971). *Northwestern Syntax Screening Test.* Evanston, IL: Northwestern University Press.

Lindblom, B., MacNeilage, P., & Studdert-Kennedy, M. (1988). *Biological bases of spoken language.* New York: Academic Press.

Logue, R., & McClumpha, S. (1970, November). *Apraxia of speech: A case description.* Paper presented at the annual convention of the American Speech and Hearing Association, New York.

Macaluso-Haynes, S. (1978). Developmental apraxia of speech: Symptoms and treatment. In D. F. Johns (Ed.), *Clinical management of neurogenic communication disorders* (pp. 243–250). Austin, TX: PRO-ED.

Marion, M., Marquardt, T., & Sussman, H. (1988). *The perception and production of rhyme in normal and developmentally apraxic children.* Unpublished manuscript, University of Texas, Austin, TX.

Marquardt, T., Dunn, C., & Davis, B. (1985). Developmental apraxia of speech. In J. Darby (Ed.), *Speech and language evaluation in neurology: Childhood disorders* (pp. 113–129). New York: Grune and Stratton.

McCabe, R., & Bradley, D. (1975). Systematic multiple phonemic approach to articulation therapy. *Acta Symbolica, 6,* 1–18.

McCarthy, D. (1972). *McCarthy scales of children's abilities.* New York: Psychological Corp.

McClumpha, S., & Logue, R. (1972, November). *Approaches to children with motor programming disorders of speech.* Paper presented at the annual convention of the American Speech and Hearing Association, San Francisco.

McDonald, E. (1964). *Articulation testing and treatment: A sensory motor approach.* Pittsburgh: Stanwix House.

Milisen, R. (1954). A rationale for articulation disorders [Monograph supplement]. *Journal of Speech and Hearing Disorders, 4,* 5–18.

Miller, J. (1981). *Assessing language production in children.* Austin, TX: PRO-ED.

Morely, M. E., & Fox, J. (1969). Disorders of articulation: Theory and therapy. *British Journal of Disorders of Communication, 4,* 151–165.

Nemoy, E. M., & Davis, S. F. (1954). *The correction of defective consonant sounds.* Magnolia, MA: Expression Co.

Nicolosi, L., Harryman, E., & Kresheck, J. (1978). *Terminology of communication disorders: Speech, language, and hearing.* Baltimore: Williams & Wilkins.

Plante, E. (1988, November). *MRI findings in children with specific language impairment.* Paper presented at the annual convention of the American Speech-Language-Hearing Association, Boston.

Rosenbek, J. C., Hansen, R., Baughman, C. H., & Lemme, M. (1974). Treatment of developmental apraxia of speech: A case study. *Language, Speech and Hearing Services in Schools, 5,* 13–22.

Rosenbek, J. C., & Wertz, R. T. (1972). A review of fifty cases of developmental apraxia of speech. *Language, Speech and Hearing Services in Schools, 3,* 23–33.

Scripture, M. K., & Jackson, E. (1927). *A manual of exercises for the correction of speech disorders.* Philadelphia: F. A. Davis.

Shriberg, L., & Kwiatkowski, J. (1980). *Natural process analysis: A procedure for phonological analysis of continuous speech samples.* New York: John Wiley.

Smartt, J., LaLance, L., Gray, J., & Hibbett, P. (1976). Developmental apraxia: A Tennessee Speech and Hearing Association subcommittee report. *Journal of the Tennessee Speech and Hearing Association, 20,* 21–39.

Snyder, D., Marquardt, T., & Peterson, H. (1977). Syntactical aspects of developmental apraxia. *Human Communication, 2,* 151–158.

Sparks, R., & Holland, A. (1976). Method: Melodic intonation therapy. *Journal of Speech and Hearing Disorders, 41,* 287–297.

Stoel-Gammon, C., & Dunn, C. (1985). *Normal and disordered phonology in children.* Austin, TX: PRO-ED.

Suga, N., O'Neill, W. E., Kujirai, K., & Manabe, T. (1983). Specificity of combination-sensitive neurons for processing of complex biosonar signals in auditory cortex of the moustached bat. *Journal of Neurophysiology, 49,* 1573–1627.

Sussman, H. M. (1986). A neuronal model of vowel normalization and representation. *Brain and Language, 28,* 12–23.

Sussman, H. M. (1988). The neurogenesis of phonology. In H. Whitaker (Ed.), *Phonological processes and brain mechanisms* (pp. 1–23). New York: Springer-Verlag.

Sussman, H. M. (1989). The neural coding of relational invariance in speech: Human language analogs to the barn owl. *Psychological Review, 96,* 631–642.

Templin, M. (1957). *Certain language skills in children.* Minneapolis: University of Minnesota Press.

Templin, M., & Darley, F. (1969). *The Templin-Darley tests of articulation* (2nd ed.). Iowa City: University of Iowa.

Van Riper, C. (1978). *Speech correction: Principles and methods.* Englewood Cliffs, NJ: Prentice-Hall.

Vargha-Khadem, F., Watters, G. V., & O'Gorman, A. M. (1985). Development of speech and language following bilateral frontal lesions. *Brain and Language, 25*, 167–183.

Walton, J., Ellis, E., & Court, S. (1962). Clumsy children: Developmental apraxia and agnosia. *Brain, 85*, 603–612.

Wechsler, D. (1975). *Wechsler intelligence scale for children–Revised.* New York: Psychological Corp.

Weeks, R. A., & Madison, C. L. (1985). Screening test of developmental apraxia of speech: Validity and reliability. *ASHA, 27*, 82.

Werker, J. F., Gilbert, J., Humphrey, K., & Tees, R. C. (1981). Developmental aspects of cross-language speech perception. *Child Development, 52*, 349–355.

Werker, J. F., & Tees, R. C. (1984). Cross-language speech perception: Evidence for perceptual reorganization during the first year of life. *Infant Behavior and Development, 7*, 49–63.

Williams, R., Ingham, R. J., & Rosenthal, J. (1981). A further analysis for developmental apraxia of speech. *Journal of Speech and Hearing Research, 24*, 496–505.

Yoss, K. A., & Darley, F. (1973, November). *What happens to children with developmental apraxia of speech? A follow-up of fifteen cases.* Paper presented at the annual convention of the American Speech and Hearing Association, Detroit.

Yoss, K. A., & Darley, F. (1974a). Developmental apraxia of speech in children with defective articulation. *Journal of Speech and Hearing Research, 17*, 399–416.

Yoss, K. A., & Darley, F. (1974b). Therapy in developmental apraxia of speech. *Language, Speech and Hearing Services in Schools, 1*, 23–31.

Young, E., & Hawk, S. (1955). *Moto-kinesthetic speech training.* Stanford, CA: Stanford University Press.

ACKNOWLEDGMENT

We are indebted to Suzanne Wolff for aid in the analysis of the case study data included in this chapter.

Author Index

Abbs, J., 69, 142, 194, 195
Abkarian, G., 5, 30, 105, 206
Aboitiz, F., 351
Adam, P., 69
Adams, M. R., 323
Adams, R. N., 55
Adams, S., 204
Ahern, M., 204
Ainsworth, T., 167
Ajamani, A., 60, 68, 75
Alavi, A., 44
Albert, M. L., 30, 219
Albert, N., 30
Alexander, M. P., 68, 70, 219, 287
Alfonso, P. J., 322, 323, 325
Alfrey, A. C., 229
American Academy of Neurology, 301, 305
Aminoff, M. J., 295
Andrews, B., 224, 229
Andrews, G., 223, 232
Aram, D., 243, 349, 350, 353, 356, 363
Arbit, E., 68
Arend, R., 220, 227
Arnold, G. E., 6, 220, 279
Aronson, A. E., 72, 88, 142, 192, 222, 276, 277, 279, 284, 285, 286, 290, 291, 292, 293, 295
Arthur, G., 375
Ashby, P., 282
Aten, J., 350, 356
Attanasio, J. S., 225
Avent, J. R., 221
Axelrod, J., 281

Baba, M., 68
Babcock, E. E., 60
Bacon, M., 277
Baer, T., 324
Baird, M., 164
Baken, R. J., 328, 329, 330
Balashke, T. F., 115
Baratz, R., 229, 230
Barbeau, A., 283, 289

Barroso, A. B., 143, 144
Bartels, P. H., 301
Barton, M. M., 74
Bashir, A., 364
Bassich, C. J., 44
Basso, A., 70
Baughman, C. H., 346
Bayles, K., 190
Beaton, L. E., 282
Behrens, S. J., 247
Bell, K. R., xii, 88, 307
Bellugi, U., 351
Bennett, R., 167, 168
Benson, D. F., 44, 68, 69, 70, 72, 221, 287
Bernard, J., 165
Berndt, R., 190
Berry, M. F., 242
Berry, W., 195
Bes, A., 69
Bessoles, G., 69
Beukelman, D. R., xii, 88, 105, 206, 307, 309
Black, F. W., 74
Blakeley, R., 350, 353, 355, 361, 375, 382
Blitzer, A., 284
Bloodstein, O., 145, 146
Bloom, F. E., 117, 124
Blumstein, S., 198
Boccino, J. V., 279
Boller, F., 144
Bollier, B., 204
Bonte, F. J., 44, 60, 62, 68, 69, 74, 75
Boone, D. R., 276
Borden, G., 195, 324, 325, 328
Borovich, B., 70
Boss, P., 162
Bostwick, R., 364
Botez, M. I., 283, 289
Bottomley, P. A., 60
Bowers, D., 244
Bowman, S. N., 346, 349
Boyeson, M., 75

391

Boyle, M., 209
Bradley, D., 359
Bray, G., 160, 161
Breckenridge, J., 248
Brewer, D. W., 323, 333
Brickman, P., 158
Bril, V., 282
Brin, M., 284
Brodnitz, F. S., 277
Bromfield, E. B., 44, 61, 70
Brookshire, R. H., 23
Brown, D., 323
Brown, J. R., 142, 192, 222, 276, 277, 286, 292, 293, 295
Brown, J. W., 45, 88, 190
Brown, S., 323
Brownell, G. L., 57, 61
Brownell, H., 190
Bruininks, R., 357, 376
Brumlik, J., 286, 295
Brunner, R. J., 68, 69
Bryan, W., 155, 174
Bryant, F., 158
Buckingham, H., 188, 191, 192, 196, 199
Budinger, T. F., 57
Burchfield, J. L., 301
Burns, M., 88, 197, 198
Butler, I. J., 131
Butler, R. B., 72, 221, 222, 231
Butterworth, B., 191

Caell, A., 357
Callaway, E. A., 225
Calne, D. B., 44, 61, 69, 70, 128
Camasio, H., 249
Campbell, L. R., 351
Candy, S., 167
Cannito, M. P., 44, 68, 72, 276, 277, 281, 290, 291, 294, 295, 299, 300, 301, 303, 304, 307, 308
Canter, G., 146, 197, 198, 199, 222, 223, 236
Caplan, D., 59, 188, 191, 198, 199
Caplan, G., 155
Caplan, L., 70, 224, 226
Caramazza, A., 190
Cariski, D., 204
Carpeggiani, P., 220
Carpenter, M. B., 45, 280, 282
Carrow, E., 375, 376
Carrow-Woolfolk, E., 353

Cedarbaum, J. M., 125, 126, 127, 128, 129, 130, 131, 132, 133, 135, 138, 139, 140, 141, 142
Chapman, S. D., 305
Chappell, G. E., 345, 346, 350, 361, 362
Childers, D. G., 329
Chiueh, C. C., 61, 69, 70
Chumpelik, D., 204, 205, 363
Clark, R. G., 280
Coates, R., 68
Cohen, M. J., 351
Cohn, M., 328
Collins, M., 72, 73, 204, 206, 224
Colsher, P. L., 245, 252
Committee on Aging, 165, 167
Connor, N., 72, 295
Conture, E., 323, 333
Cooper, W., 198
Cooper, I. S., 284
Cooper, J. R., 117, 120, 121, 124
Cooper, W. E., 243, 245, 246, 247, 249, 251, 252
Corey, G., 173
Coslett, H. B., 244, 246
Cosmides, L., 243
Costello, J., 360
Coufal, K. J., 323
Court, D., 348
Court, S., 348
Crary, M. A., 345, 349, 350, 362
Critchley, M., 222, 284, 295
Cross, D. E., 323
Crosson, B., 45
Culatta, R., 219
Cullinen, W. L., 323

Dabul, B., 200, 201–202, 204
Damasio, A. R., 69, 70
Damasio, H., 69, 247
Daniloff, R., 195
Danly, M., 244, 245, 246
Dann, R., 44
Darby, J. K., 69
Darley, F. L., 5, 68, 88, 93, 142, 192, 221, 222, 277, 286, 290, 292, 293, 307, 344, 345, 348, 350, 353, 355, 361, 375, 376
Davis, B., 358
Davis, G. A., 88
Davis, S. F., 360
De Bleser, R., 68
De Villiers, J., 376

De Villiers, P., 376
Deal, J., 93, 204, 218, 225
DeBito, M. A., 148
Deck, J., 205
Dedo, H. H., 72, 276, 279, 284, 286, 290, 295
DeJong, W., 83, 54
DeLacoste-Utamsing, C., 246
Dempsey, G. L., 218
DeRenzi, E., 357, 375, 376
Derex, M. M., 69
DeSanto, L. S., 72
DeSanto, L. W., 276
Devous, M. D., 44, 60, 62, 68, 69, 74, 75, 77
Devreau, F., 224, 226, 229, 236
Diamond, I. T., 288
Diedrich, W., 342, 345, 355
DiSimoni, F., 7, 206
Dodson, L., 279
Doherty, W., 164
Donnan, G. A., 12, 226, 227, 230
Doro, J. M., 218, 225
Dowden, P. A., xii, 206
Downie, A. W., 232
Drayer, B. P., 60
Driver, L. E., 225
Dubner, R., 280, 281
Duffy, F., 64, 301
Duffy, J., 198
Dunham, M., 205
Dunn, C., 358, 381
Dunn, L. M., 353, 356
Dunn, L. M., 353, 356
Dunn, M., 156
Dworkin, J. P., xii, 5, 7, 30, 88, 105, 206

Eady, S. J., 243, 249, 251, 252
Edwards, M., 345, 349
Ekelman, B. L., 349, 363
Elliot, R. L., 229
Ellis, E., 348
Elmore, J. A., 351
Engel, J., 8
Estabrooks, N. A., 106
Evarts, E. V., 305

Fabre, N., 69
Fahn, S., 126, 128, 284, 285
Farmer, R., 172, 174
Feinstein, A. R., 5

Feldman, M., 277, 279, 288
Fennell, A., 199
Ferry, P., 348
Filstead, W., 169
Finitzo, T., 44, 64, 68, 72, 277, 299, 300
Finitzo-Hieber, T., 276, 277, 279
Fink, M., 284
Fischer, J. M., 288
Fisher, B., 209
Fisher, M., 69
Fleet, W. S., 228
Florance, C., 204
Flowers, C. R., 245, 247
Flowers, K., 69
Folkins, J., 194
Foltz, E. L., 282
Ford, J., 284
Fox, J., 348, 361
Fox, P. T., 45
Franzen, E. A., 287
Freedman, M., 70, 287, 300, 304
Freeman, F. J., 44, 72, 145, 276, 277, 279, 284, 290, 299, 300, 308, 324, 333
Freund, H., 218
Friedman, E., 162
Friedrich, F., 200
Fristoe, M., 356
Fromm, D., 199
Fukusako, Y., 198

Gacek, P. R., 148
Galaburda, A., 68, 351
Garrett, M., 186, 189
Gawle, C., 198
Gay, T., 325
Gazzaniga, M. S., 300
Gerber, K., 158
Gerling, I., 279
Gersch, F., 69
Geschwind, N., 351
Gilbert, J., 352
Gillman, A. G., 115, 120
Gilman, S., 45, 54, 55, 59, 61, 69, 125, 127
Ginsberg, A. P., 277, 290
Gintautas, J., 221
Glaser, L., 205
Glenn, C., 200
Goetz, C. J., 132, 133, 142
Goffman, E., 167, 168, 170

Goldman, M., 169, 328
Goldman, R., 355
Goldsmith, H., 323
Goldstein, J. A., 146
Goloskie, S., 245
Goodglass, H., 73, 74, 186, 190, 198, 199, 207, 219, 375
Goodman, L. S., 115, 120
Goodstein, R., 155
Gordon, W. P., 45
Gorusch, R. L., 295
Gottesman, L., 169
Gottlieb, J., 198
Gowing, P., 287
Gracco, V., 195
Graff-Radford, N. R., 243, 245, 247, 249, 252
Grafman, J., 72
Grahamjones, F., 364
Granich, M., 218
Grant, D. E., 68, 75
Gray, J., 345
Graziani, L. J., 348
Greenberg, J., 44
Greenberg, S., 157, 172, 173
Greenwald, B., 229
Grober, E., 190
Grossberg, S., 45
Groswasser, Z., 68, 71
Groswasser-Reider, I., 68
Gubbay, S., 348
Guel, A., 69
Guitar, B., 233, 234, 321
Guyette, T., 342, 345, 355

Hall, J. W., 279
Hall, S., 348
Handzel, L., 227
Hansen, R., 346
Hanson, W. R., 44, 57, 68, 69, 70, 232
Harlock, W., 68
Harnes, B., 70
Harney, J. H., 246
Harper, R. M., 8
Harr, R., 73
Harris, E., 204
Harris, M., 348
Harryman, E., 346
Hartman, D., 142, 285, 305
Hast, M. H., 288
Hawk, S., 359
Hayden, P., 323

Hays, P., 146
Hayward, R. W., 299, 302
Head, H., 220
Hedrick, D., 366
Heilman, K. M., 228, 244, 245, 246
Hekeler, R., 172, 174
Helfrich-Miller, K. R., 365
Helm, N., 30, 72, 73, 105, 206, 219, 220, 221, 222, 223, 227, 229, 230–231
Helm-Estabrooks, N., 30, 222, 229, 231, 234, 236
Henderson, G., 155, 174
Hendrick, D., 356
Herderschee, D., 69
Hibbett, P., 345
Hicks, J., 348
Hill, A. B., 113
Hill, R., 162, 164, 165
Hirose, H., 69, 199, 325
Hirschman, P., 323
Hixon, T. J., 322, 328
Hodson, B., 360, 376, 378, 381, 383
Holland, A., 205, 207, 365
Holtzapple, P., 205
Holzman, J. D., 300
Homan, R. W., 69, 70
Horner, J., 68, 73, 222, 223, 228
Horwitz, S., 344, 350, 351, 353, 356
Hoskins, B., 96, 102
Hough, M., 196
House, E. L., 281, 282, 283
Hudson, A. J., 167
Hug, L. N., 249
Hughes, O., 194
Hulstijn, W., 325
Humphrey, K., 352
Hunter, L., 199
Hutchinson, J. M., 323, 325, 326
Hyland, J., 205

Imber-Black, E., 162, 164
Ingelfinger, J. A., 114
Ingham, R. J., 344
Ireland, J., 198
Irwin, J., 360
Itoh, M., 198, 199
Izdebski, K., 276, 279, 280, 295, 305

Jackson, C., 68
Jackson, E., 359
Jackson, S., 174

Jacob, J. C., 287
Jacobs, G. A., 295
James, T. L., 60
Jankovic, J., 54, 145, 148, 283, 284, 285
Jenkins, J. J., 220
Jerger, J., 279
Jernigan, T. L., 351
Jimenez-Pabon, E., 220
Joanette, Y., 193, 196, 198, 200
Johns, D. F., xii, 5, 6, 9, 11, 30, 105, 206, 221
Johnson, J. P., 276, 277, 290
Jones, K., 162, 165
Jones, M., 169
Jones, R. K., 12–13
Jordan, L. S., 242, 256
Jürgens, U., 144, 280, 282, 283, 287, 288, 289, 290

Kaas, J. H., 288
Kahana, E., 167
Kaiser, G., 229
Kalotkin, M., 145
Kanno, I., 62
Kaplan, E., 73, 74, 190, 199, 207, 375
Kasniak, A., 190
Kastenbaum, R., 167
Kellar, L., 190
Keller, E., 193, 194, 196, 197, 200
Keller, R., 55
Kelley, A. H., 282, 288
Kelso, J. A. S., 288
Kempler, D., 44, 68, 70, 196
Kenney, M. K., 324
Kent, J., 356
Kent, R., 44, 196, 197, 198, 202, 222, 245, 246, 248, 356, 360
Kertesz, A., 68, 287
Kiml, P. J., 282, 286
Kiritani, S., 69
Kirk, S., 350
Kirk, W., 350
Kirzinger, A., 280, 287
Klawans, H. L., 132, 133, 142
Kleemeier, R., 167
Klich, R., 198
Klouda, G. V., 243, 246, 247, 249, 250, 260
Knopp, L. M., 282
Koch-Weser, J., 114
Kohn, S., 196, 197

Koller, W. C., 125, 132, 222
Kondraske, G. V., 295
Kools, J., 348, 357, 375, 376
Korn, C., 68
Kornhuber, H. H., 45, 68, 305
Kornse, D. D., 348
Koury, L. N., 168, 170
Kresheck, J., 346
Krishnamurthy, A. K., 329
Kuhl, D. E., 68, 70
Kujirai, K., 351
Kushner, D., 30
Kushner, M., 44, 61, 68, 70, 71
Kuypers, H. A., 288
Kwiatowski, J., 356

LaLance, L., 345
Lang, A. E., 128, 284
LaPointe, L. L., xii, 7, 30, 88, 200, 203, 222, 232, 257, 307
Larochelle, L., 282
Larson, C., 287
Lashley, K. S., 6
Lassen, N. A., 62
Lauterbur, P. C., 57
Lea, W. A., 243
Lebrun, Y., 223, 224, 226, 229, 236
Lechtenberg, R., 69
Lecours, A., 193, 196, 198, 200
Lee, L., 349
Leeper, L., 219
Leleux, C., 223, 224, 226, 229, 236
Lemkau, J., 158
Lemme, M., 204, 229, 346
Lester, G., 162
Levesque, M., 8
Liberman, P., 248
Lieberman, M., 167
Lindblom, B., 351
Lindeman, R. C., 287
Lindsay, D. D., 232
Litin, M. E., 276, 277, 295
Logue, R., 346, 348
Longstretch, D., 204
Lotts, D. W., 249
Louera, B., 308
Lovelace, R., 284
Low, J. M., 232
Lubinski, R., 168, 170
Luchsinger, R., 6, 220, 279
Ludlow, C., 44, 72, 295
Luper, H. L., 323

Lushene, R., 295
Luterman, D., 161
Luzzatti, C., 70
Lyon, J., 106

Macaluso-Haynes, S., 350, 361
MacNeilage, P., 198, 351
Madison, C. L., 355
Magoun, H. W., 282
Malmgren, L. T., 148
Mamelok, R. D., 115
Manabe, T., 351
Manni, J. L., 348
Manning, W. H., 323
Marin, O., 200
Marion, M., 353
Markham, C. H., 70
Maroun, F. B., 287
Marquardt, T., 349, 353, 358
Marsden, C. D., 128, 284, 285
Marshall, R., 30, 205, 209, 233, 236
Maslach, C., 173, 174
Masland, R. L., 6
Massey, E. W., 68, 73, 222, 223, 228
Mateer, C. A., 244
Matsunaga, M., 68
Mattson, R. H., 70
Mazziotta, J., 68
Mazzuchi, A., 220, 224, 226, 229
McCabe, R., 359
McCall, G., 277, 279, 284, 285, 288, 323, 330, 333
McCarthy, D., 375
McCarthy, J., 350
McClean, A. J., 229
McClean, M. D., 229
McClumpha, S., 346, 348
McCubbin, H., 162
McDonald, E., xii, 359, 379, 380, 381, 385
McDowell, F. H., 125, 126, 127, 128, 129, 130, 131, 132, 133, 135, 138, 139, 140, 141, 142
McGeer, P. L., 57
McNeil, M., 199, 205, 229
Mead, J., 328
Mefford, I., 55
Merson, R. M., 277, 290
Merzenich, M. M., 288
Messert, B., 72, 73, 224
Mesulam, M. M., 229, 230, 244
Metter, E. J., 44, 57, 68, 69, 70, 74, 232

Metz, D., 323
Meyers, R., 290
Michelow, D., 245
Milisen, R., 360
Millay, K. K., 68, 75
Miller, J., 356
Miller, L., 89, 91, 99, 102
Miller, M., 171
Miller, R. H., 54, 73
Milojevic, B., 288
Moll, K., 195
Monahan, L., 172, 174
Monoi, H., 198, 199
Monrad-Krohn, G. H., 242, 243, 244
Moore, P., 286, 295
Morely, M. E., 348, 361
Moretti, G., 220
Morningstar, D., 204
Morris, D. A., 346
Morrison, E., 168
Mosteller, F., 114
Mueller, P. R., 243, 249
Murad, F., 115, 120
Murgatroyd, S., 172
Murphy, A. T., 277
Murray, E., 322
Musselwaite, C. R., xii
Myers, P. S., 242, 253, 256
Myers, R. E., 287

Naeser, M. A., 68, 69, 70, 287, 299, 302
Nagata, K., 44, 64, 68, 74
Narita, S., 68
Nation, J. E., 243
Nekemkis, A., 158
Nemoy, E. M., 360
Nespoulous, J., 198, 199
Netsell, R., xii, 88, 243
Neuburger, S. I., 233, 236
Newhoff, M., 205
Newman, S. W., 45, 54, 55, 59, 61
Nicol, J., 245
Nicolosi, L., 346
Nies, A. S., 115
Nixon, J. V., 277
Novack, T. A., 45
Novelly, R., 70
Nowack, W. J., 72, 73, 224, 227, 230, 234, 236
Nudelman, H. B., 144
Nunnally, R. L., 60
Nurnberg, H. G., 229

Oelschlaeger, M., 44, 68
O'Gorman, A. M., 344
Oke, A., 55
Oldfield, R. C., 74
O'Neill, W. E., 351
Onstine, J., 360
Owens, R. E., Jr., 92
Ozaki, I., 68, 69

Paden, E., 378, 381, 383
Paini, P., 220
Palkovts, M., 54
Pansky, B., 281
Parma, M., 220
Parsons, C. L., 346
Pearson, J. C., 45
Pearson, J. S., 276, 277, 295
Pechadre, J. C., 282
Peled, R., 70
Penfield, W., 287
Perecman, E., 190
Perkins, W. H., 88
Peters, H. F. M., 325
Peters, T. J., 233, 234
Petersen, S. E., 45
Peterson, H., 349
Phelps, M., 68, 69, 70
Pieczuro, A., 357
Pierce, R., 190
Pines, A., 174
Plante, E., 351
Ploog, D., 144, 282, 288, 289, 290
Plum, F., 46
Poeck, K., 68
Poirier, L. J., 282
Pool, K., 44, 64, 72, 300
Porfert, A. R., 144
Posner, J., 46
Posner, M. I., 45
Potter, R., 171
Power, P., 160
Prather, E., 356, 366
Pratt, R., 282, 283, 289
Prescott, T. E., 229
Purdy, P. D., 246

Quader, S. E., 229
Quinn, P. T., 223, 224, 229

Radda, G. K., 60
Raichle, M. E., 45
Rall, T. W., 115, 120

Rao, P., 206
Rasmussen, T., 70
Rastatter, M. P., 73
Rauth, T., 167
Ravits, J. M., 279
Reich, A., 295, 323
Reis, R., 323
Reivich, M., 44
Rentschler, G. J., 225, 229, 236
Retif, J., 229
Reynolds, S., 68, 75
Riege, W. H., 70
Riemenschneider, S., 323
Rigrodski, S., 168
Rizzo, M., 69
Robe, E., 286, 295
Roberts, L., 287
Robin, D. A., 242, 243, 247, 249, 256, 258, 260
Rodnitzky, R. L., 23, 242, 256
Rogers, C., 172
Rommer, P., 62
Rosen, G., 351
Rosenbek, J., xii, 7, 30, 72, 73, 88, 196, 197, 199, 200, 202, 203, 204, 206, 221, 222, 224, 226, 227, 228, 229, 232, 233, 234, 236, 245, 246, 248, 257, 307, 308, 343, 345, 346, 348, 349, 350, 356, 361, 362, 382
Rosenberg, J., 72
Rosenberger, P. B., 145
Rosenfield, D. B., 72, 131, 143, 144, 145, 146, 147, 149, 224, 226, 284, 290, 295, 307, 308
Rosenstock, F., 169
Rosenthal, J., 344
Ross, E. D., 244, 245, 246, 247, 300, 304
Rossi, J., 169
Roth, R. H., 117, 124
Rothenberg, R., 169
Roulleau, J., 69
Rousseau, J. J., 224, 226, 229, 236
Rowland, L. P., 279
Rubens, A. B., 70, 219, 287
Rubenstein, H., 348
Rudensey, K., 171
Ruff, R. L., 68
Ryalls, J. H., 246, 247

Sackner, M., 328
Safilios-Rothchild, C., 155

Salazar, A., 72
Sasanuma, S., 198, 199
Satir, V., 162
Sawashima, M., 69, 199, 325
Schaefer, S., 72, 277, 279, 280, 281, 282, 289, 290, 299
Schecter, J., 155
Schere, K. R., 243
Schiff, H. B., 68, 70, 71
Schiller, F., 223
Schmitt, M. A., 68
Scholes, R., 245
Schuell, H., 220, 232
Schuell, M., 207
Schwartz, M., 186, 187, 188
Scripture, M. K., 359
Seemuller, E., 68
Selkirk, E. O., 243
Sessle, B. J., 280
Seth, G., 322
Shames, G., 231
Shapiro, A., 324
Shapiro, B., 244, 245, 246
Sharbrough, F. W., 279
Sharf, B., 70
Sharpe, J. A., 282
Shattuck-Hufnagel, S., 187, 188, 191
Shaw, G. L., 45
Sheehy, M. P., 284
Sherman, G., 351
Sherrington, C. S., 6
Shipp, T., 279, 280, 285, 305
Shishido, F., 44
Shriberg, L., 356
Shtremel, A. K., 232
Sidtis, J. J., 300
Siegal, A., 281
Siegel, S., 290
Silverman, D. J., 45
Simmons, N., 204, 206
Ska, B., 198
Skelly, M., 205
Smartt, J., 345, 348, 361
Smith, L. S., 60
Smutok, M., 72
Snyder, D., 349
Soares, C., 245
Solvi, P., 68
Sommers, R., 68
Sorby, W. A., 223
Sorensen, J. M., 243, 246, 251, 252
Southwood, H., 206

Sparks, R., 30, 205, 365
Speedie, L., 244, 246
Spencer, D. D., 70
Spencer, S. S., 70
Spielberger, D. C., 295, 307
Spinnler, H., 70
Springer, M. T., 323
Square, P., 68, 71, 204, 205
Square-Storer, P., 203, 205
Squire, L., 44, 69, 70
Stam, J., 69
Starch, S. A., 233
Starkweather, C. W., 323
Starosta-Rubinstein, S., 69
Statlender, S., 198
Stern, M., 44
Stevens, E., 205
Stevens, K. N., 243, 323
Stillman, R., 282
Stockard J. J., 279
Stoel-Gammon, C., 381
Stokely, E. M., 62, 69
Stone, R. E., 72, 73, 224, 227, 230, 234, 236
Storey, A. T., 281
Stott, F., 328
Strome, M., 325
Strub, R. L., 74
Studdert-Kennedy, M., 351
Suga, N., 351
Suger, G., 68
Sugishita, M., 70, 71
Sullivan, M., 209
Sussman, H. M., 351, 352, 353
Sussman, M., 156
Sutton, D., 287, 288
Sveinsdotir, E., 62

Tagawa, K., 44
Takebe, K., 68
Tallal, P., 351
Tannenbaum, R. S., 323
Tees, R. C., 352
Templin, M., 345, 353, 355, 375, 376, 381
Theodore, W. H., 44
Thibodeau, I. A., 114
Thomas, B. J., 229
Thompson, L., 165
Thompson, V. E., 288
Tikofsky, R. S., 44, 68
Till, J., 295, 323

Author Index

Tobin, A., 356, 366
Tolosa, E., 148
Tompkins, C. A., 244, 245, 247
Towne, R. L., 349
Townsend, J. J., 279
Tranel, D., 247
Traube, L., 277
Travis, L. E., 321
Traynor, C. D., 105
Trenerry, M. R., 45
Trost, J., 197, 198, 221
Tucker, D. M., 245
Tucker, H. M., 279
Tuller, B., 288
Tweedie, D., 348

Uemura, K., 44
Ushijima, T., 199, 324, 333

Vagg, P. R., 295
Valletutti, P., 157, 172, 173
Van den Berg, J., 323
Van der Gugten, J., 54
Van Hoesen, G. W., 70
Van Kleeck, A., 99
Van Lackner, D., 68
Van Riper, C., 6, 218, 221, 321, 359
Vanderheiden, G. C., xii
Vargha-Khadem, F., 344
Varney, N., 69
Versteeg, D. H. G., 54
Vickers, M, 357
Vignolo, L. A., 357
Vishwanat, B., 305
Vogel, M., 283, 289, 290
Volpe, B. T., 300
Von Cramon, D., 197, 283, 289, 290
Von Keyserlingk, D. G., 68

Wagner, H. N., Jr., 61
Walker-Batson, D., 44, 60, 68, 74, 75
Wallach, G. P., 89, 99, 102
Wallen, V., 218
Wallesch, C. W., 68
Walton, J., 348
Ward, A. A., 282
Ware, J. H., 114
Wasterlain, C., 44, 68, 69, 70
Watson, B. C., 322, 323, 325, 327, 328

Watson, H., 328
Watson, R. T., 245, 246
Watters, G. V., 344
Wechsler, D., 356
Weeks, R. A., 355
Weidner, W., 198
Weiner, A. E., 218
Weiss, B., 227
Weisshaut, R., 328
Welch, K. M. A., 60
Wendt, J., 74
Werker, J. F., 352
Wertz, R. T., 7, 30, 72, 73, 88, 200, 203, 204, 205, 206, 222, 224, 343, 345, 348, 349, 362
Weston, A., 360
Wetzel, A. B., 288
Wheelden, L. A., 145
Whitehouse, P., 190
Wilcox, M. J., 88
Williams, A., 357
Williams, C. E., 243
Williams, R., 344, 346
Williamson, P. D., 70
Wilson, C., 8
Wilson, D. H., 300
Wilson, L., 162
Winans, S. S., 125, 127
Wingate, M. E., 323
Winitz, H., 30
Wolfe, V. I., 277
Woodson, G. E., 54

Yahgmai, F., 351
Yairi, E., 221
Yorkston, K. M., xii, 88, 96, 105, 206, 307, 309
Yoshioka, H., 199
Yoss, K. A., 344, 348, 350, 361
Young, E., 359
Yule, G., 196

Zemlin, W., 321
Zervas, N. T., 70
Zhang, J. X., 8
Ziegler, W., 197
Zung, W. W. K., 295, 307
Zurif, E., 190
Zwitman, D., 277

Subject Index

Page numbers in italics refer to figures; those followed by "t" refer to tables.

Acetylcholine (ACh), 54, *55,* 117, 118t, 120–121
Acetylcholine (ACh) antagonists, 120, 122t
Acetylcholine (ACh) release blockers, 120, 122t
Acquired neurogenic dysfluency. *See* Neurogenic dysfluency
Adrenergic nerves, 117
Aerodynamic disruptions, and stuttering, 325–326
Aerodynamic measures, 329–330
AIDS. *See Assessment of Intelligibility of Dysarthric Speech* (AIDS)
Akinesia, 127
ALS. *See* Amyotrophic lateral sclerosis (ALS)
Amantadine, 136t, 140
Amygdala, *47,* 49
Amyotrophic lateral sclerosis (ALS), 28, 69, 292t, 293, *293*
Anomic aphasia, 35t, 193–194
Anticholinergics, 133, 135, 136t
Aphasia
  brain imaging and, 73–74
  classifications of, 35t
  phonological breakdown in, 191–194
  neurogenic dysfluency and, 220–221
Apraxia Battery for Adults, 200, 201, 202t
Apraxia of speech. *See also* Developmental apraxia of speech (DAS)
  brain imaging and, 70–71, 74–75
  characteristics of, 195–199
  diagnosis of, 200–202, 202t
  dysfluency and, 221–222
  effort and, 196–197
  less common errors and, 199–200
  repetition and, 199–200
  substitutions and, 197–199
  treatment for, 203–208

Arthur Adaptation of the Leiter Performance Scales, 375
Articulation tests, 355–356
Assessment. *See also* Brain imaging
  of apraxia of speech, 200–202, 202t
  of developmental apraxia of speech (DAS), 355–358, 366, 367t–374t, 375–376, 378t–379t,
  of motor functions, 121–123, 295–299, 330–333, 356–357
  of neurogenic dysfluency, 223–225
  neurologist's approach to, 21–28, 26t
  of phonemic paraphasia, 200–202, 203t
  of prosodic disorders, 248–253, 249t, 251t, 252t, 254t–255t
  speech pathologist's approach to, 31–33, 33t
  for stuttering, 330–333, *331, 332, 334*
Assessment of Intelligibility of Dysarthric Speech (AIDS), 33t, 309, 311
Assessment of Phonological Processes, 369t–374t, 376
Assistive devices. *See* Prosthetic or assistive devices
Athetosis, 126–127
Attending, during communication, 94
Augmentative communication, xii
Autonomic nervous system, 116–117, 118t–119t

Ballismus, 126
Basal ganglia, *46–48,* 49, *50–51*
Basal ganglia lesions, 283–285
BDAE. *See Boston Diagnostic Aphasia Examination* (BDAE)
BEAM. *See* Brain electrical activity mapping (BEAM)
Biofeedback, 234, 321, 325, 326–337

401

Boston Diagnostic Aphasia Examination (BDAE), 33t, 73, 74, 207, 208, 371t, 375–376
Bottom-up processing, 89
Bradykinesia, 127
Brain
  basal ganglia, *46–48*, 49, *50–51*
  brain stem, 45–47, *46–48*
  cerebellum, 47–49
  cerebral lobes, 49–53, *52*
  chemical neuroanatomy of, 54–55, *55–57*
  diencephalon, 49
  functional neuroanatomy of, 45–53, *46–48*, *50–52*
  lesion loci and spasmodic dysphonia, 279–290
  neurotransmitters, 116–124, 118t–119t, 122t–123t
Brain electrical activity mapping (BEAM), 44, 64, *66*, 72, 300–305, *303*, 304t
Brain imaging
  brain electrical activity mapping (BEAM), 44, 64, *66*, 72, 300–305, *303*, 304t
  case studies, 73–76
  clinical use of, 64–68
  and disordered premotor organization for speech, 70–71
  limitations of, 68
  magnetic resonance imaging (MRI), 8, 27, *28*, 44, 53, 58, *60*, 66–67, 69, 72, 75–76, *76*, 299–300, *300*, 301t, *302*
  magnetic resonance spectroscopy (MRS), 44, 60–61, 67
  neurologist's use of, 27, *28, 29*
  overview of, 7–8
  positron emission tomography (PET), 8, 44, 61, 67, 69, 70, 71
  research findings with, 44–45, 68–73
  single-photon emission tomography (SPECT), 8, 44, 61–64, *62, 63, 65*, 67, 69, 70, 73–75
  and spasmodic dysphonia, 71–73, 299–305, *300*, 301t, *302, 303*, 304t
  and stuttering, 73
  x-ray computed tomography (CT), 8, 27, *29*, 44, 56–58, *59*, 66–67, 69, 71, 72, 73
Brain stem, 45–47, *46–48*

Brain stem lesions, 279–282
BRAINMAP, 64
Broca's aphasia, 35t, 195–196, 199, 200, 221, 246, 287
Bromocriptine, 137t, 140–141
Bruininks-Oseretsky Test of Motor Proficiency, 356, 371t, 376
Bulbar palsy, 292t, 293, *293*
Burnout, of speech-language pathologists, 171–172, 173–175, 175t

CADL. *See Communicative Abilities in Daily Living* (CADL)
CAIDS. *See Computerized Assessment of the Intelligibility of Dysarthric Speech* (CAIDS)
Carrow Elicited Language Inventory, 370t, 372t, 375, 376
Case studies
  apraxia of speech, 206–208
  brain imaging, 73–76
  developmental apraxia of speech (DAS), 366–385, 367t–374t, 377t–379t
  dysarthria, 104–107, *107*, 176–178
  prosodic disorders, 258–268, *259, 261, 263–267*
  roles of neurologist and speech pathologist, 33–39
  spasmodic dysphonia, 308–311
CAT scan, 58. *See also* X-ray computed tomography (CT)
Catecholamines, 121
CBC. *See* Complete blood count (CBC)
Cerebellar ataxia, 69, 292t, 293, *293*
Cerebellum, 47–49
Cerebral cortex lesions, 286–288
Cerebral lobes, 49–53, *52*
Cerebral palsy, 357
Cerebrospinal fluid (CSF) studies, 26t, 27
Choline uptake inhibitors, 120, 122t
Cholinergic nerves, 117
Cholinesterase inhibitors, 121, 123t
Cholinomimetics, 120, 122t
Chorea, 126, 128–130, 129t, *293*
Cognition and cognition tests, 348, 356
Communication
  arbitrary relationship between words and referents, 96–97
  assumptions about listeners, 100–101

breakdowns in, 190–194
case study on, 104–107, *107*
cooperation in communicating, 101
developmental apraxia of speech
(DAS) and, 345–350, *347*, 355–356
discourse knowledge, 102–104
dysarthria and, 154–159, 169–171
effort in, 196–197
everyday discourse, 102–103
of intention, 100
job-related discourse, 103
joint and mutual attending, 94
levels of meaning in language, 97–98
listener's perspective, 98
metalinguistic processing, 96–99
models of language production, 186–195, *187–189*
phonology, 93–94
from planning to production, 194–195
primary-level pragmatics, 94–96
prosody, 242–243
repetition in, 199–200
secondary-level pragmatics, 99–102
semantics, 91–92
substitutions in, 197–199
syntax and morphology, 92–93
top-down characteristics of primary level of language processing, 91–96
top-down characteristics of secondary level of language processing, 96–104
top-down versus bottom-up processing, 89–91
topic initiation, maintenance and shifting, 94–95
turn-taking, 95–96
Communicative Abilities in Daily Living (CADL), 33t, 207
Complete blood count (CBC), 24–26, 26t
Computed tomography. *See* X-ray computed tomography (CT)
Computerized Assessment of the Intelligibility of Dysarthric Speech (CAIDS), 105
Computerized axial tomography (CAT scan), 58. *See also* X-ray computed tomography (CT)
Conduction aphasia, 35t, 193, 208, 210
Contextual Facilitation, 360t
Contrast Therapy, 360t

Corpus callosum lesions, 246–247, 260, 262, *263–265*
Counseling. *See also* Treatment
for prosodic disorders, 256
for spasmodic dysphonia, 307
CSF studies. *See* Cerebrospinal fluid (CSF) studies
CT. *See* X-ray computed tomography (CT)

DAF unit. *See* Delayed auditory feedback (DAF) unit
DAS. *See* Developmental apraxia of speech (DAS)
Decarboxylase inhibitors, 139–140
Delayed auditory feedback (DAF) unit, 231–232, 233–234
Denver Auditory Phoneme Sequencing Test, 350, 356
Developmental apraxia of speech (DAS). *See also* Apraxia of speech
adapted therapy approaches for, 363–366
articulation tests and, 355–356
assessment of, 355–358, 366, 367t–374t, 375–376, 378t–379t,
case study on, 366–385, 367t–374t, 377t–379t
characteristics of, 345–350, *347*
childhood aphasia distinguished from, 357
cognition and, 348, 356
description of, 342–343
differential diagnosis of, 357–358
etiology of, 343–345, 350–353
goals of treatment, 358
language and, 349–350, 356
Melodic Intonation Therapy (MIT) for, 365
neuromorphology theory of, 15
prognosis for, 350
PROMPT system for, 363–364
prosody and, 346, 348
rhyming and, 353–355
screening for, 355
sensory deficits and, 350, 356–357
speech and, 345–346, *347*
stimuli during treatment, 361
structure of treatment sessions, 361
teaching hierarchy during treatment, 361–362
theoretical framework for, 350–358

therapy principles and procedures for, 358–363, 359t–361t
Touch-Cue Method for, 364
treatment for, 358–366, 378–385, 379t
volitional nonspeech movements and, 348
Developmental Test of Visual Motor Integration, 368t
Diagnosis. *See* Assessment
Diencephalon, 49
Digital subtraction angiography (DSA), 8
Discourse knowledge, 102–104
Disordered speech motor control. *See also* Assessment; Pharmacologic therapies; Treatment; names of specific speech motor disorders
case studies, 33–39
cross-disciplinary perspective on, 7
disorders of movement, 124–143
disturbances of premotor disorganization of speech, 11–13, 70–71
dysfluency as component of, 221–223
generalized movement disorders affecting speech, 8–11
historical perspective on, 4–6
and history of patient, 21
hyperkinetic movement disorders, 125–127, 128–133, 129t
hypokinetic movement disorders, 127, 133–143
idiopathic speech-specific disorders, 13–15
laboratory tests used for, 24–28, 26t
monitoring physiologic events, 14
neurologic causes of, 25t
and neurologic diagnosis, 24
and neurologic examination, 21–23, 22t
neurologist's approach to management of, 21–31
and referral to speech pathologist, 30–31
review of nervous system function, 7–8
speech motor control, 143–149
speech pathologist's approach to management of, 31–33, 33t
speech pathologist's preparation and, 19–20

top-down approach to management of, 9–10
Dopamine, 54–55, *56,* 121
Drug therapies. *See* Pharmacologic therapies
Drug-induced chorea, 130
Drug-induced parkinsonism, 142
DSA. *See* Digital subtraction angiography (DSA)
Dysarthria
and arbitrary relationship between words and referents, 96–97
assumptions about listeners and, 100–101
brain imaging and, 75–76
case study on, 104–107, *107,* 176–178
communication of intention and, 100
compliance to therapy, 158
cooperation in communicating and, 101
discourse knowledge and, 102–104
dysfluency and, 222
everyday discourse and, 102–103
impact on family, 160–165, *163,* 166t
impact on individual, 154–159
institutionalization of dysarthric individual, 165, 167–171
job-related discourse and, 103
joint and mutual attending and, 94
and levels of meaning in language, 97–98
listener's perspective and, 98
metalinguistic processing and, 96–99
overview of, 88–89
phonology and, 93–94, 154–155
primary-level pragmatics and, 94–96
probe questions for, 159, 159t, 165, 166t
psychosocial impact of, 10–11, 155–157
secondary-level pragmatics and, 99–102
semantics and, 91–92
spasmodic dysphonia compared with, 290–294, 292t, *293*
speech therapy for, xii
and speech-language pathologist, 171–175, 175t
as stress, 157–158
syntax and morphology and, 92–93
top-down characteristics of primary level of language processing, 91–96

and top-down characteristics of
secondary level of language
processing, 96–104
and top-down versus bottom-up
processing, 89–91
topic initiation, maintenance and
shifting and, 94–95
turn-taking and, 95–96
types of and symptoms of, 34t
Dysfluency, terminology of, 218–219.
See also Neurogenic dysfluency
Dystonia, 128, 292t, 293, *293*

EEG. See Electroencephalography (EEG)
Effort, in communication, 196–197
EGG. See Electroglottography (EGG)
Electroencephalography (EEG), 64, 67–68, 75
Electroglottography (EGG), 324–325, *324*, 329, 330–337, *331, 332, 335, 336*
Electromyography (EMG), 28, 234, 324
EMG. See Electromyography (EMG)
Epilepsy, 69, 70, 75, 225
Epinephrine, 54, 117, 118t, 121
Epithalamus, 49
Evaluation. See Assessment
Extralaryngeal motor functions, in spasmodic dysphonia, 294–295, 294t–298t, 299
Extrapyramidal motor system, 124–125, 284

Family, and dysarthric individual, 160–165, *163*, 166t
Frontal lobe, 49, 50, 51–53, *52*

Gilles de la Tourette syndrome. See Tourette's syndrome
Global aphasia, 35t
Goldman Fristoe Test of Articulation, 355, 367t
Goodman and Gillman's "The pharmacological basis of therapeutics," 115
Grammar, See Syntax

History of patient, 21
Huntington's disease, 49, 69, 70, 128–130, 129t, 292t
Hyperkinesia and hyperkinetic movement disorders, 125–127, 128–133, 129t

Hyperkinetic drug-induced movement disorders, 132–133
Hyperreflexia, 127
Hyperthyroidism, 125
Hypokinesia and hypokinetic movement disorders, 127, 133–143
Hypothalamus, 49

Illinois Test of Psycholinguistic Abilities, 350
Imaging technologies. See Brain imaging
Institutionalization of dysarthric individual, 165, 167–171
Instrumentation
advantages and disadvantages in treatment of stuttering, 326–328
aerodynamic measures, 329–330
for disordered speech motor control, 14
and identification of abnormalities, 330–333, *331, 332, 334*
laryngeal monitoring, 329
respiratory monitoring, 328–329
for stuttering, 14, 320–338
Integral Stimulation, 360t
Intention, communication of, 100

Kaufman Assessment Battery of Children, 372t

Laboratory tests, 24–28, 26t
Language. See Communication
Language production, models of, 186–195, *187–189*
Laryngeal disruptions, and stuttering, 323–325, *324*
Laryngeal monitoring, 329
Left hemispheric lesions, and prosodic disorders, 245–246, 262, 266–268, *266, 267*
Lesions
of basal ganglia and related structures, 283–285
of cerebral cortex and its projections, 286–288
of corpus callosum, 246–247, 260, 262, *263–265*
in left hemisphere, 245–246, 262, 266–268, *266, 267*
of limbic system, 288–290
of medulla, 279–282

of midbrain, 282-283
of peripheral nerve, 279
and prosodic disorders, 244-247,
  258-268, *259, 261, 263-267*
in right hemisphere, 244-245,
  258-260, *259, 261*
and spasmodic dysphonia, 279-290
Letier Performance Scales, 368t
Levodopa, 135, 137t, 138-140
Limbic lobe, 50
Limbic system lesions, 288-290

Magnetic resonance imaging (MRI)
  brain white matter visualized with, 53
  case studies, 75-76, *76*
  clinical use of, 66-67
  description of, 58, *60*
  and neurological disorders affecting motor speech systems, 69
  purpose of, 8, 27, *28,* 44
  and spasmodic dysphonia, 72, 299-300, *300,* 301t, *302*
Magnetic resonance spectroscopy (MRS), 8, 44, 60-61, 67
McCarthy Scales of Children's Abilities, 371t, 375
Medications. *See* Pharmacologic therapies
Medulla, 45, *46,* 47
Medulla lesions, 279-282
Meige syndrome, 128, 147, 284
Melodic Intonation Therapy (MIT), 205, 365
Mental retardation, 348, 357
Mental Status Examination in Neurology, 74
Metabolic screening, 26t, 27
Metalinguistic processing, 96-99
Midbrain, 45, *46, 47*
Midbrain lesions, 282-283
Minnesota Test for the Differential Diagnosis of Aphasia (MTDDA), 33t, 207-208, 210-211
MIT. *See* Melodic Intonation Therapy (MIT)
Mixed transcortical syndrome, 35t
Monamines, 54-55, *56-57*
Morphology, 92-93
Moto-kinesthetic Speech Training, 359t
Motor Speech Evaluation, 200
Movement, disorders of, 124-143

MRI. *See* Magnetic resonance imaging (MRI)
MRS. *See* Magnetic resonance spectroscopy (MRS)
MTDDA. *See* Minnesota Test for the Differential Diagnosis of Aphasia (MTDDA)
Multiple Input Phoneme Therapy, 205
Multiple Phoneme Approach, 359t
Multiple sclerosis, 69
Myasthenia gravis, 143

Neologisms, 192, 193
Nerve conduction velocities (NCV), 28
Neuroanatomy. *See also* Autonomic nervous system; Brain; Parasympathetic nervous system; Sympathetic nervous system
  basal ganglia, *46-48,* 49, *50-51*
  brain stem, 45-47, *46-48*
  cerebellum, 47-49
  cerebral lobes, 49-53, *52*
  chemical neuroanatomy, 54-55, *55-57*
  diencephalon, 49
  extrapyramidal motor system, 124-125
  functional neuroanatomy, 45-53, *46-48, 50-52*
  lesion loci and spasmodic dysphonia, 279-290
  of normal speech motor output, 143-144
Neurogenic dysfluency
  aphasia and, 220-221
  categories of, 218
  characteristics of, 11-12
  clinical reality of, 219-220, 222-223
  as component of motor speech disorders, 221-223
  differential diagnosis of, 223-225
  features of, 225-228
  nonvascular etiologies of, 229
  prosthetic or assistive devices for, 13
  psychogenic dysfluency versus, 224-225
  terminology concerning, 218-219
  treatment of, 230-236, *235*
  vascular episodes and, 226-229
Neuroimaging technologies. *See* Brain imaging
Neurologic diagnosis, 24

Neurologic examination, 21–23, 22t
Neurological disorders affecting motor speech systems, 69–70
Neurologists
  approach to patient management, 21–31
  case studies on, 33–39
  and history of patient, 21
  laboratory tests used by, 24–28, 26t
  neurologic diagnosis, 24
  neurologic examination, 21–23, 22t
  referral to speech pathologist by, 30–31
  treatment provided by, 28–30
Neuromuscular junction, 117, 120–121, 122t–123t
Neuropharmacology. *See* Pharmacologic therapies
Neurotransmitters, 54, 116–124, 118t–119t, 122t–123t
Noninvasive instrumentation. *See* Instrumentation
Norepinephrine, 54, 55, *57,* 117, 118t, 121
Northwestern Syntax Screening Test, 349
Nursing homes, 165, 167–171

Occipital lobe, 49, *52,* 53
Olivopontocerebellar degeneration, 141

Paired Stimuli, 360t
Palilalia, 222, 231
Paraphasias, 195–196. *See also* Phonemic paraphasia
Parasympathetic nervous system, 116–117, 118t–119t
Parietal lobe, 49, 50, *52,* 53
Parkinsonian syndromes, 141–142
Parkinsonism-plus syndromes, 141
Parkinson's disease, 49, 55, 69, 70, 130, 132, 133–141, 134t, 136t–137t, 222, 230–231, 292t, *293*
Periaqueductal gray, 144, 289
PDR. *See* Physician's Desk Reference (PDR)
Peabody Picture Vocabulary Test, 356, 368t, 371t
Peptides, 54
Peripheral nerve lesions, 279
PET. *See* Positron emission tomography (PET)

Pharmacologic therapies
  abbreviations of terms associated with dosages, 116t
  for chorea, 130
  for disorders of movement, 124–143
  and drug-induced chorea, 130
  and drug-induced parkinsonism, 142
  for dystonia, 128
  and hyperkinetic drug-induced movement disorders, 132–133
  for hyperkinetic movement disorders, 128–133, 129t
  importance of, 112–113
  for myasthenia gravis, 143
  for neurogenic dysfluency, 230
  neurotransmitters and, 116–124, 118t–119t, 122t–123t
  for parkinsonism-plus syndromes, 141
  for Parkinson's disease, 133, 135, 136t–137t, 138–141
  principles of therapeutics for, 113–115
  sources of drug information, 115–116
  for spasmodic dysphonia, 147–149, 310
  for stuttering, 144–146
  substitutions and, 197–199
  for tic disorders, 131
  for tremor, 131–132
Phonemic paraphasia
  characteristics of, 195–199
  communication breakdown and, 191–192
  diagnosis of, 200–202, 203t
  effort and, 196–197
  less common errors and, 199–200
  repetition and, 199–200
  treatment for, 208–211
Phonetic Placement, 359t
Phonology, 93–94, 154–155, 187–188, *188–189,* 190–191, 200
Physician's Desk Reference (PDR), 115
Pons, 45, *46, 47*
Positron emission tomography (PET), 8, 44, 61, 67, 69, 70, 71
Postencephalitic parkinsonism, 141–142
Pragmatics
  primary-level, 94–96
  secondary-level, 99–102
Progressive supranuclear palsy (PSP), 141

408   Subject Index

PROMPT system, 204–205, 363–364
Prosodic disorders
  assessment of, 248–253, 249t, 251t, 252t, 254t–255t
  case studies of, 258–268, 259, 261, 263–267
  caused by cerebral injury, 244–248, 258–268
  caused by left hemispheric lesions, 245–246, 262, 266–268, 266, 267
  caused by lesions of corpus callosum, 246–247, 260, 262, 263–265
  caused by right hemispheric lesions, 244–245, 258–260, 259, 261
  treatment of, 253, 256–258
Prosody
  assessment of prosodic perception, 253, 254t–255t
  assessment of prosodic production, 248–253, 249t, 251t, 252t
  communicative functions of, 243
  definition of, 242–243
  developmental apraxia of speech (DAS) and, 346, 348
Prosthetic or assistive devices, for neurogenic dysfluency, 230–232
Pseudobulbar palsy, 290, 292t, 293, 293
PSP. *See* Progressive supranuclear palsy (PSP)
Psychogenic dysfluency, 224–225
Psychosocial impact of dysarthria, 10–11, 155–157
Pyramidal tracts, 52

Repetition in communication, 199–200
Respiratory disruptions, and stuttering, 321–322
Respiratory monitoring, 328–329
Respitrace, 328–329, 330, 331, 333, 334
Reynell Developmental Language Scales, 356
Rhyming, 353–355
Right hemispheric lesions, and prosodic disorders, 244–245, 258–260, 259, 261
Rigidity, 127

Screening Test for Developmental Apraxia, 355, 356, 369t, 375
SD. *See* Spasmodic dysphonia
Self-rating of Depression Scale, 307

Semantic paraphasia, 190, 192–193
Semantics, 91–92, 187, *188, 189,* 190
Sensory and motor functioning tests, 356–357
Sensory deficits, 350
Sensory-Motor Approach, 359t
Sequenced Inventory of Communication Development, 356, 366, 367t
Serotonin, 54, 121, 124
Serum metabolic tests, 26t, 27
Shy-Drager's syndrome, 141
Single-photon emission tomography (SPECT)
  case studies, 73–75
  description of, 61–64, *62, 63, 65,* 67
  and neurological disorders affecting motor speech systems, 69, 70
  purpose of, 8, 44
  and spasmodic dysphonia, 72
Spasmodic dysphonia
  and basal ganglia and related structures, 283–285
  case study on, 308–311
  and cerebral cortex lesions, 286–288
  description of, 146–147, 276–277
  dysarthrias compared with, 290–294, 292t, *293*
  extralaryngeal motor functions in, 294–295, 294t–298t, 299
  lesion loci and, 279–290
  and limbic system lesions, 288–290
  and medulla lesions, 279–282
  and midbrain lesions, 282–283
  neural imaging in, 71–73, 299–305, *300,* 301t, *302, 303,* 304t
  neurobiological interpretations of, 277–278, *278,* 305–308, *306*
  neurogenic model of, 13–14
  and peripheral nerve lesions, 279
  treatment for, 147–148, 307–308
Spastic dysphonia. *See* Spasmodic dysphonia
Spasticity, 127
SPECT. *See* Single-photon emission tomography (SPECT)
Speech-language pathologists
  academic preparation of, 19
  approach to disordered speech motor control, 31–33, 33t
  burnout of, 171–172, 173–174
  case studies on, 33–39
  clinical preparation of, 19–20

coping with stress and burnout, 174–175
efficacy of, 30–31
helping relationship and, 172
probe questions for, 175, 175t
referral by neurologist to, 30–31
stress of, 172–173
stress of dysarthria therapy on, 171–175, 175t
Speech motor control, xi, 143–149
Speech motor disorders. See Disordered speech motor control; and names of specific disorders
Speech motor output, normal, 143–144
Speech Pattern Remediation, 360t–361t
State-Trait Anxiety Scale, 307
Steele-Richardson-Olszewski syndrome, 141
Stress
 of dysarthric individual, 157–158, 159t
 of family of dysarthric individual, 160–165, 166t
 of dysarthria therapy on speech-language pathologists, 171–175, 175t
Stuttering
 advantages and disadvantages of instrumentation for, 326–328
 aerodynamic disruptions and, 325–326
 aerodynamic measures for, 329–330
 and brain imaging, 73
 historical perspective on, 6
 identification of abnormalities, 330–333, *331, 332, 334*
 laryngeal disruptions and, 323–325, *324*
 laryngeal monitoring for, 329
 neurogenic stuttering, 218–219
 neurological basis of, 9, 11
 noninvasive instrumentation in treatment of, 320–338
 pharmacologic therapies for, 144–146
 respiratory disruptions and, 321–322
 respiratory monitoring and, 328–329
 treatment for, 233–234, 333–337, *335, 336*
Stuttering. See also Neurogenic dysfluency
Substitutions, in communication, 197–199

Subthalamus, 49
Successive Approximation, 360t
Sympathetic nervous system, 116–117, 118t–119t
Syntax, 92–93, 187, *188, 189,* 349

Tardive dyskinesia, 132–133
Templin-Darley Test of Articulation, 345, 355, 370t, 375, 376, 377t–378t
Temporal lobe, 49, 50, *52,* 53
Test of Auditory Comprehension of Language, 370t
Tests of Apraxia, 371t
Thalamus, *47* 49, 55
Therapy. See Treatment
Tic disorders, 126, 130–131
Top-down approach to treatment for dysarthric speech
 arbitrary relationship between words and referents, 96–97
 assumptions about listeners, 100–101
 case study on, 104–107, *107*
 communication of intention and, 100
 cooperation in communicating, 101
 discourse knowledge, 102–104
 everyday discourse, 102–103
 job-related discourse, 103
 joint and mutual attending, 94
 levels of meaning in language, 97–98
 listener's perspective, 98
 metalinguistic processing, 96–99
 phonology, 93–94
 primary level of language processing, 91–96
 primary-level pragmatics, 94–96
 secondary level of language processing, 96–104
 secondary-level pragmatics, 99–102
 semantics, 91–92
 syntax and morphology, 92–93
 top-down versus bottom-up processing, 89–91
 topic initiation, maintenance and shifting, 94–95
 turn-taking, 95–96
Topic initiation, maintenance and shifting, 94–95
Touch-Cue Method, 364
Tourette's syndrome, 131
Traditional Articulation Therapy, 359t
Transcortical motor aphasia, 35t, 287
Transcortical sensory aphasia, 35t

Traumatic midbrain dysphonia, 290
Treatment. *See also* Counseling;
  Pharmacologic therapies
 of apraxia of speech, 203–208
 compliance to therapy in dysarthric
   clients, 158
 Contextual Facilitation, 360t
 Contrast Therapy, 360t
 for developmental apraxia of speech
   (DAS), 358–366, 378–385, 379t
 for dysarthria, 88–108
 institutionalization of dysarthric
   individual, 165, 167–171
 Integral Stimulation, 360t
 Melodic Intonation Therapy (MIT),
   365
 Moto-kinesthetic Speech Training,
   359t
 Multiple Phoneme Approach, 359t
 for neurogenic dysfluency, 230–236,
   235
 by neurologist for disordered speech
   motor control, 28–30
 noninvasive instrumentation in
   treatment of stuttering, 320–338
 Paired Stimuli, 360t
 of phonemic paraphasia, 208–211
 Phonetic Placement, 359t
 PROMPT system, 363–364
 of prosodic disorders, 253,
   256–258
 Sensory-Motor Approach, 359t
 for spasmodic dysphonia, 147–148,
   307–308
 by speech pathologist for disordered
   speech motor control, 31–33, 33t
 Speech Pattern Remediation,
   360t–361t
 stress of dysarthria therapy on
   speech-language pathologists,
   171–175, 175t
 for stuttering, 233–234, 333–337,
   335, 336
 Successive Approximation, 360t
 Touch-Cue Method, 364
 Traditional Articulation Therapy, 359t
Tremor, 125–126, 131–132
Turn-taking during communication,
  95–96
Tyrosine, 121

Verbal paraphasia, 192–193
Visi-Pitch, 335, 337
Vocal Feedback Device, 231
Volitional nonspeech movements, 348

*Wechsler Intelligence Scales for
  Children–Revised,* 356
Wernicke's aphasia, 35t, 192, 193, 196,
  208, 246
Wilson's disease, 27, 34t, 69

X-ray computed tomography (CT)
 case studies, 73
 clinical use of, 66–67
 description of, *29,* 56–58, *59*
 and disordered premotor organization
   for speech, 71
 and neurological disorders affecting
   motor speech systems, 69
 purpose of, 8, 27, 44
 and spasmodic dysphonia, 72